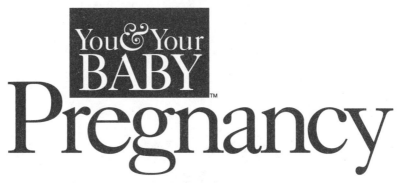

Pregnancy

The ultimate week-by-week pregnancy guide

D0167585

Dr. Laura Riley, OB/GYN

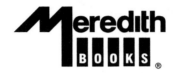

Editor:
Stephanie Karpinske

Senior Associate Design Director:
Ken Carlson

Marketing Product Manager:
Gina Rickert

Meredith Books
1716 Locust Street
Des Moines, Iowa 50309–3023
www.meredithbooks.com

You & Your Baby is a trademark of Meredith Corporation

First Edition. Printed in the United States of America.
Library of Congress Control Number: 2005929470
ISBN: 0-696-22221-3

Dr. Laura Riley

Life is an exciting whirlwind for Dr. Laura Riley, who is an author, the medical director of labor and delivery at Massachusetts General Hospital in Boston, and dedicated mom to daughters Natalie and Lauren. She is also assistant professor of obstetrics, gynecology, and reproductive biology at Harvard Medical School.

Dr. Riley has been committed to serving pregnant women for 15 years. At Boston City Hospital she focused on high-risk pregnant women, with an emphasis on HIV disease. In 1995 she joined Massachusetts General Hospital, where she currently practices, to focus on high-risk pregnancy with an emphasis on infectious disease complications of obstetrics. She has participated in numerous research projects: Her current project, sponsored by the National Institutes of Health, investigates epidural-related fever.

Dr. Riley is a consultant to the Centers for Disease Control (CDC). She has been on several major committees at the American College of Obstetricians and Gynecologists (ACOG); most recently she was chair of the Obstetric Practice Committee, which drafts guidelines for obstetric care in the United States. She has been quoted extensively in national

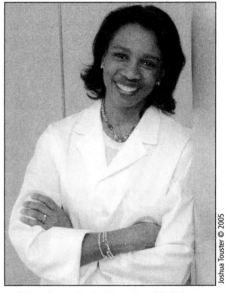

Joshua Touster © 2005

publications, including the *Wall Street Journal, Newsweek,* and the *New York Times,* and has appeared on NBC's *Today* and CBS's *The Early Show.* She has published articles in scientific journals and peer-reviewed websites.

Dr. Riley is a graduate of Harvard University. She received her medical degree at the University of Pittsburgh, completed an internship and residency in obstetrics and gynecology at the Magee-Womens Hospital of University of Pittsburgh, and completed subspecialty training in maternal fetal medicine at Brigham and Women's Hospital and in infectious disease at Boston University Medical Center.

acknowledgments

I thank my children, Lauren and Natalie; my husband, Scott; my aunts; and my parents for their support and encouragement throughout this project. My pregnancies, which were easy, my breastfeeding experiences, which were hard, and my obstetrician, whom I adored, have contributed immensely to my clinical practice and this book. The content for this book also came in part from my experiences with many great women who had low-risk pregnancies, high-risk pregnancies, joyous outcomes, and sad ones. I thank all of my patients for sharing those experiences with me.

Of course, creating a project of this scale would be an overwhelming task to face alone. Fortunately I have had the pleasure of working with two very gifted writers, Alice Lesch Kelly and Holly Robinson, who have helped me develop and refine this book.

It's also my good fortune to have trained with extraordinary obstetricians over the years whose collective wisdom is reflected here—Drs. Harger, Mueller-Heubach, Edelstone, Rulin, Caritis, Frigoletto, Heffner, and Greene. My partners, the "original" Massachusetts General Hospital obstetrical team, and our current group of obstetricians and midwives are comprised of smart, dedicated physicians and nurses whose insights permeate this work.

A special acknowledgment to Margie Noone, R.N.; Fredda Zuckerman, LICSW; Chris Stalinski, R.N.; Courtney Craig, R.N.; Lori Pugsley, R.N.; Maureen Tully, R.N. IBCLC; C.C. Martin; Dr. Jeffrey Ecker; Dr. Sandy Tsao; Dr. Thomas Toth; Dr. Kristen Eckler; Dr. Andrea Torri; Dr. Lisa Leffert; Dr. May Pian-Smith; and Dr. Suzanne Nash for their expert editorial contributions.

Finally, I owe a special thanks to Dr. Carol Major, Associate Professor of Obstetrics and Gynecology at University of California Irvine, for her thorough review and invaluable input on this manuscript.

Contents

contents

Your due date

When is your baby due? That's one of the first questions you'll get asked after you announce your pregnancy. To determine that date, your health care provider will start by asking you the first day of your last normal menstrual period (LNMP). She will add 266 days, or 38 weeks, to that date. (Why 38 weeks? It's the length of the average pregnancy from the point of conception.) She will then tack on yet another 14 days because that's the average number of days between the start of your last normal menstrual period and ovulation.

Calculate your due date. You can estimate your own due date in a simpler way: Figure out the first day of your last normal menstrual period and add exactly 9 months and 7 days to that date. For example, if the first day of your last menstrual period was January 3, you would add 9 months and 7 days to that date. Your due date would be October 10.

Better yet, use the *You and Your Baby: Pregnancy* due date wheel to help you make an even more accurate estimate of baby's arrival.

No matter what the due date is, hold off on printing your baby announcements until after the baby arrives. Babies have a will of their own, and your due date is not completely predictable. In fact, the actual medical term for a pregnancy due date is an "estimated date of delivery," or EDD.

Why the emphasis on estimated? You may be unsure of the date of your last menstrual period, for instance, or you may have irregular periods. It's also possible that you don't ovulate in the middle of your cycle but much sooner or later than that magical, "average" 14th day.

In fact, even if you do have periods that run like clockwork and you know exactly when you had intercourse, calculating your due date is still an inexact science. Sperm can take three days to travel through your fallopian tube to meet up with your egg, so the date of conception isn't always the same day you had intercourse. In addition, just as children grow at different rates after birth (remember that really tall girl in the first grade or the short boy on the high school basketball team?), they grow at different rates in utero too. Your health care provider will probably caution you that your due date is only an approximation. After all, only about 5 percent of all babies are born on their predicted due dates!

your belly button sore? This is where you'll find the answers.

Your partner

Although this section doesn't appear every single week, I've made a point of covering the relationship issues that come up most often in my practice. For instance, how can you stay close if you have no interest in sex, but your partner seems oblivious to the fact that your early weeks of pregnancy consist of sleepiness and morning sickness? How can you get your partner more involved with housework and older children now so that you won't be swamped once the baby arrives? My goal is to keep you communicating constructively with your partner throughout your pregnancy so that the two of you can be a more loving and effective parenting team.

Special concerns

These columns are printed in tinted boxes to indicate that they describe concerns that aren't common to all pregnancies, such as gestational diabetes, asthma, and lupus. You'll find statistics, current research, and the latest options pertaining to these special concerns.

Labor, delivery, and beyond

Following the week-by-week pregnancy sections, you'll find comprehensive information about what actually happens in a delivery room—and essential survival tips for every new parent.

Labor and Delivery. What are the stages of labor? What happens if there's a complication? Here you'll find clear explanations of the moments you're looking forward to most but perhaps feeling nervous about too.

Feeding Options. The most current research available on infant nutrition is available here, as well as a no-guilt explanation of the pros and cons of feeding your baby by breast or by bottle.

Bringing Baby Home. Once you bring your baby home, you'll probably wish you had an instruction manual. Here I offer a thorough minicourse on taking care of yourself as well as your baby. Check here if you're breast-feeding and have sore nipples or if you need help managing your baby's sleep-and-wake cycles so that you can get some rest too.

Prenatal Appointment Sheets. Use the handy fill-in-the-blank sheets in the back of this book to keep track of questions you want to ask your own health care provider and to note the information you get during your prenatal visits. I've listed the questions that come up most often in my own practice, but feel free to add your own as well.

Glossaries. Use the glossaries on prenatal testing, newborn screening tests, and labor and delivery terms as a quick reference for your own health and your baby's during pregnancy and the first few months after birth.

Week-by-week sections

You and Your Baby: Pregnancy includes a separate chapter for each week—from 1 to 40—of your pregnancy. Within each week, you'll find the following sections:

Your Baby

Look here for fascinating facts on fetal development, including how big your baby is at every week of pregnancy, when your baby's vital organs begin functioning, how babies practice breathing and swallowing in the womb, and why your child already loves the sound of your voice before he even meets you.

Your Body

From wondrous moments—such as your baby's first movements—to minor miseries—like having to use the restroom in the middle of every movie—your body changes during each week of pregnancy. I'll tell you how and why these changes occur. I'll also provide solutions to common pregnancy complaints and offer the latest research highlights on topics that might affect your health or your baby's. In these sections of the book I also describe the various labor positions you can practice ahead of your due date, ways to recognize when you're in labor, safe pain relief options, and what to expect if your baby comes too early—or late.

Your Self

Pregnancy and childbirth transform every aspect of your life, from the way you eat to the choices you make in your work, home, and relationships. In these sections I catalog the complex lifestyle questions of expectant mothers, offering information and insights on a broad array of topics: How do you ride that hormonal roller coaster? How can you negotiate a longer maternity leave at work? What are the most important things to buy for the nursery? Whatever changes are happening in your life, rest assured that you'll find sensible advice here.

Diet & Exercise

Do you really have to stop drinking coffee completely? Can you keep jogging? What can you eat to reduce heartburn and constipation? Whatever questions you may have about diet and exercise during pregnancy, you'll find practical answers and solutions here—without the guilt. (As a busy working mother, I know how important those small indulgences can be!)

Common Questions

No question is silly when you're pregnant and worried. I've addressed the most common ones here. What makes a pregnancy high-risk? Why is

How to use this book

If you're reading this book, then you have a lot on your mind. You may be thinking about becoming pregnant, or perhaps you've just had a positive pregnancy test. You may even be halfway through your pregnancy already but still eagerly learning all you can about this momentous journey. After all, pregnancy is as much about giving birth to a new identity—you as a mom!—as it is about giving birth to a healthy baby.

As a practicing obstetrician, and as a mother myself, I know firsthand that every pregnant woman's medical and emotional journey is unique. Your concerns will be different each week as your baby grows and your body changes rapidly to support that growth. For that reason I have organized this book into week-by-week sections—starting with week 1 and going through week 40—that are organized into three trimesters. Each week provides the most commonsense, up-to-date approach on every aspect of maternity. After week 40, you'll find a detailed chapter on labor and delivery, along with a special section dedicated to the weeks following your baby's birth.

Get started. You can read the book chronologically, starting with whatever week of pregnancy you're in right now. Or you can go directly to the topics that interest you with the help of the indexes at the front and back of the book and within each trimester. The multiple indexes are meant to help you locate information quickly and easily, but the one in the back of the book is the most inclusive, so check that one if you're looking for something very specific.

As you read through each week, you may notice that I've included some of the same topics in several different sections of my book. Why? As you know from chats with other women, expectant moms don't all experience the same things at the same times in their pregnancies. It's also important to know that some key symptoms—vaginal bleeding or abdominal pain, for instance—may mean something completely different in the early weeks of pregnancy than in the final weeks.

Take a peek at these babies. Before you begin reading, go ahead and flip to the astonishing section of color photographs in the book. They chronicle fetal development in precise detail. You'll want to refer to these photographs over and over again as your own pregnancy progresses so you can visualize just how your own baby is growing.

as your pregnancy progresses or pick out topics that apply to your pregnancy.

It is important to remember that no single book can answer all of your questions. In this book, my goal is to provide you with enough information to address common concerns, to put the complicated issues into perspective, and to jump-start conversations with your own doctor. Often there are different ways to accomplish the same goal. Always talk to your own doctor about the approach that's best for you and your baby.

Ask questions, questions, and more questions! As you go to each prenatal visit, never be afraid to ask as many questions as you want. As an obstetrician I am thrilled when my patients come to their prenatal appointments prepared with a list of questions. The prenatal visits are opportunities to learn about pregnancy, delivery, caring for a newborn, and getting to know your provider's pregnancy care philosophy. It is also fun to keep track of the same things that your provider is monitoring, such as your weight, your blood pressure, and the baby's heartbeat. Prenatal visits are informative for both mother and doctor; if you ask questions and share information, you'll make the most of your time together. (To get you started, I've written down some of the most common questions I get asked; see the "Questions for Your Doctor" section that starts on page 405.)

Choose your sources of medical information wisely. As a new mom, you'll also likely seek information from sources other than your doctor. If you do, remember that not all sources of medical information are trustworthy. Much of what you find on the Internet or hear from a stranger in the grocery store may be dangerous or inappropriate for your situation. Rest assured that *You and Your Baby: Pregnancy* has been carefully researched and reviewed by top medical experts. You're getting the best of what I've learned during my residency and fellowship training and in treating my own patients.

Welcome to the grand experience of becoming a mom. I hope this book becomes your treasured companion as you embark on the wondrous journey of having a baby.

Laura Riley
Obstetrician and mother of Natalie, 10, and Lauren, 13

Dear Moms-to-be,

Having a baby is an amazing journey. To this day, I can remember exactly where I was and what I felt when I found out I was pregnant with my first child. My first thoughts were: Will it be a girl or a boy? An artist? A scientist? After the initial shock passed, more practical questions flooded my brain. Will my child be healthy? Can I really work all 9 months? How will I survive the labor marathon?

As a mother of two darling girls—and as an obstetrician who has delivered more than a thousand babies—I know firsthand that the physical and emotional changes you'll experience during pregnancy and delivery may seem overwhelming at the outset. But while you may have concerns, remember that this is also a time of great joy and celebration. That's why I've written *You & Your Baby: Pregnancy.* I wanted soon-to-be mothers to have the most up-to-date medical information available as well as practical tips on choosing names and weathering everything from morning sickness to fashion emergencies.

The more you know, the better you'll feel. When I was pregnant, I had the luxury of sharing my experiences with my patients who were also expecting. We shared the wonders of the first ultrasound, regaled each other with stories of labor, and then tiredly discussed the dramas of taking care of a newborn. I want this book to have that same sense of camaraderie and easy sharing of information. I want you to know that there are many things you can do to make this journey easier and safer. I want you to understand exactly what's going on with your body because knowledge provides comfort.

Much of what the medical community knows and recommends for new moms is guided by science—either from years of observation or through cutting-edge research. I've distilled that information into easy-to-understand language that doesn't require a medical degree to decipher. While some of these topics will never appear on your pregnancy radar screen, others may be vitally important for you. So jump right in and start reading. Tackle the book in order, week by week,

life before birth

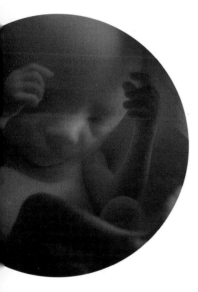

Although you know your belly is expanding day by day—and some days you can feel your baby stretching and moving about—don't you wish you could see clearly what's going on inside your body? These incredible photographs, such as this one of a baby at 24 weeks into the pregnancy, document a baby's journey at its earliest stages.

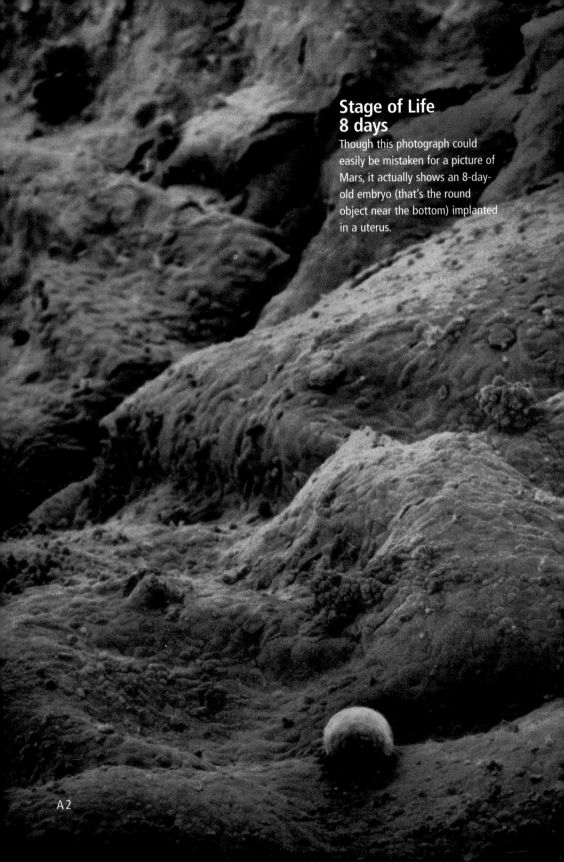

**Stage of Life
8 days**

Though this photograph could easily be mistaken for a picture of Mars, it actually shows an 8-day-old embryo (that's the round object near the bottom) implanted in a uterus.

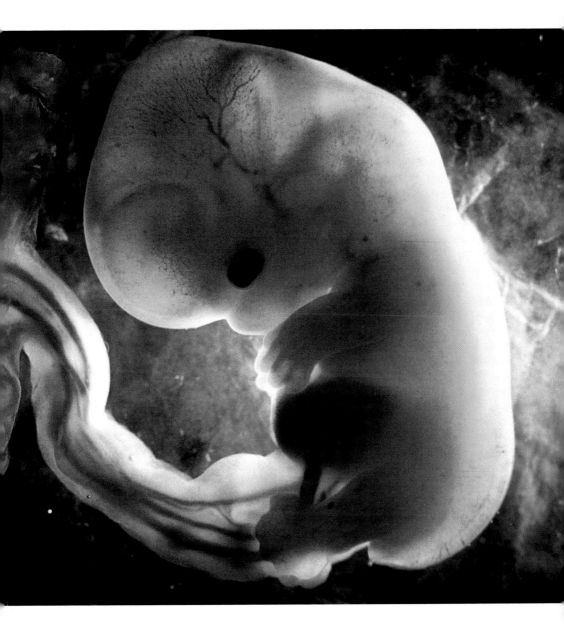

Stage of Life
46 days

This embryo—which is less than 1 inch long—gets all the sustenance it needs from the blood that journeys to and from it through vessels in the umbilical cord.

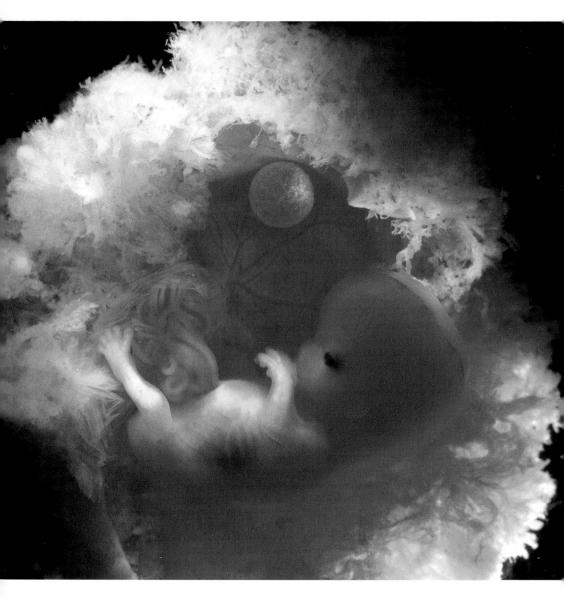

Stage of Life
13 weeks

This baby has just been through
an ultrasound exam and is taking
a nap in this photograph. The
round object above the baby's
head is the yolk sac.

Stage of Life
17 weeks

It's easy to count 10 toes and 10 fingers on this fetus, and facial features are also becoming more defined. The amniotic fluid that surrounds the fetus gradually increases throughout pregnancy to allow the baby to move about.

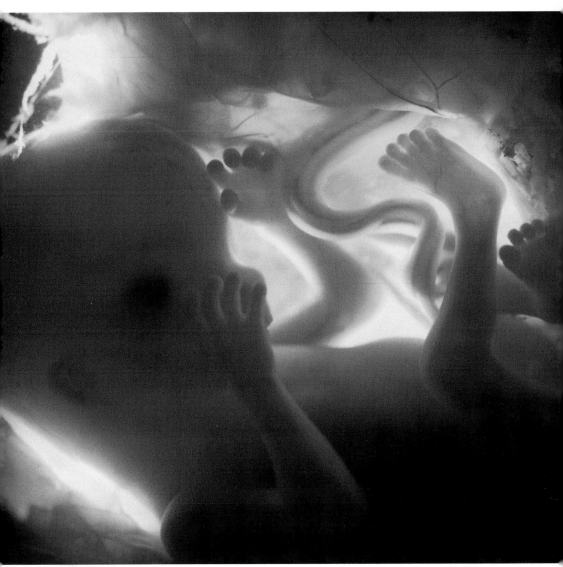

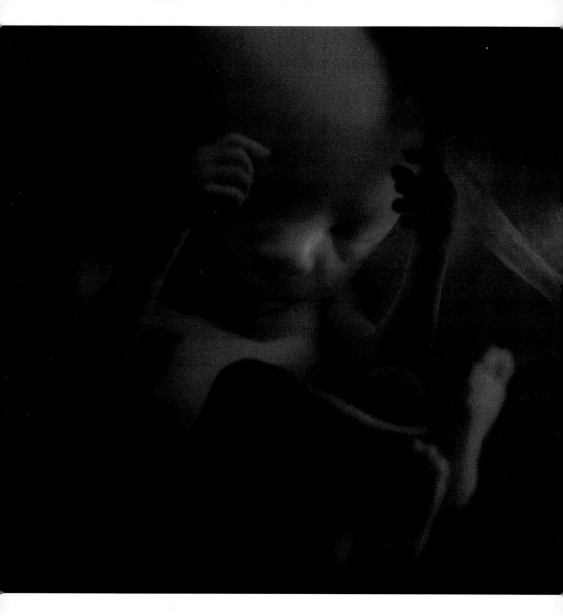

Stage of Life
24 weeks

My, how you've grown! By now the
baby is almost 12 inches long and
weighs a little over 1 pound. There's
still a lot of growing to do, however,
in the next 16 weeks! A full-term
"average" baby usually weighs
between 6 and 8 pounds at birth.

Stage of Life
27 weeks

Those cheeks aren't quite as
chubby as they'll be at birth (this
baby will still gain about 4 pounds
before it enters the world), but the
face is completely developed. The
eyes even open and shut.

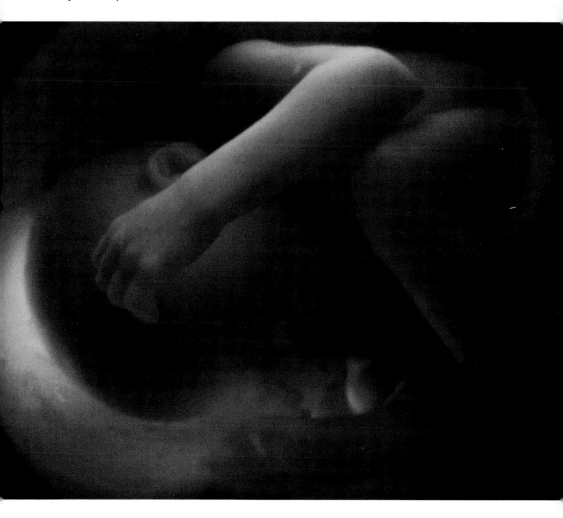

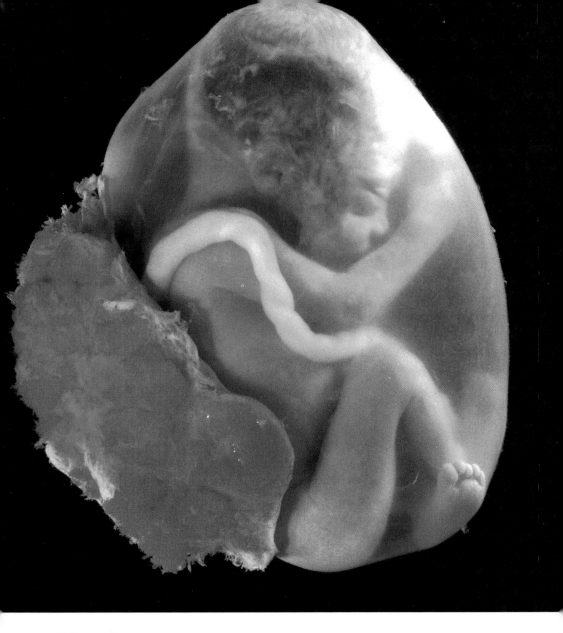

36 weeks

It won't be long now until this baby is born. During the next few weeks, the baby's lungs will finish developing; they are the last organ that needs to mature. By now the baby has learned to suck in preparation for feeding and may have even started sucking his or her thumb!

the.1st trimester

1

Although no one would guess by looking at you that you're pregnant, the miracle of life has begun inside you. As your baby grows from a few tiny cells into a fully formed infant, you'll experience a natural process that is as wondrous physically as it is emotionally. This is a crucial time in your baby's development, and your body is working overtime to produce hormones and additional blood cells. What's really exciting is that by the end of this 1st trimester, your baby will actually look like a baby, complete with eyelids, a nose, a mouth, arms, and legs. Your sweet little baby will be able to move too. It will be a while before you see your beautiful baby, but the journey is well under way!

In this section

Weeks 1 through 4

Weeks 1 and 2

Even if you don't feel a thing (yet!), you're experiencing the amazing transformation of your egg into an embryo. Though the terms used to explain your body's changes during the first couple of weeks of pregnancy may sound clinical, they are a necessary part of describing the complex process of a baby's growth.

During week 1, your body sheds its uterine lining (that's when you get your period) and prepares to make a new one that's a hospitable nest for a fertilized egg. Meanwhile, about a thousand of your eggs make their way down the road to maturity. Only about 20 of those eggs will ripen inside fluid-filled sacs known as follicles, and then only one of those follicles will develop, ovulate, and rupture, allowing the egg (ovum) to start its trip down your fallopian tube during the 2nd week of pregnancy. (If two or more rupture, you may have twins, triplets, or more.)

Of course there can be no baby without a fertilized egg—and that requires your partner's sperm. Typically, of the millions of sperm ejaculated into your vagina, only a few hundred will make it into your fallopian tube. Then the race is on, as the sperm swim upward toward the descending egg. Sperm can live inside a woman's body for as long as six days. Once an egg is released from the ovary, it must be fertilized within 12 to 24 hours. If the egg is not fertilized, it will simply pass through your body with menstrual flow.

How the sperm attaches to the egg is a marvel of biological engineering. Because your eggs have tough, protective shells, each sperm has a sticky structure at one end that allows it to attach to the egg's shell and tunnel right through it, taking along a tidy package of genetic material. Once one sperm penetrates the egg's lining, your egg is fertilized.

Conception typically takes place between days 14 and 17 of a regular 28-day menstrual cycle. It can take up to three days for the sperm to meet up with your egg in the fallopian tube, so the date of intercourse isn't always the same day your baby was conceived. (Remember those cautionary tales in high school health class?)

Week 3

Your fertilized egg, which is now called an embryo, continues moving down the fallopian tube, growing larger as cells divide. If the egg implants in the fallopian tube, you will have an ectopic pregnancy (see "Ectopic pregnancy," page 37), but this is a rare occurrence. More commonly, the embryo cruises down the fallopian tube just fine, growing into a solid ball of about 200 cells by the time it enters your uterus about four days after conception. The embryo usually bounces around in the uterus for a few days until it finds a suitable spot to implant in the lining.

Week 4

Don't be nervous if you experience a little spotting this week. The embryo burrows into your uterine lining as part of the implantation process, and this sometimes causes a small amount of bleeding. That's normal. Your baby's cells continue to multiply, and the placental tissue grows, inhabiting the lining of the uterus and establishing contact with your circulation, which will supply more blood to your growing baby. The placenta also produces estrogen, progesterone, and hCG (human chorionic gonadotropin), which is often referred to as the "pregnancy hormone."

Although your baby is still a microscopic cluster of cells at this point—you can't even see it on an ultrasound—three different essential cell layers are already beginning to develop. Their names are probably familiar from biology class: the ectoderm, which will become your baby's nervous system, hair, and skin; the endoderm, which will form your baby's gastrointestinal tract, liver, pancreas, and thyroid; and the mesoderm, which eventually develops into your baby's skeleton, connective tissue, blood system, urogenital system, and muscles.

Your Body

Clues that you're pregnant

A missed period will probably be your first physical sign of pregnancy. That's because instead of shedding its lining, the uterus is building up its lining to prepare for the implantation of the fertilized egg. Soon after your first missed period, you may also notice that your breasts feel sore and that you're more tired than usual.

Getting proof of pregnancy

A home pregnancy test kit, which you can buy at any drugstore, is a simple, fast, and private way to confirm that you're expecting. It works by testing your urine for the hCG hormone that's produced during pregnancy. If the test detects a certain level of hCG, it will show a positive result, confirming that you are pregnant.

However, if the test is negative, you may still be pregnant. You may have done the test too early, before there is enough hCG in your urine. Wait a few days and repeat the test. If it is still negative and you haven't gotten your period, something else may be happening in your body. Certain medications and illnesses can cause you to skip a period, as can

Moms-to-be with diabetes

Having preexisting diabetes when you get pregnant will make your pregnancy more complicated. However, you'll minimize the risk to your baby if you work closely with your endocrinologist and obstetrician. The key is controlling your blood sugar levels. According to the March of Dimes, if a woman with diabetes has well-controlled blood sugar levels before conceiving, her chances of having a healthy baby are nearly the same as those of a woman without diabetes.

Women with preexisting diabetes do have a higher chance of miscarriage and of having a baby who has birth defects. They also have a greater risk of having a very large baby—10 pounds or bigger—who is more likely to be injured during delivery than a smaller baby. Such problems tend to occur in women whose blood sugar is out of control; that's why blood sugar control before and during pregnancy is absolutely crucial. (If you take oral diabetes medications, your doctor will probably switch you to injected insulin because it is not known if oral diabetes medications taken in the 1st trimester can cause birth defects.)

Taking folic acid before conception and during the first few weeks of pregnancy is even more important for women with diabetes than for women without diabetes because babies of diabetic women have an increased risk of birth defects. It's best to check with your doctor about folic acid before you conceive; women with diabetes may be advised to take a higher-than-normal dose. (Don't do this without your doctor's recommendation.)

Note: Preexisting diabetes is different from gestational diabetes, which occurs during pregnancy and usually ceases after delivery. (See "Gestational diabetes," page 231.)

excessive exercise, low body weight, early menopause, birth control pills, or stress.

After testing positive on a home pregnancy test, some women like their doctors to confirm their pregnancies. Your doctor can perform a simple blood test that can detect hCG in even smaller amounts than a home pregnancy kit can.

Important first steps
There are many months to go before you hear your baby's sweet cry, but as soon as you know that you're pregnant—or better yet, before you start trying to conceive—it's important to consider how your lifestyle or personal habits affect your baby's growth. A baby's brain and organs begin to develop very early in pregnancy, and behaviors such as smoking, drinking alcohol, and using certain medications and street drugs can cause irreparable harm to a developing fetus.

A nutrient-rich diet is also important early on, and it's especially important that you get adequate amounts of the vitamin folic acid. Start taking folic acid supplements as soon as possible (see "Folic acid reduces birth defects," page 26) if you're not already taking them.

Get off to the right start by calling your primary care physician or prenatal provider now to schedule a prenatal appointment. (Your first visit will likely be scheduled around week 10.) Good medical care during pregnancy is crucial for the health of you and your baby, and a doctor can help you make the critical lifestyle changes that are important for your baby's growth.

The fatigue factor

The good news is that you'll feel much more energetic by the start of your 2nd trimester. The bad news? You're going to be very tired until then. Tasks that used to take you minutes seem to drag on forever. Why? Your body is concentrating on the important task of creating your baby, and that puts tremendous demands on it, especially during the 1st trimester. Because your body is working so hard, you are likely to feel fatigued. In fact you may need as much as 10 or 11 hours of sleep each night in order to feel refreshed.

When fatigue strikes, listen to your body. Go to bed early at night, sleep late in the morning, and take naps in the afternoons. If you work and can't get naps on weekdays, set aside time for extra sleep on the weekends. You may feel like a hibernating bear, but that's both normal and common.

Your hormones' wild ride

You may have thought that the phrase "raging hormones" applies only to teenagers in love. Guess again.

During the first few weeks and months of pregnancy, you'll be producing hormones in ways and amounts that are new to your body. These hormones influence you in a variety of ways and cause a wide range of possible effects, including moodiness, headaches, fatigue, breast soreness, complexion problems, and changes in hair and nails. Most of these changes are relatively minor. If something starts to bother you in a major way—for example, if you develop migraines, depression, or irritating complexion changes—talk with your doctor; you may benefit from medication to treat these problems. Although some medications are dangerous during pregnancy, others can be taken safely. Always get your doctor's approval before taking any medication, whether it's over-the-counter (OTC) or prescription.

Your Self

Reactions to being pregnant

No matter how prepared you thought you and your partner were for parenthood, the reality of being pregnant may leave you alternately joyful, panicked, optimistic, resentful, giddy, or grief stricken about the approaching loss of freedom and increase in responsibility. Don't be surprised if your moods are all over the place during the first few months of pregnancy. Hormone surges can certainly influence your roller-coaster ride of emotions, as can fatigue and anxiety.

It's natural to feel worried about delivery, your job, your baby's health, your transition to motherhood, financial demands, and other concerns. You'll look at everything with a new and different perspective. One or both of you may worry that you're not ready for parenthood after all. Understanding, resolving, and appreciating these thoughts and feelings are essential parts of growing into parenthood together.

A certain amount of anxiety is normal, but if you find yourself worrying excessively, discuss your fears with your partner, a family member, or a trusted friend. If high levels of anxiety continue, consider seeing a therapist or social worker. Your doctor can refer you to a good one who is familiar with pregnancy-related issues.

Telling your partner

Should you surprise your partner with the news of your pregnancy over a romantic, candlelit dinner? Or should you do the home pregnancy test when your partner is with you? Only you know the best way to share your pregnancy news. In some couples, the woman determines whether she is pregnant and then shares the news with her partner. If your pregnancy was unplanned, how you make the announcement may depend on whether your partner will view the news as a wonderful surprise or a worrisome development.

Whatever your situation, understand that your partner may react differently from the way you might expect. Men don't experience pregnancy the same way as women, and they may respond with less emotion than you might hope. (See "Your partner: How men react to pregnancy," page 30.) Give your partner room to digest the news in the way that is best for him.

Sex

Though it may seem like pregnancy has thrown your entire life into upheaval, one thing that doesn't have to change right now is your sex life. Unless your doctor has told you to refrain from intercourse, having sex won't harm the baby. Some couples even report that lovemaking is more enjoyable during pregnancy because there's no need to take birth control pills or fiddle with diaphragms or condoms. You may have more or less interest in sex than usual; both are normal. Likewise, your partner's libido may change during your pregnancy. Be open with each other about changes in your sexual desire.

If you have any reason to believe that your partner has been exposed to a disease that can be transmitted sexually, practice safe sex or abstain from sex. If you think you may have been infected with a sexually transmitted disease, see your doctor so you can get treatment.

Work and fatigue

Most healthy women work throughout their pregnancies without any adverse impact on their babies. The only pregnancy-related symptom that is likely to impact your job performance during your first four weeks is fatigue. If you feel tired at work, go to bed early and get more rest during the night. Or if there is a sofa or comfortable chair at work, take a catnap at lunch. (Ask a coworker to wake you up or bring an alarm clock so you don't sleep all afternoon.)

Try not to rely on your favorite double latte to stay alert. Although studies show that moderate caffeine consumption is probably safe during pregnancy, too much may not be safe. Limit your daily caffeine to 300 mg (milligrams), keeping in mind that the caffeine content of 8 ounces of coffee can average 64–288 mg. Remember that the type and amount of beans used to make the coffee determine the caffeine content, and some coffee shops and restaurants make strong brews that contain more caffeine than you'd expect. Also keep in mind that tea, cola, chocolate, and chocolate milk contain caffeine. (See "The buzz about caffeine," page 43.)

Workplace hazards

A pregnant woman needs to look at her workplace with new eyes. What may have been a safe environment for you prepregnancy may now pose harm to your developing fetus. Look around. Does your work require you to use or be near solvents, paints, paint thinners, cleaning products, fumes, pesticides, chemicals such as lead and mercury, carbon monoxide, benzene, or formaldehyde? Is there a chance that you'll be exposed to

radiation? Do you work in a dental, medical, or veterinary office where you are exposed to nitrous oxide, which has been shown to cause birth defects? If so, you will need to take steps to protect your baby. (See "What hazards should I worry about at work?" page 69.)

Two other working conditions can impact pregnancy: lifting and standing. If your job requires you to lift heavy objects or stand most of the day, talk with your doctor about whether these activities put your baby at risk.

Diet & Exercise

Prenatal vitamins

If your typical lunch before you got pregnant consisted of a candy bar and a low-calorie soda, it's time to give your diet a makeover. An important first step is to take a daily prenatal vitamin, which will ensure that your body gets the vitamins and minerals it needs to create a healthy baby. Prenatal vitamins include folic acid, iodine, iron, vitamin A, vitamin D, zinc, and calcium.

Remember that a vitamin pill is no substitute for a healthy diet. Aim to eat a diet rich in fruits, vegetables, non-fat dairy foods, whole grains, lean meats, and safe fish. (See "Safe fish," page 86.)

Folic acid reduces birth defects

Scientists have discovered that the risk of neural tube defects—which are birth defects of the spine and brain—plummets when a woman gets adequate amounts of folic acid before and during pregnancy.

Folic acid, also known as folate, is a B vitamin that is found in foods such as fortified breakfast cereals, leafy greens, oranges and orange juice, black beans, asparagus, spinach, and lentils. However, to ensure that you get the amount needed to prevent neural tube defects, your doctor will recommend that you take a prenatal vitamin or a multivitamin with 400 mcg (micrograms) of folic acid every day. It's best to start taking prenatal vitamins before you conceive, but if you haven't, start taking them today. Folic acid is particularly important during these first weeks of pregnancy. You can buy prenatal vitamins at most stores, but check with your doctor to see which one he or she recommends. Or ask the pharmacist at your local drugstore.

Doctors sometimes prescribe additional folic acid supplementation to women who are at extra high risk of delivering babies with birth defects, such as women who have had babies with neural tube defects or women who have diabetes or epilepsy. Be warned, though, that you should take only as much folic acid—or any supplement—as your doctor recommends. Megadoses of certain vitamins and minerals can harm your baby.

The role of calcium

Calcium is one of the major building blocks of bone and teeth. It also contributes to the development of the baby's circulatory system, nervous system, and muscles. Your body needs an ample supply of calcium to help build your baby. If it can't get enough from your diet, it will take calcium from your bones, weakening them and increasing your chance of osteoporosis later in life. Dairy foods are the best source of calcium. Aim to get 3 servings of low-fat or non-fat milk or yogurt each day. If you can't tolerate dairy, use a calcium-fortified equivalent, such as soymilk. (See "Your 1st trimester diet," page 41.)

It's time to get moving

All you want to do is curl up on the couch all afternoon, right? Although you may think you're too tired for this

Epilepsy

Women with preexisting epilepsy can sustain a pregnancy and deliver a healthy baby. However, your pregnancy must be closely monitored, and your drug regimen may need to be adjusted. Some types of medication used to treat epilepsy increase the risk of birth defects such as cleft lip/palate, so it is crucial for women with preexisting epilepsy to consult with their doctors before conceiving. Changes in medications, vitamin supplements, and diet may be necessary.

reminder, here it is: Staying active during pregnancy does many good things for you. It gives you energy, helps keep your weight in check, reduces your risk of gestational diabetes, builds stamina for labor and delivery, and elevates your mood. However, to gain these benefits, you must exercise safely.

Before you start exercising, get your doctor's approval. Your doctor will probably give you a thumbs-up unless you have a high risk of premature labor or you've been diagnosed with heart disease, an incompetent cervix, placenta previa (see page 268), or preeclampsia (see page 253). If you are having bleeding during this pregnancy, your doctor may advise you to hold off on exercising. Some women who are carrying multiples are concerned about exercise, but exercise should be fine as long as the pregnancy is not considered high-risk.

If you are already an exerciser, stick with the fitness regimen you followed before you became pregnant. Even athletes and others who exercise vigorously can, in many cases, continue their activity during pregnancy, according to guidelines from the American College of Obstetricians and Gynecologists (ACOG). As the months go by and your body gets larger, you may have to decrease your intensity level. Talk with your doctor about what makes sense for you.

If you haven't exercised recently, choose an activity that won't overtax your body, such as walking or swimming. Now is not the time to take up an extreme sport. Aim to exercise for at least 30 minutes a day, most days of the week. If 30 minutes is too much, start with 10 minutes and gradually work up to 30 minutes or more. If you find it difficult to block off 30 minutes each day for exercise, schedule three 10-minute sessions throughout the day.

Avoid any activities that put you at high risk for injury, such as horseback riding or downhill skiing. Contact sports in which you may receive a blow to your abdomen, including ice hockey and soccer, are out. Finally, forgo scuba diving; it is not safe for the baby's circulatory system.

Are you exercising too hard?

Use the "talk test" as a yardstick for how vigorously to exercise. Here's how it works: While you exercise, you should be able to talk without losing your breath. If you're not sure whether you're exercising too hard, try singing "Happy Birthday." If you can't make it all the way through, slow down. If you experience any alarming symptoms, such as shortness of breath, bleeding, light-headedness, or chest pain, call your doctor.

A cure for morning sickness?

You'll probably be tempted to skip exercise if you have morning sickness. Lying down might seem like a better idea than being up and around, yet for some women, the opposite is true. When morning sickness strikes, they feel better if they go outside for a walk in the fresh air. Others find relief when they swim or do yoga. Since every pregnancy is different, it's worthwhile for you to try exercising even when you have morning sickness. If exercise makes you feel worse, take the day off.

Smoking and alcohol use

Smoking tobacco of any kind or drinking alcohol during pregnancy is dangerous. Smoking robs your developing baby of oxygen and can cause developmental abnormalities, premature birth, miscarriage, and low birthweight. Babies born to mothers who smoked while pregnant have more colds, ear infections, and upper respiratory infections than babies with nonsmoking mothers. They also have a greater risk of SIDS (sudden infant death syndrome).

If you smoke, now is the time to stop. Ask your doctor about smoking-cessation resources in your area. If you can't quit completely, cut down as much as possible; keep in mind that even a few cigarettes a day can potentially harm your baby. If your partner or other family members smoke, ask them to quit or to smoke outdoors in a place where you won't be exposed to the smoke. Research shows that even secondhand smoke can be harmful to a developing fetus.

Now is also the time to stop drinking. Alcohol can cause your baby to be born with fetal alcohol syndrome, which is characterized by

---

Obesity

Obese mothers have a higher risk of miscarriage, preeclampsia, gestational diabetes, cesarean deliveries, complications during childbirth, and difficulty with breastfeeding. Their babies are at increased risk of being born with neural tube defects and a high birthweight, and they are more likely to be overweight later in life.

That said, if you are obese there are steps you can take to boost your chances of having a healthy baby:

Eat well. This isn't the time to diet, but it's a perfect time to cut down on sugary desserts, fried foods, salty snacks, and fast food. Consider meeting with a registered dietitian (RD); many health insurance plans cover RD bills. A dietitian can help you design a healthy diet that is not too high or too low in calories.

Exercise. Even a short walk every day can make a difference. Start by walking a few minutes a day, gradually lengthening your walks. Focus on time, not speed. If you don't like walking, try swimming, riding a stationary bike or recumbent bike, or exercising with a workout video designed for obese people.

Talk with your doctor about weight gain during pregnancy. The standard recommendation for obese women is to gain 15 to 25 pounds, but your doctor may give you different advice.

Take your prenatal vitamins daily. Because your baby has an increased risk of neural tube defects, it's essential that you take your folic acid without fail.

mental retardation, growth restriction, and facial abnormalities. Alcohol is particularly dangerous to your fetus during the 1st and 2nd trimesters, when the baby's organs are developing. If you can't stop drinking, seek help immediately.

Common Questions

Q. How does family health history affect a pregnancy?

A. Some health problems are more likely to occur in certain families, racial groups, or ethnic groups. Certain diseases are linked to specific genes. Tay-Sachs disease, sickle-cell anemia, and cystic fibrosis are three such examples. In addition, your baby's risk of developing diseases such as diabetes, seizure disorder, or mental retardation may be higher if someone in your family has had them.

In order to assess your baby's risk of developing or inheriting diseases, your doctor will ask you about your family's health history. The more complete you can be in giving specific details, the better; find out as much health information as possible from relatives, both on your side and your partner's. If necessary, your doctor may recommend that you see a genetic counselor for further discussion and, possibly, genetic testing.

Your doctor will also ask you about your own health and sexual history, as well as your partner's. It's important to tell your doctor everything, even if it's embarrassing. If you've had previous pregnancies, abortions, or sexually transmitted diseases, or if you've used street drugs, or if your partner uses drugs or has a sexually transmitted disease, your doctor needs to know. Your health and sexual history may affect your pregnancy, so be completely honest. Rest assured, there is nothing you can tell your doctor that he or she hasn't heard many times before.

Q. When should I tell my other child or children that I'm pregnant?

A. That depends on your child's age. A toddler may not understand the concept of a new brother or sister until you bring one home from the hospital. You may want to wait as long as possible to share the news with a preschooler because the idea of waiting several months for a new sibling can frustrate children of that age. Elementary school children can be told right away.

Be prepared for your child to be less than excited about the arrival of a new sibling. The news might make your child feel threatened, unloved, or angry.

These feelings are normal. Give your child space to share worries and fears. Offer reassurance that you have enough love for all of your children. Be honest and explain that a new baby will take up a lot of your time; then emphasize that you'll still have time for your older child or children. You might want to squeeze in some special outings together before the baby is born.

Your partner: How men react to pregnancy

Your girlfriends jumped for joy when you told them your good news, so why did your partner barely look up from the newspaper? Men don't always react to pregnancy the way women do. While many are over-the-moon excited, particularly if the pregnancy is planned and happily anticipated, others are flooded with worries. The best way to help your partner feel more comfortable about your pregnancy is to understand that men and women often look at pregnancy differently. Don't criticize him if he doesn't react the way you think he should. Give him space to experience the pregnancy in his own way. There are often legitimate reasons for men's reactions; for example, consider the following:

Men can't experience the pregnancy the way you do. Sure, the man contributes half of the conception equation, but after supplying the sperm, the man's body is no longer part of the pregnancy. Both physically and emotionally you will feel more, from morning sickness and labor pains to first kicks and hiccups. Because of this, your partner may feel less attached to the pregnancy than you do, especially before you start to show. He may also feel left out because everyone is paying attention to you.

Men worry, even if they don't tell you. Even if your partner doesn't mention it, he may be worrying about what pregnancy will do to your lives. He may feel anxious about upcoming expenses, your health insurance coverage, the pain that you'll feel during pregnancy or delivery, what life will be like with three rather than two, and the effects of pregnancy on your sex life. If you are planning to quit your job to stay home with your baby, he may feel more pressure because he'll be the sole breadwinner.

Men question what type of dad they'll be. For some men, fatherhood is something they have looked forward to for years and feel well equipped to handle. Others may feel apprehensive. If a man was abused, abandoned, bullied, or ignored by his father, he may wonder whether he can be a good father to his child. He may fear that he will make the same mistakes his father made. Talk with him about his worries. Reassure him that you will work together to solve problems and that he'll most likely be an excellent father, even if his own father wasn't.

If you find that pregnancy brings up issues that are too difficult for the two of you to handle on your own, talk with a social worker, marital counselor, or therapist. It's best to tackle these issues now, because after your baby is born, you'll have less time and energy to focus on each other.

Week 5

Your Baby

The inside story

It's difficult to imagine, but this week your baby is still tinier than the "I" at the start of this sentence. Even so, exciting changes are taking place each day. Your embryo now looks less like a ball and more like a curled tube. One end of it will eventually become your baby's head; the other, your baby's bottom. Between those two ends, the spinal cord is forming, and by the 5th week there will be a series of bumps along your baby's back. This is the start of your baby's central nervous system.

Like a baby chick, your baby has a pear-shape yolk sac filled with fluid that will help nourish him. Blood moves to the wall of the yolk sac by your baby's primitive heart, where it circulates and then is returned. Your baby's heart is only a small tube now, but by next week it will have right and left chambers.

Other major organs are also developing rapidly. Your baby's brain has divided into two lobes by the start of this 2nd month of life, and his respiratory system will first appear as a groove behind his face. It will keep growing downward as your baby develops, branching 23 times along both sides of his body as the lungs finish forming.

The arms and legs are tiny buds, and minuscule, paddle-shape hands may even show finger buds. Your baby will finally be visible to the naked eye.

Your Body

Bigger breasts

If you've always longed for a bigger bust, your wish is about to be granted. Most women's breasts swell an entire cup size during the first 12 weeks of pregnancy, and you can expect to gain at least two cup sizes by the time you deliver your baby. In fact, your breasts will ultimately account for 2 pounds of your pregnancy weight.

Breast sensations in early pregnancy range from a slight, pleasant tingling to such acute discomfort that you wince and pull away when your partner reaches for you. This swelling and sensitivity are due to your body's increased production of estrogen and progesterone, the hormones responsible for increasing the blood flow to your breasts in preparation for nursing.

Your breasts may start to look different too. Within a few weeks, they will probably start to darken around the areolae (the pigmented areas around your nipples) as tiny glands grow and prepare for breast-feeding. These glands secrete a lubricating oil and may start to look bumpy around your nipples. You may also notice a map of blue veins across your breasts, experience occasional shooting pains, or have a persistent throbbing sensation. Most of your dis-comfort will subside after the 1st trimester. Meanwhile, soothe sore breasts beneath warm (not hot!) showers or compresses. You can also tame aches by wearing a soft, stretchy cotton bra to bed. (See "Finding a good pregnancy bra," below.)

Will your breasts look the same after pregnancy? Probably not. However, the amount your breasts sag or suffer from stretch marks is mainly due to genetics, so it's not really worth worrying about. Wearing comfy, supportive, well-fitting bras day and night may help minimize sagging and stretch marks. Staying within the limit of your recommended weight gain will also help because additional excess pounds stretch the skin more.

Finding a good pregnancy bra

If your cups runneth over and your bras leave marks on your skin, splurge at the lingerie store for a few pretty, extra-supportive bras in a larger size. (The truth is that there's really no such thing as a maternity bra; the bras many women turn to for support in late pregnancy are actually nursing bras.) What style is going to be most comfortable? Some women insist on underwires for extra support—and to make the most of their new curves— while others switch to bras with wide, soft cotton bands beneath their breasts. Look for bras with multiple closures that can grow with you and choose wider straps to take some of the strain off your shoulders. Avoid inner seams that might irritate sensitive nipples. For sleeping or at home, you can wear cotton sports bras. Beware, though: Tugging sports bras over your head can be a real pain, so look for bras that go on more easily.

Frequent urination

As early as your 5th week, your uterus will begin to expand, putting increas-ing pressure on your bladder. Even immediately after a trip to the bathroom, you may still feel that maddening urge to urinate because of the added pressure from your uterus. Look on the bright side—at least you're getting exercise as you return (again and again) to the toilet.

Although it may be tempting to cut back on your fluid intake to reduce bathroom visits, don't. This could cause you to feel light-headed.

One additional note: Pain or burning during urination is absolutely not a normal pregnancy hurdle. This is a sign that you may be suffering from a common bladder infection known as cystitis, a condition sometimes accompanied by a fever. See a health care provider who can test your urine for bacteria and prescribe a pregnancy-safe medication.

Complexion problems

For some lucky women, pregnancy provides a beauty treatment for skin that trumps anything you can buy in a jar. That added blood volume coursing through your body brings a flush to your cheeks, and rising hormone levels cause the skin glands to produce more oil, making your skin supple and shiny. The total effect is a lovely pregnancy "glow."

Unfortunately, many women skip that glow and battle skin problems instead. Hormone changes can cause skin to misbehave, so it's slick one minute and scaly the next. Here are some strategies for coping:

Oily skin. If your body's unique mix of pregnancy hormones is especially strong, you may find yourself with acne like you haven't seen since high school. Although many over-the-counter (OTC) topical acne medications are safe for you to use, avoid creams that contain retinol, benzoyl peroxide, or antibiotics. Always ask your prenatal provider before using any OTC medications just to be sure. You should also stay away from prescription acne medications, including vitamin A-derivative lotions such as Accutane, Retin-A, Differin, and Tazorac.

Clear your shelves of any topical cleansers, makeup, or moisturizers that contain chemical exfoliants made with salicylic acid. Chemical exfoliants that don't contain salicylic acid are safe to use and can help remove dead skin cells.

What else can you do? Because most pregnancy acne is caused by pores clogged with oil, keep your pores clear with mechanical exfoliants. (Mechanical exfoliants are products that may contain synthetic beads or ground-up nutshells, which help scrub away dead skin.) Choose a nondrying daily cleanser and wash your skin with a gentle, oatmeal-base facial scrub a few times a week to further clean pores and remove dead skin. You can also try clarifying masks. For a home remedy, beat two egg whites into soft peaks, apply them to your face, and rinse after 15 minutes. Use oil-free makeup and oil-free sunblock and carry blotting papers to sop up excess oily shine.

Dry skin. How can you possibly suffer from acne breakouts one month and dry skin the next? Simple: As your hormones naturally fluctuate, so will your skin's appearance.

To cope with flaking skin, boost your water intake to stay hydrated. Topical creams moisturize your skin from the outside, but water helps hydrate your skin from the inside. Remove dead skin cells with a gentle scrubbing cleanser, such as one that contains oatmeal.

Apply baby oil or a scent-free moisturizer twice a day, preferably when your skin is damp, to seal in moisture. Another good trick is to shower for no more than 10 minutes in warm (not hot) water and use a mild moisturizing cleanser and a light body oil while you're in the shower. You can make a moisturizing mask at home by cooking oatmeal until it's thick, letting it cool, and patting it onto your face. Let it dry for 20 minutes; then rinse with warm water. Body balms and a room humidifier also leave skin smoother and more supple, and wearing natural fabrics such as cotton will allow your skin to breathe.

Some skin medications to avoid

Because of their proven association with birth defects, do not use these dermatologic medications during your pregnancy:

- Fluconazole, an antifungal agent
- Tetracycline, an antibiotic often prescribed for acne
- Minoxidil, a hair-promoting agent
- Isotretinoin, prescribed for severe nodular acne

Genetic screening

Your provider may recommend that you be screened through blood tests to determine whether you're a carrier for a particular genetic disorder, depending on your racial background and family history. Genetic screening tests are optional, and the decision to have them is yours. You may decline the screening. Or you may agree to the tests so that you can be as informed as possible about the potential effects of genetics on your unborn baby's health. If you and your partner should discover that you carry genes that put your child at greater risk for a potentially life-threatening disease, your provider will likely advise you to have a genetic test such as chorionic villus sampling (CVS) (see "1st trimester tests," page 92) or

amniocentesis (page 126) to find out if your baby has the illness. This will help prepare you ahead of time to either offer your child the best medical help available or terminate the pregnancy. The most common of these inherited disorders include:

Tay-Sachs disease, Canavan disease, and familial dysautonomia. If you are of Eastern European Jewish (Ashkenazi) descent, the American College of Obstetricians and Gynecologists recommends that your health care provider offer carrier screening for Tay-Sachs disease, Canavan disease, and familial dysautonomia. All of these diseases affect a baby's central nervous system, are incurable, and may be associated with a shortened life span.

Cystic fibrosis (CF). This disease most commonly affects breathing and digestion. Individuals with CF are born with an abnormal protein that prevents chloride from passing normally in and out of certain cells, including cells lining the lungs and pancreas. As a result, these cells produce a thick, sticky mucus and other secretions, making it difficult to breathe, causing frequent lung infections, and harming digestion.

About 1 in 30 Caucasians is a carrier of CF. Although it is more common in Caucasians, all racial groups are affected by this disease.

CF is usually treated through special diets, medications that contain pancreatic enzymes to aid digestion, daily respiratory therapy, and mucus-thinning medications. Depending on the severity of the disease, individuals with CF may die in childhood or live past their 40s.

Thalassemia. This describes a group of blood diseases, most of which are different forms of anemia (a deficiency of red blood cells). Your health care provider may test for this if your routine blood work indicates that thalassemia is a possibility. The two main types are alpha and beta thalassemias, named according to which part of hemoglobin (a protein that carries oxygen) is lacking.

Some forms of thalassemia are more severe than others. It can occur worldwide but is more common in people of Greek, Italian, Middle Eastern, African, or Asian descent.

Some children with thalassemia appear healthy until early childhood, when they grow slowly and appear listless; others may die in utero. Children with thalassemia major, a severe form of the disease, may need to have blood transfusions and antibiotics for life.

Sickle-cell anemia. This is a disease caused by abnormal hemoglobin, the red blood cell protein that carries oxygen from the lungs to other parts of the body. There are several types of sickle-cell anemia, depending on which genes a child inherits from his parents. Some people affected by sickle-cell anemia lead normal lives, while others suffer severe complications. Infants and young children with sickle-cell anemia are more prone to serious bacterial infections. Individuals with sickle-cell anemia

may also suffer from pain crises, stroke, vision problems, slow growth, and acute chest syndrome (similar to pneumonia).

Sickle-cell anemia affects mostly African-Americans; approximately 1 in 12 is a carrier. It is much less common in other racial groups.

Children affected with sickle-cell anemia may be treated with antibiotics to prevent infection. Other symptoms of the disease are treated as they arise; for instance, there are now medications used to treat painful episodes, and individuals at an increased risk of stroke may have regular blood transfusions to decrease the risk.

Miscarriage

A miscarriage is defined as the loss of a pregnancy before the 20th week. It is usually preceded by heavy bleeding and cramping. According to the American College of Obstetricians and Gynecologists, one in five pregnancies ends in miscarriage; more than 80 percent of miscarriages occur in the first 3 months of pregnancy. The actual number of miscarriages may be higher, however, because so many occur in the first few weeks of pregnancy, before a woman knows she's pregnant or before a pregnancy could be detected.

No matter how early you miscarry, you may feel shock, profound sadness, and anger. The dramatic drop in estrogen after a miscarriage can cause weepiness, but most women feel a deeper sadness as well.

That grief is often made worse by the fact that miscarriage is so often dismissed as "a bad period" or a pregnancy that "wasn't meant to be," even by the most well-meaning friends and family members.

Many women also suffer from guilt following a miscarriage, convinced that they did something to cause it. Was it that hour you spent lifting weights at the gym? The computer terminal at work? The glass of wine you had at dinner? No. Remember that the vast majority of miscarriages are attributed to random chromosomal abnormalities. For the small number of women (4 percent) who suffer more than one miscarriage, there may be a medical cause that can often be identified and treated.

It's important to find emotional support following a miscarriage. Give yourself time to go through the four stages of grief—denial, anger, depression, and acceptance—before trying to get pregnant again. Acknowledge

Bleeding and spotting: What's normal and what's not

Nothing is scarier than finding blood on your underclothes or sheets when you're pregnant. Yet light bleeding or spotting affects nearly one-third of all pregnancies, and it is not necessarily a sign that something is wrong. Spotting after intercourse can be common for a small percentage of pregnant women, for instance, and bleeding may sometimes be caused by reasons that have nothing to do with pregnancy, such as infections, trauma, or tears to the vaginal wall.

Only about half of women who bleed during pregnancy will go on to lose their babies due to miscarriage. Still, it's important to notify your health care provider if bleeding occurs. When you call, be prepared to give information about the amount of blood lost and a description of how you're feeling overall. You should insist on being seen if you have any vaginal bleeding that makes you feel faint or soaks through a sanitary pad. You should also be seen if the bleeding is persistent or accompanied by pain or a fever.

Some other common causes for bleeding during pregnancy include the following:

Implantation bleeding. About 4 weeks into your pregnancy, you might have some spotting or light bleeding as the embryo implants into the uterine wall. This is called implantation bleeding and is perfectly normal. However, it can be confusing because this small amount of blood usually appears at about the same time your period was due. Implantation bleeding is not associated with any risk to the fetus, but it can be scary if you've already had a positive pregnancy test.

Threatened miscarriage. Vaginal bleeding during pregnancy is sometimes called a "threatened" miscarriage. Basically it means that you've had some heavier bleeding, but an ultrasound shows that the fetus is still alive inside the uterus. This bleeding can be caused by infection, physical trauma, medications, subchorionic hematoma, or an abnormality in the fetus. It can also happen for no reason at all, whether you're a sedentary software programmer or a competitive snowboarder.

how painful it is and communicate that pain to someone you trust. Recognize that your partner will be grieving for this loss as well and tune in to his needs. Finally, remember that in most cases, even women who have endured successive miscarriages go on to have healthy babies.

Possible causes of miscarriage

The following are all possible causes of miscarriage:

Chromosomal problems. During fertilization the sperm and egg each bring 23 chromosomes together to create 23 perfectly matched pairs of chromosomes. This is a complex process, and a minor glitch can result in a genetic abnormality that prevents the embryo from growing.

Researchers blame genetics for most miscarriages. As you age, these glitches are more likely to occur. (See "When you're older than 35," page 78.)

Hormone imbalance. About 15 percent of all miscarriages are attributed to unbalanced hormones. For example, an insufficient progesterone level can prevent your fertilized egg from implanting in your uterus. A doctor can diagnose a hormone imbalance through an endometrial biopsy; this procedure is typically done at the end of your menstrual cycle to assess ovulation and development of the uterine lining. Treatment may include fertility drugs that can improve the quality of egg development and hormone production.

Uterine problems. Uterine fibroids may be responsible for some miscarriages; most grow on the outer wall of the uterus and are harmless. If they grow inside the uterus, fibroids can occasionally interfere with implantation or blood supply to the fetus.

Some women are born with a septum, an uncommon uterine defect linked to miscarriage. A septum is a tissue wall that divides the uterine cavity.

Also uncommon are bands of tissue within the uterus caused by scarring from surgery or second-term abortions. This tissue can keep an egg from implanting properly or may hamper blood flow to the placenta. A doctor can determine uterine defects through specialized X-rays; most can be treated.

Chronic illness. Autoimmune disorders, heart disease, kidney and liver disease, diabetes—chronic illnesses such as these cause as many as 6 percent of recurring miscarriages. If you have a chronic illness, find an obstetrician experienced in caring for women with your condition.

High fever. No matter how healthy you are normally, if you develop a high fever—a core body temperature over 102 degrees—during early pregnancy, you may experience a miscarriage. A high core body temperature is most damaging to the embryo before 6 weeks.

Ectopic pregnancy

Probably the most dangerous cause for bleeding during the 1st trimester is an ectopic pregnancy. Ectopic pregnancy occurs when your fertilized egg implants somewhere outside the uterus—usually the fallopian tube—and begins growing. ("Ectopic" means "out of place.") Typically this happens if your fallopian tube is blocked by scar tissue or has an abnormality. Eventually the abnormal pregnancy will grow and could cause the tube to rupture; if this occurs, severe abdominal pain and bleeding will result. Most ectopic pregnancies are diagnosed in time to prevent this, but in the United States the condition still causes about 50 deaths a year.

One out of every 100 pregnancies is ectopic. How do you know if you have an ectopic pregnancy? In addition to vaginal spotting or bleeding, you might suffer from abdominal or pelvic pain and vomiting. You may also have an odd pain in the tip of your shoulder, caused by internal bleeding that irritates nerves that travel to your shoulders. If you have any of these symptoms, call your health care provider immediately. You're much more likely to save your fallopian tube—and perhaps your own life—if you treat an ectopic pregnancy early.

At the doctor's office or emergency room, alert your provider to any risk factors you may have for an ectopic pregnancy. These include a prior tubal ligation, a previous ectopic pregnancy, getting pregnant with an intrauterine device (IUD) in place, having a mother who took DES (diethylstilbestrol) while pregnant with you, or infertility treatments.

(Infertility is often caused by damaged tubes, so there's a higher chance that you'll have an ectopic pregnancy if you've been infertile.) Other risk factors are pelvic infections and surgeries, such as the removal of an ovarian cyst.

In diagnosing an ectopic pregnancy, the doctor will most likely administer a blood test to check the level of the pregnancy hormone hCG. You may also have a vaginal exam and an ultrasound to check for an enlarged fallopian tube and the presence of an abnormal pregnancy. If you're not in pain, you may be monitored for several days with hormone tests and ultrasounds to confirm the diagnosis.

If diagnosed early, an ectopic pregnancy can be treated without surgery. You may be given methotrexate, a drug that will remove the abnormal pregnancy tissue. Your provider will monitor the pregnancy hormones in your blood to make sure that you are no longer pregnant. If the ectopic pregnancy is diagnosed later, or if you're in severe pain or having heavy bleeding, you may need surgery to have the tube opened and the pregnancy extracted, or you may need to have part of the fallopian tube removed.

It's scary to have an ectopic pregnancy, but you may also feel sadness because the pregnancy cannot continue. But remember this: More than half of all women who have had an ectopic pregnancy in the past go on to have one or more healthy pregnancies in the future.

Your Self

Doubts and desires

If you're not suffering from morning sickness, your jeans aren't tight, and that face in the mirror looks just like yours, then your emotional reaction to pregnancy might be simple disbelief. Are you really pregnant?

Feelings of doubt or even full-blown denial are absolutely normal. Planned or unplanned, it may be many weeks before this pregnancy feels "real." Wallow in your doubts. Use this time to explore all of the excitement, uncertainty, or perhaps grief you may feel at the prospect of having a baby. Start a pregnancy journal to catalog your hardest questions: Will this pregnancy go to term? How will motherhood affect my life? What will a new baby do to the relationship with my partner and other children?

Answers to these questions might

Most Common Birth Defects

Birth Defect	Frequency	How it's diagnosed	Treatment
Congenital Heart Defects	1 in 125 births	Through ultrasound in the 2nd trimester, then confirmed with fetal echocardiogram	Corrected with surgery during infancy, or monitored if mild
Pyloric Stenosis (obstruction in the stomach's lower opening that prevents normal digestion)	1 in 500–1,000 births	Sometimes through an ultrasound exam or through symptoms (failure to thrive, vomiting) by 2 months of age	Surgery
Congenital Hip Dislocation	1–2 in 1,000 births	At birth or in early infancy through physical exam	A diapering technique that keeps legs apart to stabilize hip joints
Cleft Lip and Cleft Palate	1 in 1,000 births	With ultrasound in 2nd trimester, or at birth	Surgery before first birthday
Clubfoot	1 in 1,000 births	Sometimes through ultrasound in 2nd trimester, but more often at birth	Exercise, a cast, or surgery
Spina Bifida (the neural tube does not close)	1 in 2,000 births	With MSAFP serum screening and/or ultrasound	Surgery, but babies may still have varying degrees of paralysis depending on where along the spine the defect occurs

depend on the day—or the minute—as hormones fluctuate and your body feels like it's being taken over. To get through this uncertain time, find activities that are engaging but relaxing. Try comic movies, a fun novel, or dinner at a new restaurant.

Confide in your partner too. This is the start of a new level of intimacy between you. If your partner tunes out when you're venting, turn the conversation around and ask him to talk. Candid communication is the surest way to help your relationship grow as your baby does. If you're a single mother, talk with family and friends, especially those who have been pregnant before.

Worrying about baby's health

As you grapple with the reality of pregnancy, you may find yourself dwelling on every single thing you might have done that could harm your baby: that extra glass (or two) of champagne on New Year's Eve, the X-ray your dentist took, the fumes you inhaled last week when you painted the guest room, that fall you took while skiing. Or you could stumble onto a newspaper article about birth defects that leaves your mouth dry with fear about your own baby's health.

Don't worry about worrying. The overwhelming majority of babies are born healthy. Paradoxically, the best way to keep your peace of mind is to reassure yourself that some worrying is OK. Relax and let your mind roam into even the darkest corners. List everything that scares you. The fact that you're anxious is actually a good sign, because it can mean that you're growing attached to your baby. The next step is to find ways to prevent these worries from festering in secret and attaining monster proportions.

Examine your fears. Instead of trying to push the fear away, drag it into a good strong light. Examine your fears and consider the worst-case scenario. In this way you may find that you already know how you'd handle a scary situation. For instance, if genetic testing showed that your child had Down syndrome or cystic fibrosis, what would you do, and why? How would you feel?

Talk to your health care practitioner. Ask about every item on your worry list. Chances are your provider can reassure you. Developing an action plan for each case may also temper your anxiety. If you embrace your fears instead of sweeping them under the rug, they can become your greatest resource, helping you plan for the future as you get to know your own heart and mind.

Search for distractions. If you're still spending a lot of time feeling anxious, take further steps to distract yourself from dire thoughts. Share your fears with your partner, friends, or a therapist. Researchers have found that people with emotional support deal better with stress.

Set aside time for yourself too. Research suggests that pregnant women who enjoy leisure activities tend to have fewer premature and low-birthweight babies. Find time to walk, see movies, have picnics, or simply lie in a hammock all afternoon with a good book.

Finally, try this relaxation technique: Lie down or lean back in a chair with your eyes closed. For 10 minutes, repeat a simple word such as "peace" or "joy" as you take deep breaths to slow your heart rate and lessen muscle tension.

When you shouldn't have sex

For most women it's safe to have sex at any stage of pregnancy. Your baby is cushioned against jouncing inside the amniotic sac and guarded against infection by the mucus plug blocking the cervix. There are only a few exceptions to this rule. Talk to your provider about any of these concerns:

- A sexually transmitted disease
- An incompetent cervix (the cervix opens prematurely)
- A history of premature labor, or signs that you're going into labor
- Placenta previa (the placenta blocks all or part of the cervix)
- Placental abruption (the placenta separates from the uterine wall)
- Ruptured membranes

Diet & Exercise

Your 1st trimester diet

If you've tried—and failed—in the past to curb your love of take-out pizza and ice cream, perhaps you simply needed the right motivation: nurturing a beautiful, healthy baby.

Eating well is especially important now. Your body uses the nutrients and energy provided by the food you eat both to build a healthy baby and to keep your body strong. A healthful diet for pregnancy is one that contains most or all of the essential nutrients your body needs and one that provides the right balance of carbohydrate, fat, and protein without too many calories.

To build your healthful pregnancy diet, choose a range of nutrient-packed foods from the following groups:

Fruits: 3–4 servings a day. Choose fresh, frozen, canned (in natural juice, not heavy syrup), and dried fruit or 100-percent fruit juice. Include at least one citrus fruit (orange, grapefruit, tangerine) each day because citrus fruits are rich in vitamin C. Limit fruit juice consumption to no more than 1 cup a day; juice is high in calories compared with whole fruit, and it does not deliver the fiber that whole fruit does. One serving equals one medium piece of fruit such as an apple or orange, or ½ of a banana; ½ cup of chopped fresh, cooked, or canned fruit; ¼ cup dried fruit; or ¾ cup of 100-percent fruit juice.

Vegetables: 3–5 servings a day. To get the greatest range of nutrients, think of a rainbow as you fill your plate with vegetables. Choose vegetables that are dark green (broccoli, kale, spinach), orange (carrots, sweet potatoes, pumpkin, winter squash), yellow (corn, yellow peppers), and red (tomatoes, red peppers). One serving equals 1 cup of raw leafy vegetables such as spinach or lettuce, or ½ cup chopped vegetables, cooked or raw.

Dairy foods: 3 servings a day. Dairy foods provide the calcium that your baby needs to grow and that you need to keep your bones strong. To get sufficient calcium, drink milk and eat yogurt and cheese. To save on calories and saturated fat, choose low-fat or non-fat dairy products. If you are lactose intolerant and can't digest milk, choose lactose-free milk products, calcium-fortified foods, and beverages such as calcium-fortified soymilk. One serving equals 1 cup of milk or yogurt, 1½ ounces of natural cheese such as cheddar or mozzarella, or 2 ounces of processed cheese such as American.

Protein: 2–3 servings a day. Select lean meats, poultry, fish, and eggs prepared with minimal amounts of fat. Beans (pinto, kidney, black, garbanzo) are also a good source of protein, as are lentils, split peas, nuts, and seeds. One serving equals 2–3 ounces of cooked meat, poultry, or fish, which is about the size of a deck of cards; 1 cup of cooked beans; 2 eggs; 2 tablespoons of peanut butter; or 1 ounce (about ¼ cup) of nuts.

Whole grains: 3 servings a day. It is recommended that you eat a minimum of six servings of grains per day; at least 50 percent of those grains should be whole grains. Whole grain breads, cereals, crackers, and pasta provide fiber, which is very important during pregnancy. Eating a variety of fiber-containing foods helps maintain proper bowel function and can reduce your chances of developing constipation and hemorrhoids. As often as possible, select whole grain foods over those made with white flour. For example, eat whole wheat bread rather than white bread. One serving equals 1 slice of bread, 1 ounce of ready-to-eat cereal (about 1 cup of most cereals), or ½ cup cooked cereal, rice, or pasta.

Calorie totals

Depending on height and activity level, pregnant women need about 2,500 calories a day, according to the American Dietetic Association (ADA). If you are underweight, overweight, or pregnant with multiples, you may need a different number of calories to sustain a healthy pregnancy. If you fall into one of those categories, talk with your doctor or a registered dietitian for advice on how to plan a healthy diet.

Read food labels

If you haven't paid attention to labels on food, start now. Use nutrition facts labels to select foods that are low in sodium (salt), sugar, saturated fat, and cholesterol. The label also gives a food's serving size. Pay attention: The serving sizes are often much smaller than people realize.

Food content labels will help you steer clear of trans fat. If "partially hydrogenated" or "hydrogenated" fat is listed as one of the first ingredients, the food contains a large amount of trans fats. Choose foods with monounsaturated or polyunsaturated fats instead, but keep in mind that fat of any kind is high in calories. (See "A lesson on fats," page 217.)

The buzz about caffeine

Caffeine is the drug you consume in coffee, tea, some soft drinks, and chocolate. Like other foods and drugs you ingest while pregnant, it crosses the placenta and enters your baby's system. Caffeine can affect the fetus's heart rate and breathing; however, researchers are unsure whether caffeine harms a fetus. Some studies suggest a link between high caffeine consumption and birth defects, miscarriage, low birthweight, sudden infant death syndrome, and infertility, but others find no relation. To be safe, the American Dietetic Association recommends that pregnant women consume less than 300 mg of caffeine daily. Use the "Caffeine Levels in Popular Beverages and Foods" chart (this page) to stay within that limit.

Caffeine Levels in Popular Beverages and Foods

Coffee (8-oz. cup)	
Brewed, drip method	96–288 mg
Brewed, percolator	64–272 mg
Instant	48–192 mg
Tea (8-oz. cup)	
Brewed, major U.S. brands	33–144 mg
Brewed, imported brands	40–176 mg
Instant	40–80 mg
Brewed iced tea (12-oz. glass)	67–76 mg
Bottled iced tea (12-oz. bottle)	6–50 mg
Other	
Cola (12-oz. can)	34–44 mg
Diet cola (12-oz. can)	36–45 mg
Root beer (12-oz. can)	0–22 mg
Mountain Dew (12-oz. can)	55 mg
Hot cocoa (12-oz. serving)	3–32 mg
Chocolate milk (8-oz. serving)	2–7 mg
Milk chocolate (1 oz.)	1–15 mg
Dark chocolate, semisweet (1 oz.)	5–35 mg
Baking chocolate (1 oz.)	26 mg
Chocolate-flavored syrup (1 oz.)	4 mg
Red Bull Energy Drink (8.3-oz. can)	80 mg

Sources: Food and Drug Administration (FDA), American Beverage Association, National Soft Drink Association

Common Questions

Q. I've been taking prescription drugs for a chronic illness for years. Should I stop now that I'm pregnant?

A. You're right to be concerned, because right now your baby's rapidly developing organs are extremely vulnerable. However, you should never stop taking prescription medications without first consulting with your health provider. Many untreated diseases can be more harmful to your baby than the drugs that treat them.

How will a drug affect your unborn baby? It depends mainly on the characteristics of the drug, how much you take, and when you take it during your pregnancy. Your baby is most susceptible to drugs between 18 days and 55 days after conception. Before the 18-day mark, your body will usually spontaneously abort a damaged embryo. After 55 days your baby is much less apt to be harmed by anything you ingest.

Discuss your medications right away with your health care provider, who might prescribe a safer alternative or change the dose now that you're pregnant. Here's a starter list of medications that aren't safe during pregnancy. Ask your doctor about any that you take that aren't on this list:

- Some antibiotics, such as tetracycline, doxycycline, streptomycin, and kanamycin. Erythromycin estolate can affect a pregnant woman's liver function. Fluoroquinolones might hurt your baby's developing cartilage and bones.
- Antiseizure drugs such as carbamazepine and valproic acid.
- Migraine medications, including ergotamine drugs.
- Acne medications such as Accutane and other oral vitamin A compounds.
- Blood thinners such as warfarin.
- Certain high blood pressure drugs, such as ACE inhibitors captopril and enalapril.
- Ulcer medications such as Cytotec (misoprostol).
- Androgens and testosterone products such as danazol.

Q. When should I tell people that I'm pregnant?

A. You may be so tickled with your pregnancy that you can't imagine why your exciting news isn't being broadcast worldwide. You're sure everyone knows you're pregnant just by looking at you. In fact, it will be many weeks before your pregnancy shows, so whom you choose to tell, and when, is really your choice. You might be someone who tells her sister, mother, and girlfriends about every event in her life, from hair coloring to career changes. In that case, confiding in them about your pregnancy is a natural impulse. Just remember that their reactions may be different from what you expected.

After 12 weeks, the risk of miscarriage decreases, so many women will wait at least until that milestone to share their good news.

One more consideration: If this pregnancy doesn't come to term, whom, of the people you've told, would you want to tell about a miscarriage? All in all, at this point in your pregnancy, it might be wisest to tell only a select few people who you know will be the most supportive.

Your partner: understanding his sexual desires

There they are: your lovely new breasts, blooming out of your bra. They're bigger and sexier than ever. Your partner can't stop ogling you or trying to touch that tantalizing twosome. You wish he could enjoy them. After all that used to be your favorite part of foreplay.

Unfortunately there's a catch to your alluring new physique. Besides being sick to your stomach every morning—and sometimes all day—you find that your breasts are so swollen and sore that you're ready to slap your partner the minute he reaches for you.

Is your sex life ever going to be the same? No. But that doesn't mean it will be worse. Fatigue, morning sickness, mood swings, and breast tenderness may put the brakes on your sex drive during these early weeks, but they will go away soon. Let your partner know how you feel and tell him it's fine to look (but not to touch). Talk candidly about your own sexual needs. Find ways of staying close that satisfy both of you right now. In a few weeks, when the worst symptoms of morning sickness and fatigue subside, your libido may reach a new high. Sexual desire typically returns by the 2nd trimester, when many women feel lustier than ever. There are no worries about birth control, they have curvy new bodies to show off, and extra blood flow to the pelvic area, caused by hormonal changes, can produce a heightened sensitivity, making it easier to orgasm.

Week 6

Your Baby

The inside story

By your 6th week of pregnancy, your baby's heartbeat measures 150–160 beats per minute, which is about twice your heart rate. The fetus is nearly ½ inch long and looks even more like a baby.

Your baby's head is as large as the rest of his body, but his arm and leg buds are starting to lengthen. His nose is starting to show, and eyelids are forming. Your baby's eyes already have a lens at this point, as well as an iris, cornea, and pigmented retina. Your baby's spine is completely developed and has closed over at both ends. Inside his lungs, secondary branches have started to appear, and they will continue branching out after he's born. Someday these branches will connect to the 300 million tiny air sacs (called alveoli) in his lungs.

Although your blood is supplying nutrients and oxygen to your growing baby, your blood does not flow directly to him. Instead it passes through the umbilical cord to the baby via the placenta, a disk-shape organ with lots of little roots and veins. The placenta produces hormones that support the baby's growth; it also sends nutrients and oxygen to the fetus and helps excrete the baby's waste. Think of it as a glorified filter that prevents your bloodstream from ever directly mixing with your baby's; because of this filter, your baby can have a blood type that's different from yours.

Your Body

Sleep deprivation

Some women are so sleepy by their 6th week that they complain of feeling drugged. Their heads are down on their desks every few hours at work, and their feet feel as if they're encased in cement shoes. At the same time they report having trouble falling asleep at night, feeling restless when they're lying down, having to get up often to urinate, or having trouble getting comfortable. According to the National Sleep Foundation, almost 80 percent of pregnant women suffer from disturbed sleeping patterns. With all the changes their bodies are experiencing, it's not surprising.

The extreme fatigue you may be feeling is caused by high levels of pregnancy hormones coursing through your body and the energy demands of the developing fetus. Whether you're at home with small children or working outside the house, steal a half-hour nap or put your feet up. If morning is your sleepy time, rearrange your schedule to catch extra shut-eye.

Stick to your sleep and nap routines even on weekends, no matter how many errands beckon. This is a great time to cut back on that "to do" list and limit yourself to top priorities. Ask your partner to take on more responsibilities, such as the grocery shopping, so that you can rest for an hour on Saturday afternoons.

If you're feeling sleepless at night, address anything that may disrupt your sleep. Install room-darkening shades if the room seems too bright, use a white noise machine to block out distractions, and install a cool-mist humidifier to improve air quality. Be sure to go to bed and wake up at the same time every day, including weekends. Create a presleep ritual. Maybe it's listening to soft music, taking a warm bath, reading a magazine on the porch, or leisurely walking with the dog. Avoid vigorous workouts before bed, or you'll find it difficult to fall asleep. It might also help to prop yourself up with extra pillows because your head may feel more congested than usual.

Surviving morning sickness

It's a challenge to embrace your pregnancy joyfully when you're feeling nauseous or vomiting all day. You're not alone. Most pregnancies are accompanied by nausea, especially in the 1st trimester. Practitioners call it "morning sickness" because that's when it's apt to hit you hardest.

Why the tricky stomach? The rapid rise in pregnancy hormones is to blame, along with an enhanced sense of smell and sensitivity to odors. (That's why your favorite Thai restaurant may now send you scurrying to the opposite side of the street the minute you sniff the curry.)

Although it might feel like you're hurting the baby with all of this vomiting, morning sickness rarely has harmful effects. Your baby is too small for you to require extra calories yet, and your multivitamin can cover your nutritional needs (assuming that you can keep it down). There's an upside to morning sickness too. Scientists at Cornell University recently examined thousands of pregnancies and reported that morning sickness typically peaks between weeks 6 and 18 and that women who suffer from morning sickness have a higher chance of having healthy pregnancies.

Foods that work for you. You may not feel like eating at all right now, but an empty stomach will only make you feel worse because morning sickness can be exacerbated by low blood sugar. Nibble on crackers before you get up in the morning, snack on salty foods, and eat a small complex carbohydrate snack such as a whole grain muffin before bedtime so that your stomach will feel less queasy. Some women find that eating salty or tart foods, like potato chips

week 6

and lemonade, can help alleviate nausea. Watermelon may also help.

Nobody knows why certain foods work better than others, so follow this plan: If you crave a food and can keep it down, eat it. At the same time, avoid foods or smells that trigger your nausea. It might also help to eat food that is cold or at room temperature because that will cut down on odors.

Liquids. If you're vomiting often, increase your fluid intake to ten 8-ounce cups a day; that's two more than the recommended eight cups a day. Alternate watermelon ice cubes and freezer pops with glasses of water and ice chips if you're having trouble drinking enough water. Italian ice or lemon slush will also help you hydrate. Try to drink fluids only between meals; if you must drink during meals, limit the amount to keep your stomach from feeling overly full. You can also use a sports drink to replace lost electrolytes. If you're taking a vitamin supplement with iron, talk to your doctor about skipping that vitamin until you're feeling better, because iron is tough on a stomach that's already queasy.

Remedies. Unisom, an over-the-counter sleep aid, contains an antinausea ingredient, and most practitioners agree that it's safe to take during pregnancy. The American Medical Association (AMA) has approved acupuncture to treat nausea associated with pregnancy. For short-term relief you can also purchase BioBands, which are acupressure bracelets available at most pharmacies. Some women swear that ginger eases nausea, so look for ginger candies, drink ginger tea, or find a ginger ale made from real ginger.

Test out this easy acupressure technique too: Press three fingertips gently but firmly on the base of your palm, just above where you'd take your pulse on your wrist. Breathe deeply and press that area with your fingertips for a minute or more, gradually increasing the pressure until

Severe morning sickness

It's rare for morning sickness to become a serious concern. However, if you can't keep down any food or fluids for 24 hours, are steadily losing weight, or become dehydrated, it's time to call your practitioner. These symptoms can be signs of hyperemesis gravidarum, which literally means "excessive vomiting in pregnancy." It can cause dehydration severe enough for you to lose minerals crucial to you and your baby.

This condition is manageable once diagnosed and rarely has any serious long-term effects. Your caregiver will probably put you on intravenous (IV) fluids and check your electrolyte levels to make sure you have no underlying disease that might be provoking these frequent purges. Depending on your condition, you might even be hospitalized for a few days so that you can stay on antinausea medication and IV fluids. Most women feel much better after they're rehydrated and are able to use medication to stop vomiting.

you feel slight discomfort. The sensation should be the same as the feel of a mini-massage.

Nausea kit. In case you're seized by a bout of nausea in an unexpected place, keep an emergency kit handy: plastic bags, wet wipes, napkins, water for rinsing your mouth, a toothbrush and toothpaste, and breath mints. And remember: This too shall pass.

Fluid intake

You should drink at least 64 ounces of fluid a day. That's equal to eight 8-ounce glasses; drink more if you're vomiting often (see "Surviving morning sickness," page 47).

Water is best. Juices can boost your fluid intake, but they contain calories and unnecessary sugar. Caffeinated beverages like coffee and sodas aren't ideal because they are likely to make you urinate more and therefore actually lose water.

If you can't keep track of your fluid intake, fill a 64-ounce container with water and finish it by the end of the day. Stop by every water fountain you see and take a quick drink. If you're too nauseated to drink, or just dislike the taste of plain water, add a wedge of lemon or suck on ice chips.

Why so many fluids? During pregnancy your blood volume will swell 40 percent higher, accounting for about 4 pounds of your pregnancy weight. That extra blood is an essential transportation system, bringing nutrients to your baby and helping your kidneys flush extra

waste products. Added fluid intake will also lower your risk of bladder, urinary tract, and kidney infections; it also prevents constipation.

Your Self

Choosing your birth team

Though your due date may seem years away instead of mere months, now is the time to start investigating whom you'd like to deliver your baby and where you'd like the happy event to occur.

Obstetricians. In the United States, most pregnant women choose obstetricians. Obstetricians are physicians who have completed four-year residencies in obstetrics and gynecology after medical school. If you have a serious chronic illness, are carrying more than one baby, are an older mother, or anticipate other potential complications, you will certainly want to consider working with an obstetrician. You may also want to consider a perinatologist; a perinatologist is an obstetrician who specializes in the care of women with high-risk pregnancies.

Family practitioners. These physicians do obstetric training as part of their residency and may do prenatal care and low-risk deliveries.

Nurse-midwife. If yours is a relatively low-risk pregnancy, you might prefer a nurse-midwife. In most parts of the world, obstetricians deliver babies only during emergencies, and midwives handle the rest. That's increasingly true in the United States

The dangers of secondhand smoke

You already know that mothers who smoke cause harm to their unborn babies. But did you know that your baby can also be harmed by people smoking around you?

Secondhand smoke is a complex chemical mixture of more than 4,000 chemicals (more than 50 of them cancer-causing), and it's associated with a number of pregnancy complications. For instance, new research reveals that nonsmoking pregnant women who have been exposed to secondhand smoke are more likely to have babies with health problems such as low birthweight and intrauterine growth restriction (IUGR) (see "Common Questions," page 284); those babies also are more likely to have an increased risk of sudden infant death syndrome (SIDS). Furthermore, according to a recent study done by researchers at Columbia University's Center for Children's Environmental Health, children whose mothers were exposed to secondhand smoke during pregnancy scored lower on cognitive development tests at age 2 than children from smoke-free homes.

The bottom line? Even if you don't smoke, avoid being in smoke-filled rooms while you're pregnant. This is easier to do now that many restaurants and other public places have banned smoking; however, ask your friends and family members who smoke to take it outside too. If they won't, then go to a different room or head outdoors yourself so you—and your baby—get a breath of fresh air while the others light up.

too, where nationwide about 10 percent of all pregnant women now choose midwives over obstetricians.

Certified nurse-midwives complete two years of graduate work in midwifery after nursing school. Certified nurse-midwives don't accept high-risk pregnancies, and they always have a doctor on call, even for seemingly uncomplicated deliveries. In general, certified nurse-midwives use fewer medical interventions than obstetricians, though this depends on your particular provider. Several research studies in the United States show that healthy women with normal pregnancies who choose certified nurse-midwives are just as likely to have healthy births as those who choose obstetricians.

Communication is key. No matter who guides you through pregnancy and birth, it will be an essential partnership. You're going to be feeling excited, overwhelmed, joyful, anxious, and unsure—often all at once—so a good practitioner can be a welcome guide on your journey to motherhood.

Experts say that miscommunication is the reason for most conflicts between patients and their health care providers, so this is a good time in your life to learn to speak up, both for your own good and for your baby's. Prepare questions for each visit, taking notes on what your provider says so that you don't forget her answers. Answer your provider's questions honestly, get your partner involved, and speak up whenever you're unsure about a provider's advice or when your expectations have not been met.

Birthplace options

Birth options include assisted delivery at home, in a birth center, or in a hospital. Of course, where you have your baby will depend on who assists your delivery.

Home births. The American Medical Association and the American College of Obstetricians and Gynecologists both caution against having your baby at home. No matter how healthy you are or how uncomplicated your pregnancy might seem, there's always a small chance that your delivery will take a wrong turn. Consider these statistics: When researchers in Washington State compared more than 10,500 planned hospital births with more than 6,000 home births, they discovered that the rate of infant death was doubled among home births (3.5 deaths per 1,000 at home, compared with 1.7 per 1,000 in hospitals). Mothers who gave birth at home had a 50 percent higher rate of prolonged labor and a nearly 60 percent increase in the risk of postpartum bleeding. The rate of low newborn-assessment scores was also greater among babies born at home than in hospitals.

With a healthy woman and a low-risk pregnancy, a home birth would most likely be fine, especially if a certified midwife were on hand to deliver the baby. However, if you're considering giving birth at home, be aware that your midwife would not have the capability to take care of you and/or your baby during those rare, but possible, emergency situations in which your health and/or your baby's health is in danger.

Birth centers. Birth centers are a terrific alternative to home or hospital births for women with uncomplicated pregnancies who want the relative comfort of giving birth in a low-tech environment and the security of being in or near a hospital. These sites are typically decorated to look less like hospital rooms and more like bedrooms, right down to curtains on the windows and rocking chairs in the corners. Most are staffed by midwives working with physicians affiliated with hospitals that are part of or near the birth center.

Birth center staffs encourage women to manage their own births as naturally as possible. Midwives are skilled at managing pain during childbirth through controlled breathing, labor positions, and relaxation techniques. Most birth centers are also equipped to provide opioids for pain relief. However, if you want an epidural, you will have to give birth in a hospital. Look for a birth center accredited by the Commission for the Accreditation of Birth Centers, which ensures that centers have physician contacts and hospital affiliations.

Hospitals. The overwhelming majority of births in the United States take place in hospitals. Women who have no midwives or birth centers near their homes give birth in hospitals. So do those women who want the security of knowing help is at hand during emergencies and those who want the option of using pain medication such as epidurals.

Women with preexisting medical conditions such as diabetes, heart problems, and kidney conditions should choose hospital births. So should women who are older than 40, those who have had previous miscarriages, and women who have had a prior cesarean delivery. Your health care provider might also suggest a hospital delivery if your baby is disproportionately large or in a breech (butt first) position.

If you decide to give birth in a hospital, you can still plan a natural birth. Many hospitals have adopted more relaxed, homelike furnishings for their labor and delivery rooms, and many hire midwives to work alongside the obstetricians.

To ensure that things go as smoothly as possible, you and your partner should discuss your ideal birth experience with your health care provider before you go into labor. That will allow your partner to best advocate for your choices if necessary. Remember that things might not go as planned. Nature is always full of surprises, and certain hospitals still have medical intervention policies that may not always promote a natural birth. Keep the big picture in mind: The most important outcome is a healthy baby and healthy mother, not a particular type of birth.

For more information contact these organizations about obstetricians, midwives, and birth centers.

American College of Obstetricians and Gynecologists
Resource Center
P.O. Box 96920
409 12th Street, SW
Washington, DC 20090-6920
202-638-5577
E-mail: resources@acog.org
Website: www.acog.org

American College of Nurse-Midwives
8403 Colesville Rd.
Suite 1550
Silver Spring, MD 20910
240-485-1800
E-mail: info@acnm.org
Website: www.midwife.org

National Association of Childbearing Centers
3123 Gottschall Road
Perkiomenville, PA 18074
215-234-8068
E-mail: reachnacc@birthcenters.org
Website: www.birthcenters.org

Diet & Exercise

Active vs. nonactive women

Food is fuel, and active women need more fuel than sedentary women. If you exercised vigorously before pregnancy and continue to do so now, stick to eating about the same number of calories in the 1st trimester and then add 300 calories a day during the 2nd trimester. The same is true if you did not exercise vigorously before pregnancy and continue not to during pregnancy.

However, if you were active before pregnancy and are slowing down during your 1st trimester, you will probably need to eat less to avoid gaining excess weight. If you didn't exercise before but are starting a walking regimen now, you can eat a few more calories—but not much more. A 150-pound woman burns about 100 calories per mile, so don't mislead yourself into thinking that a 20-minute walk entitles you to a huge slice of apple pie. If you think you need extra calories to fuel your revved-up workouts, add something nutritious, such as a piece of fruit.

Calcium needs

Pregnant women should get 1,000 mg (milligrams) of calcium each day. Don't count on getting it all from your prenatal vitamins, however: Most contain only a few hundred milligrams. Ensure adequate calcium intake by including 3 servings of non-fat or low-fat milk or yogurt in your diet each day. Other food sources of calcium include broccoli, kale, tofu processed with calcium sulfate, and juices fortified with calcium.

Protein's power

Protein is one of the human body's building blocks. Your baby's body needs protein in order to build cells and organs, and your body needs it for a healthy placenta.

But you don't need to go wild

eating protein. It's relatively easy to get the 10 extra grams of protein that you need each day. (Pregnant women need about 60 grams of protein daily, compared with 50 grams for nonpregnant women.) In fact many Americans eat too much protein, so it's possible that you are already getting more than you need.

As you choose protein sources for your pregnancy diet, reach for foods that are low in fat, particularly saturated fat. For example, select extra-lean cuts of beef and pork and white-meat chicken without skin. Here are some protein-rich foods, along with their protein content:

- 3½ ounces of boneless, skinless chicken breast: 30 grams of protein
- 4-ounce broiled hamburger patty made with extra-lean beef: 29 grams
- 4 ounces of baked Atlantic salmon: 25 grams
- 8 ounces fat-free yogurt: 12 grams
- 8 ounces of non-fat milk: 8 grams
- 2 tablespoons peanut butter: 8 grams
- 1 egg: 6 grams

Eat your fruits and veggies

Fruits and vegetables are an important part of your diet at all times in your life, but they're particularly important during pregnancy. They deliver the nutrients that your body and your baby's body need. A vitamin pill can't take the place of these nutrient-packed plant foods, however. That's because fruits and vegetables contain compounds such as

Eating disorders

Your baby will probably weigh about 7½ pounds at birth, but your body must gain about four times that amount to be able to provide support for your growing child. Women who are underweight and gain too little weight during their pregnancies are at a higher risk for fetal and neonatal deaths, say researchers, while obese women are more likely to suffer from gestational diabetes, hypertension, and prolonged labors.

One recent study by Harvard Medical School showed that women with eating disorders of any kind are more likely to develop complications during pregnancy, are more likely to give birth to a baby with a congenital problem, and will be more apt to suffer from postpartum depression. Women who abuse laxatives, purge, or rely on diuretics to lose weight during pregnancies have more fetal abnormalities because they rob their bodies of necessary nutrients and fluids.

If you're suffering from any type of eating disorder, now is the time to get help. Tell your provider about your problem and ask for a referral to a program or therapist specializing in eating disorders. Women who address eating disorders early in their pregnancies stand a good chance of having normal, healthy babies. If you can't stop vomiting, using laxatives, starving yourself, or engaging in any other behavior related to an eating disorder, it might be best to check yourself into a hospital or other facility where your nutrition can be professionally monitored while you continue therapy.

antioxidants that can't be delivered by a pill. Fruits and vegetables also contain fiber, which helps keep your digestive system working well. Fiber helps prevent constipation, which is common in pregnancy, particularly if you're taking iron supplements.

Your exercise routine

During the 1st trimester, you can continue to exercise as you did before you conceived, provided you clear it with your doctor. If it feels like too much, slow down. This is not the time to do a no-pain, no-gain exercise routine, particularly if you have morning sickness. Fatigue may slow you down too. Listen to your body: If you feel worn out by a workout that usually invigorates you, tone it down a bit. Make a point to always drink water before, during, and after exercise to prevent dehydration.

Is one alcoholic drink OK?

It's no fun being a teetotaler at a party where everyone else is drinking and having a great time. You may be tempted to have a cocktail or a glass of wine, but it's better not to. Nobody knows for sure how much alcohol is needed to harm a fetus. Because people are genetically programmed to metabolize alcohol differently, what would be OK for one woman would be too much for another. It's best not to have any alcohol at all.

week 6

Common Questions

Q. Why don't I have morning sickness?

A. Congratulations, you're one of the lucky ones! You may worry that something is wrong with your pregnancy if you're not throwing up like your best friend or every pregnant woman you see in the movies. Be assured that plenty of women with perfectly normal pregnancies manage to escape morning sickness. In fact, a full 25 percent of pregnant women never get morning sickness, and nobody knows why. Research shows that the women likely to suffer the worst cases of nausea during these first months are those pregnant with twins or multiples, women who have a history of nausea as a side effect of taking birth control pills, women whose mothers and sisters were sick during their pregnancies, those who had migraine headaches even before getting pregnant, and women susceptible to motion sickness.

Q. Is it really that bad to gain more weight than my doctor recommends?

A. Yes. Weight gained over and above the recommended levels is not healthy. It actually increases your risk of complications. For instance, women who gain too much weight during pregnancy are more likely to have gestational diabetes or pregnancy-related high blood pressure, which can hamper your health and promote premature delivery.

Q. I'm nervous about choosing the right doctor to help me through pregnancy and delivery. How can I make the right choice?

A. Your geographic location, health insurance, friends, individual health history, and family health history will all influence which practitioner you ultimately use. However, here are some key questions to ask your potential practitioner up front.

- **Where do you deliver?** You might be looking for a facility close to home or a birth center that allows labor coaches or family members to be present during the birth. You may also be looking for a facility that has 24-hour-a-day in-hospital anesthesia coverage or one with a neonatal intensive care unit.
- **Who will deliver my baby if you're not around?** No midwife or doctor can be on call every day of the year. To increase your chances of getting the provider you want, choose a small practice. Meet the backup providers early in your pregnancy to find out if you're comfortable with them. Keep in mind, however, that some practices, especially those in large teaching hospitals, have large provider groups, and meeting with all of them may be impractical. With your partner, decide what practice model will best meet your expectations.
- **What prenatal tests do you suggest?** Ask the provider which tests she gives at each stage of pregnancy, what the risks are, and what help you'd get in making an informed decision after receiving test results. Consider whether this provider is someone who will give

you the details you need to make important decisions and who will take the time to listen to your concerns.

- **When do you recommend a cesarean delivery?** Cesarean births are necessary in some situations, so ask your provider how she makes that decision. For instance, how long will she allow you to push before performing this surgery? What is her cesarean rate? (Nationwide, it's about 27.6 percent.) Will she perform a vaginal birth if you've already had one cesarean?
- **What's your philosophy on pain management during labor?** Right now, you don't know how much pain you'll be in. However, if you're leaning toward pain management drugs such as an epidural, ask your provider how she feels about medication. The last thing you need is for someone to make you feel guilty about asking for pain relief. On the other hand, if you definitely want to experience natural childbirth, look for someone supportive of a drug-free labor and of pain management options such as massage, showers, labor tubs, or acupuncture.

- **How much authority will I have as labor progresses?** You'll have to follow the rules of whatever facility you choose, so it's important to know what those rules are ahead of time. For instance, if you want to walk around during labor, find out if IV hookups and fetal monitoring are optional or required. Also ask your provider her general philosophy on episiotomies.
- **Whom can I take into the delivery room with me?** Again, the answer to this question will depend largely on the rules of the facility you choose, so find out what they are. Your provider may also have a say, so ask to hear her philosophy on dads, children, and grandmothers in the delivery room.
- **What will happen after my baby is born?** Ask whether you'll be moved from the labor and delivery room and how long you can hold the baby following delivery. If having the baby examined in your presence is important, say so. Finally, ask how long your provider will recommend that you stay in the facility after a vaginal or cesarean birth and what sort of follow-up care she provides.

Week 7

Your Baby

The inside story

Although your baby is a mere ½ inch long and still curved as tightly as a comma, he's growing quickly. Some of the most important growth is happening in his brain, where new nerve cells are forming at the astounding rate of 100,000 per minute. As your baby's brain cells multiply, they will branch out and connect, forming the first primitive pathways for his central nervous system. By the time your baby is born, his brain will have more than 10 million intertwined nerve cells!

By now, your baby's heart rate is even faster than it was last week, and his heart tube has formed small bulges. His cells are frantically churning out the building blocks for what will become 40 pairs of muscles and 23 pairs of vertebrae radiating from his spinal column. Your baby's limb buds are starting to grow; they look like tiny flippers at this point. His outer ears are beginning to take shape, and he now has joints in his elbows, wrists, and knees. His eyelids are nearly complete too.

Your Body

Starting to feel pregnant

Finally, you may start to feel pregnant this week, even though you're still not showing. You may have trouble buttoning your most fitted clothing, especially if this isn't your first pregnancy. This is because your uterus is starting to compete for space with your other organs. The upper part of your uterus, which is called the corpus, is extremely muscular and flexible; its muscle fibers will lengthen 100 times to keep up with your baby's increasing size.

Your uterus is below your pelvic bones, so you can't feel it from the outside yet. As it continues to expand, though, it will grow upward from your pelvis and press against your abdomen from the inside, displacing your intestines and your stomach. Right now, your uterus is probably only a quarter of the way to your belly button; it will reach halfway to your belly button within the next month.

So if your uterus is still relatively small, why can't you button your jeans? Because that rush of pregnancy hormones has made you gain a little weight. In addition, you might have

week 7

some bloating because food moves more slowly through your intestines when you're pregnant, allowing your body to absorb more water so that you'll digest your food in a way that provides the most nutrients to your baby. This can make you feel some cramping sometimes, especially if you're constipated.

As long as there is no bleeding associated with the cramping, there is little reason to be concerned about a miscarriage. However, do call your health care provider if the cramping is painful or prolonged. At the very least she might be able to suggest a stool softener or other strategies for easing your bloating and discomfort.

Mood swings

Giggly, tearful, frightened, furious—during pregnancy most women experience mood swings. You can pin some of the blame for your seesawing emotions on hormonal surges, especially during this 1st trimester. However, there's much more to these wild fluctuations than revved-up body chemistry. Having a baby—whether it's your first or not—is a momentous life change. You may be stressed about finances, anxious about your baby's health, or terrified about childbirth. Besides, how can anyone expect you to be sweet, stable, and sensible when you can't get out of bed without vomiting, your clothes don't fit right, and you're too

Yeast infections

Thanks to the many hormonal changes your body is going through, you may have yeast infections more often during pregnancy. Yeast infections are caused by fungus that's normally found in the mucous membranes of your body, and they are not harmful to your unborn baby. At worst, if you have a yeast infection during childbirth, your baby may get a mild mouth infection called thrush about a week after birth, and that can be treated easily.

Meanwhile, a yeast infection can make you awfully uncomfortable. You'll usually notice a change in vaginal discharge; it will look like dry cottage cheese. You'll also feel an itchy or burning sensation in your vagina, especially while having intercourse or at night. You might also have some redness near the opening of the vagina.

To help ward off yeast infections, cut back on refined sugar, wear loose clothing and cotton underpants instead of tight clothing and pantyhose, and keep your genitals dry. (That means peeling off your wet bathing suit right after swimming.) Wear nightgowns to bed without underwear and avoid wearing pantyliners.

If you get a yeast infection during your 1st trimester, your provider will probably be able to diagnose it by examining the vaginal discharge; she may also take a sample to rule out other possible infections. She'll probably advise you to use an over-the-counter medication such as Monistat. Home remedies may also help make you more comfortable. These include adding 1 cup of cornstarch plus ½ cup of baking soda to warm baths, using cold compresses to reduce itching, and eating yogurt with live active cultures.

exhausted to cook a decent meal?

Mood swings are likely to dissipate after your 1st trimester, when your hormones settle down, your energy returns, and you become more adjusted to the idea of being pregnant. Meanwhile, choose one of your calm spells to have a conversation with your partner. Explain that your emotions sometimes take you by storm and apologize in advance for any hurtful things you might say or do when that happens. Let your partner know how best to support you when you're being steamrolled by a black mood. Sharing your moods will help you see things more clearly and objectively. Whether you're worrying about childbirth, breastfeeding, or daycare, ask other parents how they've coped. It helps to hear that others have gone through (and survived) what you're experiencing.

Finally, do whatever you can to rest and relax because stress can make pregnancy and delivery even harder. Take deep breaths when you're feeling angry or upset. Inhale deeply through your nose and count to five; then slowly exhale through your mouth as you count back down to one. Imagine a wave of warm water washing over you as you breathe in and washing your worries away as you breathe out. Splashing cold water on your face, blasting the air conditioner in your car, or opening a window for fresh air may help too. The cold temperature can momentarily wake up your system and allow you to look at things from a different perspective.

So can a change of scenery. Step out onto the front steps or duck into the bathroom for a few minutes while you calm yourself down.

Your Self

Doubts about motherhood

Although your body doesn't look that different, you're starting to think of yourself as a mother. Perhaps you're doubting your own ability to fulfill that particular role, especially if this is your first child. If you already have children, you may be wondering how you can possibly add even more responsibilities to your already overflowing plate.

Everyone has these doubts because current ideals of motherhood are so overblown. Not long ago if you kept your house reasonably clean, served dinner, and made it to school for teacher conferences, you were considered a good mother. More recently, moms are being measured against perfection: Despite the fact that more than 65 percent of mothers with young children work outside the home, media coverage promotes the ideal mother as someone who has enough time to be constantly responsive to her children while still keeping the romance in her marriage alive and regularly toning her body at the gym.

Guess what? That's a myth. No matter how many heavy, heartfelt texts are written on how to be a better, more loving, more efficient

week 7

mother-lover-worker bee, motherhood is a tough job, and there's a steep learning curve for everyone. Rest assured that you too will make the transition. Motherhood is more like a makeover than a personality transplant; you will still be you, just wiser than before.

What kind of parent will I be?

Nobody can predict what life will be like after a new baby. Even if you've had children before, every baby's birth and personality are unique. However, it may help you adjust to parenthood if you make a written list of the priorities you want to guard in your life—and the things you can let slide. This is a good time for you and your partner to talk about how you both envision life after baby. Use these questions to help jump-start your conversation:

What are your expectations of parenthood? Right now, they might be pretty abstract. Now is the time to observe the mothers in your own life—your mother, your aunt, your friends—and consider their behavior toward their children. You'll realize that every mother has both good days and bad.

What was your own childhood like? If you enjoyed your childhood and think your mom did a great job of raising you, then you've got a handy rule book. Ask her about her own transition to motherhood, and you may discover that even when she seemed most loving, she was experiencing her own doubts and fears.

How was your partner raised? Looking at your partner's family background is a great way to start talking about your doubts, ideals, and goals for your own family life. It's probably unrealistic to think that the two of you will agree about every parenting tactic. Still, talking ahead of time about life with a newborn will mean fewer surprises later. Topics to tackle may include whether to breastfeed or bottle-feed, where your newborn should sleep, who should get up at night, who's going to handle the housework, and how much you should hold your baby. You'll be a better parenting team as a result of these discussions.

When you resent your partner

If your partner never seems exhausted, nauseous, worried, or robbed of sexual desire, it's easy to feel resentful. The problem with that nasty emotion is that it snowballs over time. If you perceive pregnancy as all work for you and just a pleasant passing thought for your partner, you'll eventually start seething about every small thing your partner does (or doesn't do) and you'll drive a wedge between the two of you when you need each other most. Take the time now to focus on what makes you feel resentful. Do you wish your partner would notice how sick you are and bring you toast in bed? Are you longing for more foot massages, dinners out, or help with housework? Do you wish he were less (or more) demanding in bed?

Review your expectations and consider whether they're reasonable. What do you really want, and why? Then approach your partner as you would a friend. Tell your partner first about all of the things he is doing right, including the little things (like remembering to buy milk) and the bigger things (like refinancing the house to allow you a longer maternity leave). Have a heart-to-heart about your own expectations, vulnerabilities, and frustrations, with the goal of appreciating each other more as you bring a baby into your family.

Diet & Exercise

Your (healthy) weight gain

If you are starting your pregnancy weighing more than you'd like, don't try to diet. Dieting will rob you and your baby of needed nutrients. Focus instead on eating a healthful diet, avoiding junk food, and exercising to the extent that your doctor allows. Aim for gradual weight gain. It's best to gain a little at a time rather than load on 6 pounds in 1 week and nothing for several weeks afterward. Pay attention to the scale and these general weight-gain guidelines:

If you are a normal weight before pregnancy, gain 25–35 pounds.

If you are overweight before pregnancy, gain 15–25 pounds.

If you are underweight before pregnancy, gain 28–40 pounds.

If you are obese, gain 15 pounds or less.

Your Pregnancy Weight

Where does the weight come from? Here's a breakdown, based on a 30-pound weight gain:

Blood	4 pounds
Breasts	2 pounds
Uterus	2 pounds
Baby	7.5 pounds
Placenta	1.5 pounds
Amniotic fluid	2 pounds
Fat, protein, and other nutrients	7 pounds
Retained water	4 pounds

If you are pregnant with multiples, your weight gain will depend on several factors, including your prepregnancy weight and how many babies you're carrying. For example, a normal-weight woman who is having twins should gain 35–45 pounds.

Starting an exercise program

Here's good news for couch potatoes: Even if you've never exercised before, you can start during pregnancy, provided you have your doctor's permission. The best fitness activity for sedentary pregnant women is walking. If you start now, you can work your way up to the recommended daily fitness prescription, which is to exercise for at least 30 minutes a day most days of the week. Begin with a 10-minute walk five to seven days a week; then gradually add more minutes to your daily walks. (See "New exercisers? Get walking," page 79.)

week 7

Common Questions

Q. I'm feeling so ugly and need something to lift my spirits. Is there any kind of spa splurge that's safe?

A. At this point in your pregnancy, you may not feel beautiful. Heck, you may have trouble just getting out of bed and matching your socks in the morning. You definitely deserve a beauty treatment, and there are many safe ones from which you can choose.

Manicures and pedicures. These are a great way to feel a glimmer of glamour. Bring your own instruments to the salon or ask your aesthetician to use a fresh set. Although the chance of an equipment-borne infection is low, it's best to avoid the risk altogether early in your pregnancy. Stay away from cuticle cutting, acrylics, and any polishes that might contain dibutyl phthalate (DBP), a class of chemicals that cause developmental deformities in animals. You can use paste-on nail tips without those chemicals.

Facials and makeovers. A facial is fine as long as your aesthetician keeps it simple (cleansing, massaging, and moisturizing your skin). Things to avoid include invasive extractions, chemical peels, and electronic stimulation. If you have a makeover, avoid cosmetics that contain phthalates, the chemicals often used in deodorants, fragrances, lotions, and sprays. Chemicals in this class are used industrially as solvents and softeners; they are commonly found in pesticides, nail polish, and paint.

Hair treatments. Your new abundance of estrogen may increase the growth rate of your hair. If this happens, your hair might not shed as quickly, and it may look shinier or healthier than ever before. On the other hand, you may now wince at the sight of the black roots quickly overtaking that blond hair you've always worked hard to maintain. Your hair might be straighter and limper than usual or drier and stiff-feeling because of hormone fluctuations. What can you do?

Recent studies show no link between birth defects and hair dyes, permanents, or hair relaxants. This has led the American College of Obstetricians and Gynecologists to OK these hair treatments during pregnancy. However, be aware that the hormonal changes that affect your hair during pregnancy may also alter the way your hair reacts to the products you usually use, leaving you with surprising textures and colors. This might be a good time to consider adopting a new, flattering haircut and a more natural look. You could also try a henna rinse; this is free of noxious ammonia, peroxide, and metals. Or use a highlight that's painted on; it's less likely than all-over color to produce a disastrous effect during pregnancy.

Shaving and waxing. You can still shave or wax your leg hair during pregnancy. However, waxing may prove extra painful now because of your pumped-up blood vessels. Use leg lotions to ease fatigue. Those lovely mint-scented soaks are safe for your aching legs and feet; use water that is cool or warm, not hot (hot water dries out the skin).

Heat treatments. One of the biggest spa no-no's during pregnancy is anything involving heat treatments. Mud and seaweed wraps are totally off-limits; so is hydrotherapy because an elevated body temperature during early pregnancy may be linked to miscarriage and birth defects.

Massages. With backaches, leg cramps, and tired neck and shoulders, a pregnant woman has every reason to crave a massage. It's important to find a massage therapist licensed by the American Massage Therapy Association and familiar with techniques that are both safe and relaxing for expectant mothers. For instance, your massage therapist should have a special table with an opening or pillows that will allow you to lie on your stomach or be supported on one side without lying on your baby and feeling uncomfortable. Your belly shouldn't be massaged because it can cause uncomfortable uterine contractions.

Q. How can I get my questions answered between office visits?

A. There are many pregnancy books, online resources, classes, and support groups for expectant mothers, but your pregnancy is unique. If you don't find a satisfactory answer on your own, call your practitioner's office. If your provider isn't available, speak to the person answering the phone and ask to talk with one of the nurses or midwives in the office. They're often more available to return calls, and they can set your mind at ease about most medical problems or contact the physician if they think your question warrants another opinion.

Other good resources include:

International Childbirth Education Association and Book Center
P.O. Box 20048
Minneapolis, MN 55420
800-624-4934 (Book Center)
952-854-8660
E-mail: info@icea.org
Website: www.icea.org

National Childbirth Education Foundation
P.O. Box 251
Oxford, PA 19363
717-529-2561
E-mail: jpncef@aol.com

week 7

Sexually transmitted diseases

Being pregnant doesn't protect you from acquiring a sexually transmitted disease (STD). If you become infected with an STD during pregnancy, or if you already have one when you become pregnant, you put your own health and your baby's health at risk. Many STDs have few symptoms, so the Centers for Disease Control (CDC) suggests that all pregnant women—young or old, married or not—be tested for STDs during their first prenatal visits. Most of these diseases can be treated easily, before any harm can come to your baby. The most common include:

GENITAL HERPES SIMPLEX INFECTION

At least one-fourth of all American women have genital herpes, a sexually transmitted disease caused by herpes simplex virus. Because this virus doesn't cause symptoms in everyone, many people don't even know that they're putting their partners at risk for the infection. The initial infection often causes only general symptoms, such as fever, swollen glands, and fatigue. Only a small percentage of people who have herpes ever develop the itchy, painful blisters in the genital area that make the virus easier to diagnose.

If you know you have genital herpes, tell your provider at your first prenatal visit. If you don't have herpes but your partner does, tell your provider. Children born to mothers with active herpes infections at the time of labor run a small risk of contracting the disease themselves and may develop eye infections or sores on the skin or mouth. These infections aren't serious if treated with antiviral drugs immediately. However, herpes can morph into more life-threatening infections of your baby's brain or internal organs, so your provider will want to deliver your baby by cesarean if you have an active infection when you go into labor. If you have herpes and get frequent outbreaks, your doctor may suggest that you start taking an antiviral drug such as Acyclovir beginning at 36 weeks to prevent an outbreak at delivery.

During pregnancy it's important to protect yourself against contracting herpes for the first time. Be sure that your partner is tested, and if your partner's test is positive, use a condom; avoid intercourse if he has symptoms. You should also avoid oral sex if your partner has cold sores in his mouth; cold sores may be caused by a herpes simplex virus. Your provider might suggest that you abstain from intercourse altogether during your 3rd trimester if your partner tests positive.

CHLAMYDIA

Chlamydia affects about 10 percent of all expectant mothers. You're at higher risk for having chlamydia if you're under 25 years old or have had multiple sex partners. Only about half of all women with chlamydia experience any symptoms, which usually include a burning sensation while urinating or a vaginal discharge. Unfortunately, whether you have symptoms or not, this infection can have devastating effects if it goes untreated. It can spread to your upper genital tract and cause pelvic inflammatory disease, ectopic pregnancy, or infertility. Your baby might become infected during delivery and contract pneumonia or eye infections as a result.

The Centers for Disease Control recommends that all pregnant women be tested for chlamydia. This is easily done by taking urine or vaginal fluid samples. If your test is positive, your provider will prescribe a safe antibiotic. She'll suggest that your partner get tested too so you can avoid passing the parasite back and forth during pregnancy.

HIV

About 160,000 women in the United States are now living with HIV, the virus that causes AIDS (acquired immune deficiency syndrome). This virus brings on symptoms that are mild at first or that can easily be mistaken for cold or flu symptoms; for this reason, many women don't realize that they're infected. The Centers for Disease Control is now recommending that all pregnant women be offered testing for HIV at the first prenatal visit.

Whether or not you suspect that you're infected with HIV, it's wise to have the test for your baby's sake. Expectant mothers with the virus can now get treatment, which is usually a combination of medications, to prevent passing the infection to their unborn babies. New drugs make it possible to reduce the risk of passing HIV on to your baby to less than 2 percent; the risk jumps to 25 percent in mothers who are untreated. Women with advanced HIV may need cesarean deliveries to further protect their babies from contracting the virus.

If you do not get tested in early pregnancy, your provider may ask you again during labor if you'd like to be tested using a rapid HIV test. If you test positive, your baby will have the benefit of medications to prevent transmission during delivery.

Week 8

Your Baby

The inside story

By the end of your 2nd month of pregnancy, your baby will measure just under 1 inch, and he will weigh in at half an ounce. Yet his central nervous system and major organs will be nearly complete. His heart has four chambers, and by now his heart rate is probably a good, strong 160 beats per minute. That's a rate that you'd achieve only after a sweaty workout!

Your baby's head is more upright now, but it's still nearly the same size as his body. And his skin, although formed, is still nearly transparent. Although the genitals may start to show, it's still impossible to tell whether your child is a boy or a girl by looking at an ultrasound picture. The baby's eye structures are complete, he has tiny earlobes, and his wrist, elbow, and knee joints are visible. All in all your baby finally looks like what he is: a miniature human being. In medical terms he has graduated from an embryo to a fetus, and soon he will begin to stir.

Your baby's first ultrasound

You'll be hopping and skipping to this doctor's appointment—most women agree that an ultrasound is the one prenatal test they enjoy. An ultrasound is a painless diagnostic test that relies on sound waves, and most women will have at least one during pregnancy. Your first ultrasound will typically be done between 18 and 20 weeks, but you may have one before 12 weeks to confirm your due date. You may also have an earlier ultrasound—or more than one—if yours is a high-risk pregnancy, if you have any pain or bleeding, if you have a history of having children with birth defects, or if another prenatal test or exam shows something abnormal. In addition, you'll have additional ultrasounds if you have a chronic illness such as diabetes or a history of ovarian cysts or fibroids.

An ultrasound usually can be done in your practitioner's office or your local hospital. You will be asked to lie on your back while a technician rubs a warm gel on your belly. The gel allows the transducer (a handheld device that looks like a microphone) to slide more easily over your belly and improves the transmission of sound waves into your body. The sound waves bounce off various surfaces within your body—including your baby—as vibrations. The echoes are translated into electrical signals that are projected as pictures onto a monitor for viewing. An abdominal ultrasound poses no risk to you or your baby. In fact, there are many benefits to checking on your baby's development during pregnancy.

If you need an ultrasound early in pregnancy, it may be necessary to use a vaginal probe (a transducer placed in the vagina). This allows the technologist to view your uterus through the cervix. This method may also be used later in pregnancy to locate your placenta if it's over the cervix or to measure the length of the cervix. Vaginal probes may cause a sensation of pressure but shouldn't adversely affect your pregnancy.

Your ultrasound in the 1st trimester can show your baby's heart rate, umbilical cord, and size, as well as the placenta. It will also tell you if you have one, two, or three babies. An ultrasound in the 2nd trimester (around 18 weeks) can show details of the fetal head, face, spine, heart, abdomen, and limbs, in addition to the placenta.

The examiner is looking for physical characteristics that might indicate any abnormality. Ultrasounds can't detect all birth defects, and a normal ultrasound doesn't guarantee a healthy baby. However, ultrasound is a wonderful diagnostic tool that can help ensure that your pregnancy and your baby are both on the right track.

Your Body

Scheduling regular checkups

Whether you're seeing a midwife or an obstetrician, the goal of prenatal care is to monitor your pregnancy progress and head off problems before they become serious. Your provider will use regular office visits to teach you about pregnancy, monitor your health, perform tests, and refer you to support groups, childbirth education classes, and other services. Research on prenatal care suggests that these visits—even when you're feeling just fine—are an essential step toward having a healthy baby, so keep all of your appointments.

How often you see your provider will depend on whether your pregnancy is considered low- or high-risk and whether you have any complications. If your pregnancy progresses without problems, your provider will probably schedule prenatal visits as follows:

During weeks 4 to 28: One visit every 4 weeks

During weeks 28 to 36: One visit every 2-3 weeks

During week 36 to birth: One visit every week

Cold, flu, and allergy remedies

Most expectant moms suffering from colds, flu, or allergies wouldn't think of taking a prescription medicine without their provider's approval, yet many make the mistake of reaching for whatever over-the-counter pills or cough syrups are in their medicine cabinets. This is risky because very few of these remedies are known to be safe to use during pregnancy.

If you're sick, start with home remedies such as chicken soup, plenty of fluids, and rest. If they don't work, contact your health care provider and ask whether your over-the-counter medicine is safe to take before you use it. Remember that whatever medicine you take, your baby will be taking it too.

Here are some home remedies for each of these ailments, as well as medications generally considered safe to use in early pregnancy:

Colds. You'll most likely catch a cold sometime during your pregnancy. The safest way to treat it is by resting and drinking extra fluids. Hot fluids, such as chicken soup or decaffeinated tea, can help ease congestion. Cold compresses may alleviate headaches and muscle pain.

If you're suffering from severe nasal congestion, use saline nose drops, which are considered safe at any stage of pregnancy. Buy drops at the pharmacy or make your own at home by mixing ¼ teaspoon of salt into 8 ounces of water. Put a few drops in each nostril, wait 10 minutes, and then blow your nose. Vicks VapoRub is also a good cure for a stuffy head. You can also invest in a steam vaporizer or humidifier.

The only safe over-the-counter drug for aches associated with colds is acetaminophen (the key ingredient in Tylenol), which has a well-established

safety record in pregnancy. For severe congestion that does not respond to saline drops, your provider might also suggest a nasal spray.

For coughs ask your provider about using a suppressant called dextromethorphan, which is found in Vicks Formula 44 and Robitussin. Avoid any cough suppressant that contains iodine; iodine can cause life-threatening thyroid problems in your baby. Steer clear of aspirin and nonsteroidal anti-inflammatory drugs such as ibuprofen (the main painkiller in Motrin and Advil) and naproxen (the active ingredient in Aleve). Studies have suggested that taking these medications in the 1st trimester can raise the risk of birth defects.

Flu. Flu can be more serious during pregnancy because it sometimes results in pneumonia. Flu shots are safe for both you and your baby at any stage of pregnancy, so get one now if your pregnancy falls during flu season.

If you do contract the flu, follow the suggestions (this page) for treating cold and flu symptoms without medication. A high fever (102 degrees or higher) should be taken seriously because it can increase the risk of miscarriage. Call your provider immediately if you have a high fever and take two aceta-minophen tablets. Tepid baths or showers can help bring down a fever, as can drinking cool beverages.

Allergies. You'll certainly want to humidify your bedroom or use a facial steamer if you suffer congestion

What hazards should I worry about at work?

Take steps to protect your baby by investigating whether any substances or conditions at your workplace might prove hazardous to your baby's development. Always wear protective gear (gloves, eye mask, breathing mask), wash your hands frequently (this is good advice in any workplace), insist on thorough ventilation of your work space, and if necessary, transfer to a safer department. Workplace hazards to look for include:

CHEMICALS

Investigate your exposure to chemicals. If you're employed in the health care industry, for instance, these may include chemotherapy drugs, anesthetic gases, and ethylene oxide (used to sterilize medical equipment). These drugs are associated with miscarriage, and chemotherapy drugs may also raise the risk of birth defects. Do you work in a dental, medical, or veterinary office where you are exposed to nitrous oxide, which has been shown to cause birth defects? Does your work require you to use or be near solvents, paints, cleaning products, fumes, pesticides, chemicals such as mercury, carbon monoxide, benzene, or formaldehyde? Other chemicals to avoid include organic solvents—nail-polish remover, paint thinner, certain types of alcohol—because some research indicates that expectant moms exposed to these solvents during the 1st trimester are more likely to have babies with birth defects. You're most likely to be exposed to these solvents if you're a factory worker, graphic designer, or laboratory technician. Workers in semiconductor plants are also exposed to high levels of glycol ethers, which can raise the risk of miscarriage. Ask your employer for the Material Safety Data Sheets (MSDS) for the products you use or contact the Occupational Safety and Health Administration (OSHA).

IONIZING RADIATION

Laboratory researchers who use instruments that emit ionizing radiation are at greater risk for miscarriage, and their babies may suffer birth defects as a result of the exposure. X-ray technicians and their babies are also at greater risk. The American College of Obstetricians and Gynecologists recommends that pregnant women avoid this type of radiation.

LEAD

Lead is associated with an increased risk for miscarriage and pregnancy-induced hypertension. Lead exposure also puts your baby at risk for birth defects and neurological problems. If you work in an industry that uses lead, limit your exposure.

FOR MORE INFORMATION about the effect of workplace hazards on reproductive health and the federal laws that protect the health, safety, and employment rights of pregnant women at work, contact the National Institute of Occupational Safety and Health: 800-35-NIOSH or www.cdc.gov/niosh.

week 8

because of allergies. You can also ask your provider about taking antihistamines such as chlorpheniramine, which has a long history of use by pregnant women and may not be associated with side effects. Your doctor may also prescribe inhaled steroids, especially for severe seasonal allergies.

When to call the doctor. There are a few reasons to call your health care provider right away:

- If you come down with influenza. Your doctor might want to treat it with antiviral medications.
- If your fever stays higher than 102 degrees after you take acetaminophen.
- If you have trouble breathing.
- If you feel contractions or if you see bleeding.

Your Self

Work smart, work safe

If you work outside the home, talk to your provider early on about any medical conditions or work-related factors that could influence how—and how long—you stay on the job. In general, this will depend on your health, your age, how the pregnancy is progressing, any problems you've had during prior pregnancies, and the type of work you do. Avoid working more than 8 hours a day, five days a week, and take advantage of all available lunch and rest breaks.

Sitting for long periods. If you have to sit at a desk for long periods of time, empty your bladder at least every few hours and get up and stretch every hour or so to reduce the potential for back pain, varicose veins, and blood clots. Use a chair that has adjustable armrests and good support for your lower back and bring a small pillow if you need it. Sit with your feet up on a footrest. This will take more strain off your back and reduce swelling in your feet.

Standing for long periods. If you have a job that requires you to be on your feet all day, sit for 15 minutes every hour or so. Instead of standing in one place, put one foot on a box or low stool to help ease the pressure on your back. Wear support hose and shoes with low heels.

Work stresses. If your work is especially physical, hazardous, or stressful, talk with your doctor about whether your job duties will put your baby at risk. For instance, are you required to do any heavy lifting, standing, or walking? During your 1st trimester, your provider might suggest cutting back on your hours or duties. And if you have trouble with balance as your pregnancy progresses, you might want to stop working during the last few weeks. In addition, if you're exposed to potential hazards, such as toxic substances or X-rays, your provider might suggest that you request a reassignment to an area that's safer for you and your baby.

Just as high levels of stress aren't good for your baby, they're not good for your health either, so it's important to organize your work schedule so that you can rest more during the day and keep regular hours. Work out interpersonal problems as well, because they can add to stress on the job.

Health concerns. If you have a chronic illness such as kidney disease or diabetes, or any pregnancy-induced conditions like back problems or high blood pressure, you might have to cut back on your work hours or quit completely. You may also have to stop working sooner if you're carrying multiples or have any pregnancy history that could cause complications during your current pregnancy.

Scary and weird dreams

Pregnancy dreams are often like weird movies in living, breathing, scary colors. They may be the strangest dreams you've ever had. Wacky imagery in dreams—talking kittens, car crashes, sex with the next-door neighbor—is extremely common when you're pregnant. A combination of hormones and disrupted sleep forces you to spend more time in lighter, dreamy REM sleep than in deeper, dreamless states. And waking more often means you're more likely to remember your dreams.

In the 1st trimester, visions of baby animals and other small creatures (especially aquatic ones) are common, perhaps because you'll soon be required to take care of someone small and fragile. Erotic dreams about former lovers, movie stars, and even neighbors are also common because, it's theorized, you're approaching a

major life transition that will forever close doors to the past.

Many pregnancy dreams are filled with terrible images. You might dream about giving birth to a baby without hands or wake up feeling certain that you tossed your newborn off a moving train. These images are natural extensions of the anxious feelings you may have during the day about whether your baby will be born healthy and whether you'll be a good mom. If you wake up feeling disgusted by a dream of wearing a tent for a dress or bleeding in public, you may be insecure about your changing body.

Diet & Exercise

Your need for iron doubles

Iron is a mineral that's essential to the manufacture of red blood cells, and once you're pregnant your body needs twice as much iron as normal. Without enough iron you'll develop iron deficiency anemia. Babies born to extremely anemic mothers have a higher chance of low birthweight and preterm birth. Anemia can also make you feel sluggish and tired.

Prenatal vitamins do contain iron, but it may not be enough for some women. If your iron levels are low, your doctor will prescribe an iron supplement in addition to your prenatal vitamin. If your doctor prescribes extra iron, keep in mind that supplemental iron can contribute to constipation. Drinking plenty of water and eating high-fiber foods can help.

To get enough iron in your diet, eat high-iron foods such as lean red meat, fish, poultry, dried fruits, spinach, beans, and iron-fortified cereals. Vitamin C helps maximize your body's absorption of iron, so eat some vitamin C-rich foods such as orange juice or strawberries along with your nonmeat iron source.

Are you really eating for two?

Wouldn't it be nice if pregnancy gave you permission to eat twice as much? According to that old saying, a pregnant woman is eating for two. If you do the math, however, you'll find that you're really only eating for about one and a fraction of another. So put down the nachos and the candy bars—you need only about 300 extra calories a day during pregnancy. If you eat for two, you'll gain way too much weight.

Spend your extra calories wisely on nutritious foods. Here are some healthful 300-calorie choices:

- 1 cup of non-fat fruit yogurt and a medium apple
- A baked potato with skin, topped with an ounce of low-fat cheese and ½ cup each of broccoli and cauliflower
- 1 piece of whole wheat toast spread with 2 tablespoons of peanut butter
- A turkey sandwich: 2 slices of whole wheat bread, 2 ounces of lean turkey, and lettuce and tomato
- 1 flour tortilla (7-inch), ½ cup refried beans, ½ cup cooked broccoli, and ½ cup cooked red pepper
- 1 cup of beef-and-bean chili sprinkled with ½ ounce of cheddar cheese
- 1 cup of raisin bran cereal with ½ cup non-fat milk and a small banana

Environmental toxins at home

Although you're more likely to be exposed to environmental toxins on the job than at home (see "What hazards should I worry about at work?" page 69), there are still some substances you may routinely use at home that you should now avoid. These include:

Chemical insecticides. If your neighborhood is being sprayed—for mosquitoes, for example—visit someone away from the spraying area. Stay away for a few days until the fumes are gone because certain insecticides have been linked to birth defects. Avoid using insecticides at home too. If you must spray your home or apartment for insects, close all pantry and cabinet doors to avoid contaminating food. Stay out of the house until the fumes are gone; after the chemicals have dissipated with the help of fresh air, they are no longer a danger to you or your baby.

Paint and paint removers. Most paints manufactured today, including latex, no longer contain harmful lead or mercury, so you can probably paint safely. Yet consider the risks: Balancing on a ladder can be dangerous, and the repetitive motion

Toxoplasmosis

If you change cat litter, work in a garden, or eat raw meat, you're at risk for a toxoplasmosis infection, unless you're already immune. This infection is caused by a parasite called *Toxoplasma gondii*. Although it poses little risk to you, you could pass the infection on to your unborn baby, with serious consequences that include severe illness or death. Talk to your provider about your risk factors and testing. The test results may be difficult to interpret, so your doctor may send you to a specialist. If an infection is confirmed, you can be treated with antiparasitic drugs to lower the risk to your baby.

How do you know if you have toxoplasmosis? You probably won't detect it on your own, although some people experience symptoms similar to the flu. That's why it's important to let your practitioner know if you have risk factors. Your practitioner may do a blood test to see if you've been exposed to the parasite, and he will repeat the blood test if necessary. To avoid toxoplasmosis in pregnancy:

- Avoid eating undercooked meat or unwashed fruit and vegetables.
- Don't rub your eyes or face when preparing food.
- Keep your cat inside so it doesn't come into contact with the parasite and never let your cat eat uncooked meat.
- Ask another person to change the cat litter box.
- Wear rubber gloves if you must clean the cat litter box and wash your hands afterward.
- Use work gloves when gardening and wash your hands afterward.
- Keep your children's sandbox covered when not in use to prevent cats from using it as a litter box.

of using a roller or brush can be hard on your back. If you must paint, open the windows. Stay away from oil-base paints, which may contain solvents. Avoid using any paint removers or thinners because most of these are extremely toxic.

Household cleaners. Avoid dry-cleaning fluids and oven cleaners because they are known toxins. There is no known correlation between other common household cleaners and pregnancy problems, so go ahead and disinfect your counters and toilets. However, if the product has a strong odor, avoid breathing it in directly and wear rubber gloves when using any cleaner.

Lead. Exposure to lead can increase your risk of pregnancy-induced hypertension or miscarriage. High lead exposure is also associated with birth defects and neurological problems in infants. One common source of lead exposure during pregnancy is tap water; check with your local Environmental Protection Agency (EPA) to see how your home's tap water measures up. Invest in a filter or use bottled water for drinking if you suspect your water contains lead. It's best to use cold water for drinking or cooking because hot water leaches more lead from pipes. Another source of lead exposure is food or drink contaminated by lead-lined pottery or china. If you have pitchers or dishes that are handmade or imported, they may contain lead, so use them for display, not for serving or eating food. To avoid exposure to paint containing lead, postpone any plans for renovating an old home.

Common Questions

Q. What questions should I ask during my first prenatal visit?

A. No matter how silly you feel about a question, ask anyway. You can rest assured that someone else has asked the question before. Besides, your provider's job is to help you relax. If she isn't answering your questions with patience, humor, and enough detail to inform you without scaring you, then it's time to find another provider. Write down your questions ahead of time so that you'll remember them when you meet with your provider. You probably already have a list that's growing, so add these questions to it:

- How much weight should I gain, given how much I weigh now?
- Should I be concerned about any hazards at work, such as lifting, stress, or chemicals in my environment?
- I'm worried! Did I hurt my baby when I (you fill in the blank)?
- What sexually transmitted diseases are you testing me for? Should I have any other tests?
- Should I be worried about these (you fill in the blank) that I'm feeling?
- What exercises should I be doing, given my current fitness level?
- What prenatal screening tests do you suggest I have, given my age and medical history?
- How can I reach you between visits?
- Where can I find childbirth classes?
- Is it all right if I bring my partner or friend to prenatal visits?
- I've already had a cesarean delivery. Could I have a vaginal birth this time?

Q. Are microwave ovens safe?

A. All of those myths about the dangers of microwave ovens were born out of a fear of radiation exposure. However, new studies show that the radiation emitted from a microwave oven is negligible. It's extremely unlikely that using one could cause any harm to you or your baby. If it makes you feel better, go ahead and stand to one side as you zap, but there's really no need.

Week 9

Your Baby

The inside story

You're already starting your 3rd month, and though you can't feel them yet, your baby is actually starting to make small movements. The baby's nerves and muscles are starting to be in good working order, and she can now bend her arms!

Your baby's rapid growth continues, but the furious rearrangement of cells has nearly stopped. Soon your baby will no longer need the yolk sac that once provided blood cells, because her bone marrow, liver, and spleen are starting to take on that task. In fact, almost all of the organs are beginning to function. Her liver is secreting bile, and her pancreas is producing insulin.

By now your baby's heartbeat is about 160–170 beats per minute. That's about as fast as the human heart rate ever gets! She's slightly over an inch long, and she will more than double in length before the end of this month.

If you could see your baby, you'd discover that her arms and legs have lengthened even more now, and her fingers and toes are better defined. You'd also see that her head is more rounded and more upright on her developing neck. The plates of her skull are forming. Her eyes are still on either side of her head, but they are starting to move forward as her head grows. The tip of her nose has formed, her ears are continuing to form, and she now has tubes leading from her throat to her lungs.

Your Body

Changes in taste and smell

One whiff of a stranger's perfume makes you gag. Or the pungent food you loved just weeks ago now turns your stomach. Tastes and smells may intensify while you're pregnant, but not every woman experiences this. In fact, some doctors doubt whether it's a real phenomenon. Still, if your senses sharpen, avoid the things that bother you and be thankful that your senses will return to normal after your baby is born.

Sore nipples

Nipples and breasts tend to feel sore during this part of pregnancy, thanks to the action of pregnancy hormones such as estrogen. There's not much that will relieve your achiness other than avoiding tight clothes and other irritants; anything that touches your

week 9

breasts (including your partner) can exacerbate soreness. Hang in there: The soreness should cease within the next couple of weeks.

Flatulence

Hormones such as progesterone enable your body to expand as your baby grows. Unfortunately, those hormones also slow the rate at which food moves through your digestive system. This can result in heartburn, constipation, and most embarrassing of all, flatulence.

Passing gas during pregnancy is normal and shouldn't be treated with over-the-counter anti-gas medications. Avoiding gas-producing foods such as beans and cabbage can help; so can eating small meals rather than large feasts. Don't fret too much if you pass gas in the company of other people. Anyone who has had a baby understands what you're going through.

Tracking your weight

Every time you have an appointment with your obstetrician, you'll be asked to get on the scale. You may feel embarrassed by these regular weigh-ins, but what you weigh matters, both to you and to your baby. Here's why: Gaining too much or too little weight can complicate your pregnancy. Too little weight can result in a baby who is too small; too much weight can lead to a big baby who is difficult to deliver. Gaining a large amount of weight also increases your risk of gestational diabetes, high blood pressure, prolonged labor, complications during

delivery, and cesarean delivery. Women who gain a lot of weight during pregnancy feel less comfortable, and of course, the more you gain during pregnancy, the more you'll need to lose after your baby is born.

Your Self

Your first OB exam

Will your baby be a Taurus or a Gemini? You'll find out at your first prenatal exam, when your obstetrician will calculate your official due date. The exam, which is typically scheduled around week 9 or 10, will likely include the following:

Complete medical history. Your doctor will ask about your health, details of any past pregnancies, your partner's health, and the health of your family and your partner's family.

Physical exam. Your height, weight, and blood pressure will be measured and recorded. Your doctor will discuss any chronic health problems you may have and how they will affect or be affected by your pregnancy. She will perform a complete physical exam that includes checking your thyroid and breasts and listening to your heart and lungs. She will also perform an internal exam, checking your cervix, ovaries, vagina, and uterus.

Calculation of your due date. Your due date is based on the date of the start of your last period. An average pregnancy is 40 weeks (280 days) from the first day of your last normal menstrual period (LNMP). (Keep in

Common Prenatal Lab Tests

Type of test	What it tests for	Why it's needed
Blood type	Determines whether your blood type is A, B, AB, or O	It must be in your medical record in case you need a blood transfusion.
Rh factor	Determines if your blood is Rh-negative or Rh-positive	If you are Rh-negative and your partner is Rh-positive (his blood may be tested too), your pregnancy will require closer monitoring.
Hemoglobin/ hematocrit	Indicates vitamin B_{12}, folate, or iron deficiency	If you're low in iron, you may need an iron supplement in addition to the iron you get in your prenatal vitamin. Low iron levels are not unusual, particularly if you've had one or more children already and the interval between your pregnancies is short.
Syphilis	Checks for this sexually transmitted bacterial infection	An infected mother can pass it to her newborn baby and cause birth defects.
Hepatitis B	Detects this viral infection of the liver	Half of all people who have hepatitis B don't have any symptoms. Left untreated, it can cause life-threatening liver diseases. Treatment can prevent the virus from passing to your baby.
HIV	Tests for the presence of this virus that attacks the body's immune system and leads to AIDS	A pregnant woman who is infected with HIV can transmit it to her fetus while she is pregnant or during delivery. Antiviral medications taken throughout pregnancy can protect the baby.
Urine culture	Tests for presence of bacteria	Bacteria in the urine, if not treated with antibiotics, may lead to a kidney infection.
Pap test	Checks for cancerous or pre-cancerous cells in the cervix	This is a regular preventive exam, done only if you haven't had one recently.

week 9

mind that 40 weeks is average. A normal pregnancy can last anywhere from 37 weeks to 42 weeks.)

If your periods are irregular or you don't know your LNMP, then your due date will be based on your earliest ultrasound.

Laboratory tests. See "Common Prenatal Lab Tests" (above) for the kinds of tests your doctor may perform. Most are performed by analyzing blood or urine samples.

A discussion about genetic testing. Depending on your medical history

When you're older than 35

Age matters in pregnancy. The older you are, the more challenges you may face. Many women over 35 have normal pregnancies and normal deliveries, but statistics show that more problems arise when you're an older mother.

For example, older women are more likely to have chronic health problems such as high blood pressure, heart and kidney problems, autoimmune diseases, and type 2 diabetes, which complicate pregnancy. They also have a higher risk of having a miscarriage or a baby with a genetic disorder. In addition, older women tend to tire more quickly than younger women, although a healthy diet and a regular fitness regimen can be energizing.

Older mothers are usually offered more tests during pregnancy, including amniocentesis and chorionic villus sampling.

Age makes a difference in the delivery room too. Cesarean delivery rates go up in the over-35 set for a variety of reasons.

Finally, older mothers are more likely than younger mothers to have conceived with the help of assisted reproductive technology because fertility rates fall as women age. These pregnancies are more likely to require close monitoring and cesarean delivery than naturally conceived babies.

This gray cloud does have a silver lining, however. Mothers over 35 have accumulated more life experience and are often more financially secure than younger women, both of which come in handy when you're raising a child.

and ethnic background, your doctor may talk with you about doing tests for cystic fibrosis; Tay-Sachs and Canavan disease (if you're an Ashkenazi Jew); and sickle-cell anemia if you're black.

A schedule for future appointments. Ask your provider about upcoming tests and when you should schedule your regular appointments.

Prenatal vitamins. Ask your provider for a prescription, if you aren't already taking them. Or head to a local drugstore to buy prenatal vitamins over the counter. Ask the pharmacist if you aren't sure which kind to buy.

Healthy-pregnancy information. Your doctor may give you advice or a handout sheet about diet, exercise, weight, and over-the-counter medications that are safe during pregnancy. You may also get contact information for when your doctor's office is closed.

Diet & Exercise

Crucial vitamin C

This vitamin, which is found in foods such as citrus fruits and juices, tomatoes, red and green peppers, strawberries, mangoes, papayas, cantaloupe, and spinach, is needed for the development of connective tissue, wound healing, immune function, and iron absorption. Vitamin C helps

Sample 10-Week Walking Program for Beginners							
Week	SUN	MON	TUES	WED	THUR	FRI	SAT
1	10 min.	10 min.	10 min.	off	10 min.	10 min.	off
2	10 min.	10 min.	10 min.	10 min. (or off)	10 min.	10 min.	10 min. (or off)
3	10 min.	15 min.	10 min.	15 min. (or off)	10 min.	15 min.	10 min. (or off)
4	15 min.	15 min.	15 min.	15 min. (or off)	15 min.	15 min.	15 min. (or off)
5	15 min.	20 min.	15 min.	20 min. (or off)	15 min.	20 min.	15 min. (or off)
6	20 min.	20 min.	20 min.	20 min. (or off)	20 min.	20 min.	20 min. (or off)
7	20 min.	25 min.	20 min.	25 min. (or off)	20 min.	25 min.	20 min. (or off)
8	25 min.	25 min.	25 min.	25 min. (or off)	25 min.	25 min.	25 min. (or off)
9	25 min.	30 min.	25 min.	30 min. (or off)	25 min.	30 min.	25 min. (or off)
10	30 min.	30 min.	30 min.	30 min. (or off)	30 min.	30 min.	30 min. (or off)

build strong bones, teeth, and skin. It is also a potent antioxidant; it destroys free radicals, which are molecules that can damage cells.

Because vitamin C is a water-soluble vitamin, the body cannot store it. That means you must replenish your vitamin C stores every day. To ensure that you have the vitamin C you and your baby need, eat at least one vitamin C-rich food every day.

New exercisers? Get walking

Is high school the last time you saw the inside of a gym? Have you always sat on the sidelines cheering while others played sports? If you have never exercised, fear not: You can start during pregnancy. Intense sports are out, but if you have your doctor's approval, you can begin a fitness walking program.

You may not think of walking as exercise, but it is in fact a very effective fitness activity, particularly during pregnancy. The list of all the great things walking does goes on and on. It burns calories, tones your muscles, increases circulation, and prevents constipation. What's more, it reduces the risk of heart disease, diabetes, high blood pressure, colon cancer, depression, and anxiety. It helps control weight; it builds and maintains healthy bones, muscles, and joints; and it promotes psychological well-being. And if that's not enough, it also enhances the quality

week 9

of your sleep, reduces stress, and improves self-esteem.

How to start. The first step in a walking program is to walk as fast as you can for 45 minutes straight, right? Wrong! The first step is to focus on one thing and one thing only: making walking a daily habit. That means starting with 10-minute walks five to seven days the first week, even if you are fit enough to walk much longer. After you've worked 10-minute walks into your daily schedule, try adding 5 minutes to two or three walks a week, gradually working your way up to 30-minute walks five to seven days a week. If you increase your time and feel like it's too much, go back to the previous week's schedule.

It's important not to do too much too soon. If you overexert yourself, your muscles will feel sore, and you may feel discouraged. Add minutes to your workouts gradually.

The foundation of a good program. Here are some tips concerning how to build a walking program:

- Start by buying a good pair of shoes. Specially designed walking shoes are important because they support the walking motion in a way other shoes do not. Choose a walking shoe with good support, a moderate amount of cushioning (more if you're overweight), a roomy toe box, and a low, beveled heel that accommodates the heel-to-toe roll of walking. Have your feet measured, because foot size can change during pregnancy. Try on shoes at the end of the day, when your feet are at their largest. Find a style that fits well in the heel. Resist the temptation to buy shoes that are too big; they'll slip off your heels as you walk.
- Dress for success in comfortable clothes. Layers are best—you can peel them off one by one if you get too warm.
- As you walk be mindful of your posture. Contract your abdominal muscles, keep your chest open and lifted, let your shoulders drop down, and breathe deeply with your chest. Keep your head in line with the vertical line of your spine and keep your chin parallel to the ground.
- Walk at a comfortable speed and with a natural stride length.
- Breathe rhythmically and mindfully. Allow your breathing to fall into rhythm with your steps. Enjoy the feeling of taking deep, full breaths.
- Stay hydrated. Drink a glass of water before your walk and take water with you.
- Plan your walking routes with restrooms in mind in case nature calls while you're exercising.
- Consider using a pedometer. It's an inexpensive way to measure your steps, and it provides motivation and a sense of accomplishment. Aim for 10,000 steps each day.

Pelvic rocking helps back pain

Your back is subjected to substantial strain as you gain weight during pregnancy. As your belly grows larger, it pulls your spine forward. If you have weak back and abdominal muscles, this pulling can cause low-back pain during the latter part of your pregnancy.

Pelvic rocking is an exercise that helps strengthen muscles in the back and abdomen, which will help support your back and prevent back pain later in your pregnancy. To do it, lie on the floor or a firm bed with your knees bent and your feet flat. Begin to rock your hips in a gentle, rhythmic way. Lift your hips and roll them as if you're doing slow hula hooping or belly dancing while lying down. The point of the exercise is to work your abdominal muscles while squeezing your butt muscles at the same time, strengthening both for the sake of your back.

It's safe to do this exercise until week 24. After that avoid lying flat on your back because your growing uterus can press down on blood vessels and decrease blood circulation.

Constipation

Though it may be embarrassing to talk about, having trouble moving your bowels is a common problem throughout pregnancy. Infrequent stools or hard, dry stools occur for two reasons: Pregnancy hormones slow the movement of food in the digestive system, and the iron in your prenatal vitamin can cause constipation. Do your best to address constipation because too much pushing can cause hemorrhoids or exacerbate any you already have.

Preventing constipation is one more good reason to get out and walk: Exercise often helps move things along. Occasionally prenatal vitamins will cause diarrhea, but constipation occurs far more frequently. Don't stop taking your prenatal vitamin; you and your baby need the nutrients it provides. If iron is causing constipation that doesn't improve with changes in diet and exercise, your doctor may want to prescribe vitamins with less iron.

To alleviate and prevent constipation, drink up! Aim for eight to ten glasses of water a day and eat plenty of high-fiber foods. Here are some ways to be sure you're getting the recommended 25–35 grams of fiber each day:

- Start the day with a whole grain cereal that contains at least 5 grams of fiber per serving. Top your cereal with wheat germ, raisins, banana slices, or strawberries, all of which are good sources of fiber.
- Eat raw vegetables. Cooking vegetables can reduce fiber content by breaking down some fiber into its carbohydrate components. When you do cook vegetables, microwave or steam them until they are tender, not mushy.
- Go easy on fruit and vegetable juices. They provide far less fiber than whole fruits and vegetables.
- Leave the peels on. Much of a fruit or vegetable's fiber is in its skin, so if you peel it, you're throwing fiber away. Always wash unpeeled fruits and vegetables

week 9

with warm water to remove dirt and bacteria.

- Use beans instead of—or in addition to—meat. Fiber-rich beans and lentils are a tasty addition to soups, stews, and salads. If you don't like the way they feel in your mouth, mash them up.

Common Questions

Q. Can I go in a sauna or hot tub?

A. Stay out of hot tubs and saunas. Raising your body temperature over 102 degrees can harm your baby, and if you spend more than a few minutes in a hot tub or sauna, your body temperature may climb that high. It's best to avoid them during pregnancy. Electric blankets are fine, though—they don't get hot enough to cause trouble.

Q. What kind of prenatal vitamins should I take?

A. Prenatal vitamins are available over-the-counter (OTC) in your local drugstore or by prescription. OTC vitamins are fine provided they are labeled as "prenatal vitamins." Whether you choose prescription or OTC may depend on what kind of prescription coverage your health insurance offers. If it covers prescriptions, you can save money by using prescription vitamins. If it doesn't, you'll probably end up paying less if you buy OTC vitamins.

When you're shopping for vitamins, you may notice that some brands are fortified with omega-3 fatty acids. Emerging data suggest that omega-3 fatty acids may help prevent preterm labor; however, this data is preliminary, and more studies must be done to determine whether there is a cause and effect. Check with your provider or dietitian about whether omega-3 fatty acid supplements are right for you.

Week 10

Your Baby

The inside story

Your baby is still so tiny that he has plenty of room to move and groove in your warm, protective amniotic fluid. He's now approaching 2 inches in length. If you could see him, you'd be pleased to note that his body is more in proportion; his head doesn't seem as large in comparison to the rest of him. You'd see that his ankles and wrists have formed, and his fingers and toes are now visible too.

An ultrasound taken now would probably show that the yolk sac is separate, and the umbilical cord from the placenta to your baby would be visible. Your baby's intestines are still part of the umbilical cord, but they're starting to move into his abdomen and will soon be covered by skin.

As for his organs, several more are starting to function. His thyroid gland—the master switch for controlling his body's own unique chemistry—is now operating. His pancreas is making digestive enzymes, and his gallbladder is secreting bile; these functions will be essential for eating and digesting his own food after birth.

Your baby's lung tissue is continuing to develop, and his bones are forming, even in his fingers and toes. Cells in the tiny hollows of his bones will soon start making blood cells, a function that until now has been the job of his liver and spleen. His face is starting to look more human; he may even have his first permanent tooth buds, and he will soon be able to open his mouth and move his tongue. It won't be long before he's sticking that adorable pink tongue out at you!

Your Body

When will I look pregnant?

Strange as it seems, this is likely to be the one time in your life that you look forward to gaining weight. So when will you really start to show? That depends on your size and whether you've been pregnant before. On average, women start to show around week 20 or so. It can be earlier for smaller, thinner women and later for larger, heavier women. Also, if you've had a baby before, you'll probably start to pop out in the next few weeks.

Even though you aren't showing yet, your body is definitely changing. You may be noticing that your pants are a little tighter around the waist. You may not have gained any weight, but organs in your abdomen are starting to shift around to make room for your baby's growth.

When none of your clothes fit

Caution! Fashion emergency ahead! You're about to enter a dreaded between-time of dressing for pregnancy: You're too big for your own clothes but not ready for maternity clothes. During the next few weeks, you may find yourself staring into your closet and scratching your head, wondering what to wear. That's no problem when you're hanging around at home in sweatpants and a T-shirt, but if you need to look good for work or social events, you'll have to find something else to wear.

Don't worry, this crisis won't last long. Before you know it, you'll be all decked out in maternity clothes. Until then consider these smart, transitional outfit ideas:

- Buy a pair of pants and a skirt in the next size up. If you're a size 10, buy a 12. Because you'll be living in these clothes for a couple of weeks, choose a neutral color. That way you'll draw less attention to the fact that you're wearing the same skirt or slacks every day.

- Wear loose tops that don't require tucking and sweaters that come to the hip. Draw attention away from your belly with a colorful scarf or trendy new necklace.
- Dress in layers. Many women find that they feel warmer than usual during pregnancy. If you wear layers, you'll be able to peel off some of your clothing to cool yourself down.
- Raid your partner's closet. He may have a shirt or sweater that's perfect for your new figure.
- If you have to wear a skirt or dress, buy some maternity pantyhose. The tops are stretchy and will fit throughout your pregnancy.
- Leave the belts in your closet. They'll squeeze your belly, and if you wear them with tucked-in tops, you'll draw attention to your thickening waistline.
- Top off your outfit with a figure-hiding blazer or jacket.
- Invest in a good pair of flat shoes. This is no time to be tottering around on high heels. Buy only a pair or two at this point because your feet may grow larger during your pregnancy.

Corpus luteum cysts

Like many medical terms, "corpus luteum cyst" sounds scarier than it actually is. Each month, a clump of cells called the corpus luteum forms in the ovary and then disintegrates. If it fails to disintegrate, the clump turns into a cyst. Occasionally a corpus luteum cyst will cause pain or discomfort on one side of your abdomen, or it can bleed. Most of the time, women don't know they have these cysts unless they show up on an ultrasound. In the vast majority of cases, they resolve by the 2nd trimester.

Asthma

Preexisting asthma can make pregnancy a little more complicated, but if you keep it under control, you and your baby should be fine.

Asthma is a condition in which the airways of the lungs become blocked by muscle spasms, accumulation of mucus, and swelling of the airway walls. During an asthma attack, your chest feels tight, and you experience wheezing, shortness of breath, chest pain, and/or cough. Asthma can be triggered by allergens such as pollen, mold, animal dander, feathers, and dust. Some women with asthma find that their symptoms improve during pregnancy, while some find that their symptoms worsen. Others find that pregnancy doesn't change their asthma symptoms.

Uncontrolled asthma can lead to complications that include increased risk of perinatal mortality, preeclampsia, preterm birth, and low birthweight.

Many asthma medicines are considered safe for pregnant women. Doctors prefer to prescribe inhaled medications because they have a more localized effect and only small amounts enter the bloodstream. However, certain oral medications can also be used.

Your Self

Why sex is better (or worse)

As with so many other things during pregnancy, you can thank (or blame) your hormones for your changing interest in sex. For some women, pregnancy brings out a newfound sensuality and heightened interest in lovemaking. They may delight in their increased cleavage and feel more connected to their bodies as life grows inside them. For other women it's the exact opposite. Pregnancy makes them feel awkward and clumsy, and they may have far more desire for an extra hour of sleep than a romp in the hay. Some women feel sensual one day and distant the next as their hormone levels bounce up and down.

All these responses are normal. If you have no interest in sex, be patient. It will probably get better in the 2nd trimester, when you're less tired and feel better. If your libido has increased, take advantage of it while you can. You'll have to abstain for six weeks after delivery, and finding time for sex can be a challenge when you have a new infant in the house.

Your hair and skin

You thought you put it all behind when you left high school, but here it is again: pimples, oily skin, and blotchiness. Pregnancy affects every inch of your body, including your hair and skin. These changes are caused by—you guessed it—pregnancy hormones. Some women develop a rosy, healthy glow; for everyone else, looking in the mirror is enough to cause a downward mood swing.

If your skin starts giving you

trouble, don't automatically reach for the medications you used before pregnancy. Talk with your obstetrician about which skin treatments are safe because some can cause birth defects. If you do have a skin product in your medicine chest that worked well for you before pregnancy, take it with you to your next appointment and ask your doctor's opinion about its safety. (See "Common Skin Problems in Pregnancy," pages 194–195.)

Diet & Exercise

Safe fish

Fish is a four-star food. It's an excellent source of protein, it is very low in saturated fat, it's rich in omega-3 fatty acids (which help build and maintain a healthy brain and nervous system), and with a few exceptions, it's low in calories. It can even help keep your heart healthy.

Now the bad news: According to the U.S. Food and Drug Administration (FDA), nearly all fish and shellfish contain traces of mercury. For most adults the amount of mercury consumed when eating fish poses no health danger. For pregnant women, however, mercury in fish can be dangerous because it can harm a baby's developing nervous system. For that reason the FDA and the Environmental Protection Agency (EPA) advise pregnant women, nursing mothers, women who might become pregnant, and young children to avoid some types of fish and eat other fish and shellfish that are lower

Spider veins

There's no getting around it: Spider veins are unattractive, annoying, and an unfortunate part of pregnancy. These threadlike red or blue lines are simply enlarged blood vessels. They can appear anywhere on your body and are most common on the breasts, belly, face, and legs. Sometimes several develop in one area, making a pattern like a spiderweb—thus the name spider veins. Occasionally spider veins cause pain or a burning sensation; usually they're painless. Not everyone gets spider veins, but they tend to run in families.

Spider veins can sometimes be prevented by wearing support hose, keeping your weight at a normal level, exercising regularly, wearing flat-heeled shoes, and eating a high-fiber diet, according to the American Academy of Dermatology (AAD). Staying out of the sun helps prevent spider veins from appearing on the face.

Spider veins can be treated with laser therapy or with a procedure called sclerotherapy, in which a dermatologist injects a liquid solution into the veins. Over a period of weeks or months, the veins turn into scar tissue and are absorbed by the body. After several treatments most people can expect a 50–90 percent improvement, the AAD says.

It's best to delay treatment until after your baby is born or until you're finished having children. This is also true for varicose veins, which are larger. (See "Varicose veins," page 124.) If you have them treated now, you may end up having to do it again.

in mercury. For more information, or to find out about fish advisories in your state, check the EPA website at www.epa.gov/ost/fish. Follow these government guidelines:

- Do not eat shark, swordfish, king mackerel, or tilefish because they contain high levels of mercury. These are large fish that live long lives. These fish pose the greatest risk because they've had more time to accumulate mercury in their bodies.
- Eat up to 12 ounces (about two meals) a week of fish and shellfish that are lowest in mercury. These include shrimp, canned light tuna, salmon, pollock, and catfish. (White tuna contains more mercury than light tuna.) Other fish that contain low levels of mercury (but not as low as the aforementioned) include anchovies, butterfish, clams, cod, crab (blue, king, and snow), crawfish, Atlantic croaker, flatfish (flounder, plaice, sole), haddock, hake, herring, jacksmelt, spiny lobster, North Atlantic mackerel, Pacific mackerel chub, mullet, oysters, ocean perch, pickerel, sardines, scallops, American shad, squid, tilapia, freshwater trout, and whiting.
- Check local advisories to determine the safety of fish caught by family and friends in your local lakes, rivers, and coastal areas. If no advice is available, eat no more than 6 ounces (one meal) of fish from local waters and no other fish

during that week. When in doubt, eat something else.
- If you eat more than the recommended amount of fish in a week, cut back during the next week or two so that you average the recommended amount per week.
- Never eat raw fish.

Listeriosis

Add this to the list of odd things you have to do during pregnancy: Heat up your luncheon meat before you eat it. Why? To prevent listeriosis, an illness caused by the *Listeria monocytogenes* bacterium. When *Listeria* makes its way to your dinner table via contaminated meat, vegetables, or cheeses, it can make you very sick. Listeriosis is not a common disease—only 2,500 people in the United States become seriously ill with it each year, according to the Centers for Disease Control (CDC)—but one in five who get it will die from the illness. Because of changes in their immune systems, pregnant women are about 20 times more likely than other healthy adults to get listeriosis.

Listeriosis can be particularly dangerous for pregnant women and their unborn babies because it can be transmitted to the fetus through the placenta even if the mother is not showing signs of illness. Listeriosis during pregnancy can result in premature delivery, miscarriage, fetal death, and severe illness or death of a newborn from infection.

Watch for flulike symptoms: a sudden onset of fever, chills, muscle

week 10

aches, and sometimes diarrhea or upset stomach. The severity of the symptoms may vary. If the infection spreads to the nervous system, the symptoms may include headache, stiff neck, confusion, loss of balance, or convulsions. If you think you may have listeriosis, contact your doctor immediately. A blood test can determine whether your symptoms are caused by listeriosis. If you have it, your doctor will prescribe antibiotics.

The best way to prevent listeriosis is to avoid or use extra caution with foods that might be contaminated with the *Listeria* bacteria. The U.S. Department of Agriculture (USDA) and the FDA provide the following advice for pregnant women:

- Do not eat hot dogs, luncheon meats, or deli meats unless they are heated until steaming hot.
- Do not eat soft cheeses such as Camembert, feta, Brie, blue-veined cheeses, and Mexican-style cheeses such as *queso blanco fresco*. The following can be safely consumed: hard cheeses, semisoft cheeses such as pasteurized processed cheese slices and spreads, mozzarella, cream cheese, and cottage cheese.
- Do not eat refrigerated pâté or meat spreads. Canned or shelf-stable pâté and meat spreads are safe to eat.
- Do not eat refrigerated smoked seafood unless it is an ingredient in a cooked dish such as a casserole. Examples of refrigerated smoked seafood include salmon, trout,

whitefish, cod, tuna, and mackerel. These are most often labeled as "Nova-style," "lox," "kippered," "smoked," or "jerky." Canned fish such as salmon and tuna or shelf-stable smoked seafood may be safely eaten.

- Do not drink raw (unpasteurized) milk or juice. Do not eat foods that contain unpasteurized ingredients.
- Thoroughly wash all fresh fruits and vegetables before eating.
- Because *Listeria* can grow even at refrigeration temperatures of 40 degrees or below, use all perishable items that are precooked or ready-to-eat as soon as possible and clean your refrigerator on a regular basis.

Why all calories aren't equal

Here's a pop quiz: Your doctor suggests that you consume about 400 calories at breakfast. Which would you choose? Option one is a 1-cup serving of raisin bran, a cup of skim milk, and a glass of orange juice. Option two is a frosted chocolate-fudge toaster pastry, a handful of chocolate candies, and a can of soda. Both have about 400 calories, but you don't have to be a dietitian to know that raisin bran makes more sense.

It's a basic fact that not all calories are equal. For the same number of calories, you can have a nutrition-packed meal or a nutritionally bankrupt meal. You'll gain the same amount of weight eating 2,500 calories a day in nutritious foods as you would with 2,500 calories a day of junk food. The difference is that if you eat a lot of junk food, you'll deprive yourself and your baby of important nutrients.

Does this mean that every meal has to be perfect and that you can never splurge? No, but for the health of your baby, make an effort to choose more good foods than bad ones.

Think of your calories like money: Each day you're given a certain number to spend. If you spend most of them wisely on fruits, vegetables, whole grains, low-fat or non-fat dairy products, beans, and lean meats and fish, you'll be able to "afford" a treat such as ice cream or candy.

Artificial sweeteners

If you have a sweet tooth (and who doesn't?), you probably have a close friendship with artificial sweeteners such as Splenda (sucralose), Equal (aspartame), Sweet One (acesulfame potassium), and Sweet'N Low (saccharin). These noncaloric products add a sweet taste to coffee, tea, soda, iced tea, and other products without adding sugar or calories.

Are these sweeteners safe during pregnancy? Yes, say the American Dietetic Association and the FDA. Currently there are no studies that show an increase in birth defects among babies whose mothers used the sweeteners.

Should you use them while you're pregnant? Do what feels right to you. If you believe they're safe, keep artificial sweeteners in your diet. If you don't trust their safety, avoid them or cut down. This will be difficult if you're a diet cola addict, but if it gives you peace of mind, it's worth it.

Common Questions

Q. What can I do if I don't have medical insurance?

A. Several programs help uninsured pregnant women get health care, including Medicaid, State Children's Health Insurance Program (SCHIP), and Healthy Start. The U.S. government's WIC program (Special Supplemental Nutrition Program for Women, Infants, and Children) provides food and nutritional assistance to low-income mothers. And most hospitals set aside funding to provide free care for needy individuals. Check with your doctor, a local hospital billing department, or your state's department of public health.

Q. Should my partner come with me to my medical appointments?

A. If the dad-to-be wants to come to your doctor's appointments—and you want him there—he's certainly welcome. He doesn't need to rearrange his schedule to come to every appointment, but there are a few he should attend:

- Your first appointment with your obstetrician. In addition to meeting your doctor, your partner can ask questions, supply details about his family's medical history, and be in on the conversation about tests such as amniocentesis (also called an amnio) and genetic screening.
- Appointments that include medical

procedures and tests. An amniocentesis is a whole lot easier when the person you love is right there with you.

- Appointments in which test results will be discussed. If your doctor has upsetting news, having your partner by your side can help, particularly if you face difficult decisions.
- An office visit toward the end of your pregnancy. During this time, your partner can ask any questions he may have about labor and delivery.

Q. How can I lift things without hurting my back?

A. Take extra care when you lift heavy objects during pregnancy. (Better yet, get your partner to take over tasks like carrying in the heavy grocery sacks.) To lift, position yourself close to the object that you want to move. Plant your feet shoulder-width apart to give yourself a solid base of support. Now, tighten your abdominal muscles and bend at the knees. Take the object into your arms and lift with your leg muscles as you stand up. Do not bend at your waist. Never lift something heavy or awkwardly shaped without help.

Your partner: 15 great ways to love you

Men often don't know how to help or best support you at this time. The next time your partner says, "Is there anything I can do for you?" hand him this list. You might even want to circle the ones that are most important to you or add your own.

1. Give her a foot massage.

2. Keep your mouth shut when she goes back for a second serving of ice cream.

3. Tell her that she's beautiful, and no, she doesn't look exhausted.

4. Do the laundry—and remember, the lingerie doesn't go in the washer with your gym shorts, and it doesn't get bleached.

5. Keep things quiet while she's napping. Put a note on the door to stop people from ringing the doorbell, give the dog a bone that will take an hour to chew, and take your other children to Grandma's.

6. Don't tattle on her at doctor's appointments. Her obstetrician doesn't have to know that she gave in to a craving and ate a box of Twinkies or a bag of potato chips big enough to feed an entire family.

7. Take walks with her.

8. Ignore her mood swings.

9. Bring her flowers—fresh if she can stand the smell, silk if she can't.

10. Since she can't drink alcohol, pop open a can of club soda instead of a beer.

11. Know what week of pregnancy she's in.

12. Learn what "Braxton Hicks" means. (See page 214 for more information.)

13. Send her off on a weekend getaway with her girlfriends and paint the nursery while she's away.

14. Put a smile on your face and say, "That's all right," when she says, "Honey, I'm just too tired tonight." And then do it again tomorrow night.

15. Even if you're kidding, don't ever, ever say, "Now there's more of you to love."

Week 11

Your Baby

The inside story

Your baby is starting to have sleeping and waking cycles, usually between 5 and 10 minutes long. You might even wake her if you cough! Your baby's body and limbs are now growing faster than her head, and she looks more and more like a tiny person. Most of her movements will be in her limbs as she starts to test her muscles, perhaps even kicking with her feet.

Your baby's ovaries are fully formed by now if she's a girl; if your baby is a boy, his testicles and scrotum are developed. However, it's still too early to distinguish your baby's sex on an ultrasound.

What else is happening? Your baby's organs are finalizing their shapes and functions. The development of her lung tissue is nearly complete, and although your circulatory system is still bringing nutrients and oxygen to your baby, her own blood supply is starting to get into the act. Meanwhile, glands in her pancreas are producing insulin and starch, and her intestines are starting to form folds in preparation for the day she'll digest food on her own.

Your baby's skin is starting to thicken as it acquires layers and becomes more opaque. Tiny hair follicles are appearing below the surface of her skin. Her jaw is starting to harden, and she has her first tooth buds, which will grow into tiny baby teeth. Her vocal cords are beginning to form too.

Your Body

Your aching pelvis

Around week 11, you may start to feel some general aches and discomfort in the area between your navel and your groin. These aches are usually nothing to worry about. As your uterus grows, your pelvic bones must shift to make room for it. Occasionally that expansion causes some discomfort. If it bothers you, two acetaminophen tablets should take care of it. Putting your feet up at the end of the day can also help. However, if pelvic discomfort is accompanied by bleeding, or if it becomes very painful, call your obstetrician.

1st trimester tests

Around this time in your pregnancy your doctor may offer to do several tests to gauge your risk of having a baby with Down syndrome or other chromosomal disorders. A screening test will show whether there is an increased risk for a chromosomal abnormality, but only a diagnostic test will give you definitive information.

Screening tests. In the 1st trimester—generally between 11 weeks and 14 weeks—you may be offered a blood test that measures PAPP-A (pregnancy-associated plasma protein-A) and free beta hCG (human chorionic gonadotropin), along with an ultrasound to measure the skin thickness on the back of the baby's neck (nuchal translucency). These measurements are then incorporated into a complicated formula that includes your age; the result tells you the likelihood that your baby has a chromosomal abnormality. This detects more than 80 percent of Down syndrome cases. The screening test will suggest a problem approximately 3–5 percent of the time.

Diagnostic tests. If that screen is positive, a chorionic villus sampling (CVS) or amniocentesis is offered in order to get a definitive answer. Remember, even in the event that the screening test suggests an increased risk for a chromosomal abnormality, your CVS or amniocentesis usually will show that the fetus has normal chromosomes.

These 1st trimester screening tests are not available everywhere, and the technique used to measure the tiny fold on the back of the baby's neck must be done by an experienced sonographer or you may get mislead-ing information. If 1st trimester screening is not available where you live, don't despair. Second trimester screening blood tests work very well and have a comparable detection rate. They are universally available. (See "Multiple marker screening test," page 125.)

Excessive salivation

This is one of the weirder parts of pregnancy: Some women find that in the 1st trimester, they salivate like crazy. It's probably connected to the nausea of morning sickness—think of how you salivate just before vomiting. There's not much you can do for it other than to wait; it usually disappears by the end of the 1st trimester.

Your Self

Worries about appearance

Some women glow with radiant beauty during pregnancy, but most have to put up with the acne, swollen ankles, stretch marks, and of course, gaining 20–30 pounds. It's no fun looking less attractive than usual, but most women chalk it up as the temporary price they have to pay to become mothers.

To make up for the swollen ankles and other annoyances, do things for yourself that make you feel pretty: Have a manicure or pedicure, buy a new outfit, have your brows waxed, or take advantage of the professional makeovers offered at department store cosmetic counters. A different

week 11

palette of makeup might make you feel much more attractive.

Maternity clothes have become more fashionable during the past few years, and most stores offer something better than the polyester tents that were once a staple. If you can't find pretty maternity clothes, buy neutral or black clothing and dress it up with accessories.

If your concerns about your appearance, especially weight gain, cause you to eat less than you should or to exercise excessively, you may have an eating disorder, and you could be putting your baby in danger. Talk with your doctor. (See "Eating disorders," page 54.)

Migraines

If you've ever had migraines, you know how debilitating they can be. Unfortunately, migraines can strike in pregnancy even if you've never had a migraine before, and they can occur more frequently in women who have had them before.

Migraine symptoms may include throbbing head pain (usually on one side of the head), nausea, vomiting, and sensitivity to light and sound. Some people experience an aura, which means they see light flashes, zigzag lines, or shimmering lights before the onset of the headache. Some experience temporary vision loss or have blind spots.

Scientists have found that migraines are often triggered by certain things, although the triggers are not the same for everyone. Some of the most common triggers of migraines include:

- Diet: aged cheese, red wine, figs, smoked fish, chocolate, monosodium glutamate (MSG), meats containing nitrates (hot dogs, bacon, salami, pepperoni), onions, nuts, peanut butter, dairy products, and foods that contain caffeine
- Environment: bright lights, smoke, changes in the weather, allergies
- Emotions: stress, anxiety
- Activity: irregular exercise, change in sleep patterns
- Hormonal activity: pregnancy, birth control pills, menstrual periods

If you get a migraine, lie down in a dark, quiet room with a cool cloth on your head. It's OK to take acetaminophen, but stay away from ibuprofen (Advil, Motrin), aspirin, naproxen (Aleve), and other nonsteroidal anti-inflammatory drugs (NSAIDs) because they can damage your baby's kidneys. Migraines usually go away in a few hours, although some last for two or three days.

If the pain is terrible and you don't feel better in a couple of hours, call your doctor. There are several kinds of medications that help relieve migraines; however, most require a prescription. Some women find that exercise and relaxation techniques help.

Here's some good news: A National Headache Foundation survey found that many women report a decrease in headache frequency and severity as their pregnancies progress. That's probably because hormone levels start to stabilize during the 2nd and 3rd trimesters.

A low sex drive

Some women feel sexier than ever during the 1st trimester. Others have the exact opposite feeling—they have zero interest in sex. If you're exhausted and nauseated, it's no surprise that you don't feel sexy or that your sex drive shifts into low gear during your 1st trimester. Your libido should pick up again in the 2nd trimester, when morning sickness is likely to be gone and you feel somewhat more energetic.

If your lack of interest in sex bothers your partner, work together to find other ways to connect. Watch a movie together, lie in bed reading, take a walk, or play board games—anything to keep you close.

Remember that this may be a difficult time for your partner because all the attention is on you and your pregnancy, making him feel forgotten. Add to that your decreased desire, and you may end up with a very cranky guy. Reach out to your partner in sensual ways even when you don't feel like carrying through. Rub his shoulders, hold hands, or give him a kiss when you pass each other in the hallway. By paying attention to him and making him feel extra special, you'll help him get through this low-libido time.

Your friends' reactions

You probably have all kinds of friends: Some have kids, some want kids but haven't started trying, some have been trying and not having any luck, some want kids but haven't found a partner yet, some don't want kids.

How your friends react to your pregnancy will probably depend on which of those categories they fit in. Friends with kids will probably be excited. You'll have more in common now because moms never run out of stuff to talk about with each other; you're joining their club, and they're happy to have you. Friends with older children may not be as thrilled as parents of toddlers because they know that you'll be preoccupied with your baby and won't be as available as you were before; despite this, they'll probably still be happy for you. They may start telling you horror stories about problem pregnancies or difficult deliveries or colicky babies. If they do and it bothers you, stop them and say that you'd rather not hear such things. And remember, most people have a flair for the dramatic, so the story of the "five-day labor" needs to be put in perspective.

The friends who want to have children but haven't started trying to conceive yet may show an intense interest in your pregnancy. They may think of your pregnancy as a dress rehearsal for theirs. These may be the friends you can count on to exercise with you or accompany you to a medical test that your partner can't make. Share as much as you feel comfortable sharing with them.

Friends without children—singles and couples who want to remain childless—will think of your pregnancy as a mixed blessing. They're happy for you, but they wonder whether a baby will leave you any time for shopping, going to movies, and doing all the other things you've usually done together. This is a valid concern. Many couples who have a baby suddenly find they have little in common with their childless friends. Your friends are raving about the latest exhibit at the art museum, and you're raving about the great diaper prices at the nearby warehouse store. This is tough for everyone, and some friendships don't survive it. Others go into a dormant period that lasts until your baby is older and you have more time for socializing.

If you have a friend who is experiencing infertility, your pregnancy may make it difficult for her to spend time with you. Being with you may be a constant reminder that she can't have what she wants so much—a baby—and you can. It may be particularly difficult for her if you conceived easily. Every time someone else gets pregnant, an infertile woman feels more sadness and regret that she is not pregnant.

Think carefully of an infertile friend's feelings. Instead of springing the news of your pregnancy on her at a party full of people, for example, call her and tell her privately, in case it's difficult for her to hear. And if she starts to avoid you, be patient and don't hold it against her.

Diet & Exercise

Food cravings and aversions

Should you listen to your body? That depends. If you're craving sweets, it's fine to have a bit of chocolate once in a while, provided you don't overdo it on calories. (Here's a tip for chocolate lovers: Instead of squandering a few hundred calories on an ordinary grocery-store chocolate bar, buy yourself some of the very best chocolate you can find and have a small taste every day.) It's a myth, however, that your body is telling you something with its cravings or aversions or that pregnant women crave foods that contain nutrients they need. The fact is the foods you are likely to crave—most commonly, snack or junk foods such as french fries, pizza, salami, ice cream, pickles, cookies, or candy—don't have much nutritional value.

If you crave nonfood items such as clay, cornstarch, laundry starch, or coffee grounds, tell your doctor right away. This is a condition called pica, and it can be dangerous for you and your baby.

As for aversions, if you are repulsed by, say, meat, it's fine to avoid it, as long as you get your protein from another source. It's also fine to give in to a junk food craving occasionally. However, don't let cravings become an excuse for poor eating, and don't let aversions keep you from getting the nutrients you and your baby need.

Is sushi OK?

Say good-bye to sushi and sashimi and any other dishes that include raw fish. That's because raw fish can transmit parasites, bacteria, and viruses, including the viruses that cause hepatitis. Some restaurants serve sushi that's made with cooked ingredients, and that's fine to eat. (See "Safe fish," page 86.) If the only fish on the menu is raw fish, order rice and vegetables instead.

MSG concerns

MSG (monosodium glutamate) is a food additive that has been blamed for a wide variety of ailments, including headache, nausea, diarrhea, dizziness, and tightness of the chest. However, there is no evidence that it negatively affects a pregnant woman or her fetus. That said, it's probably best to avoid eating foods that contain a lot of MSG because it is high in

sodium, which can cause water retention and aggravate high blood pressure.

Should you go organic?

You want the best for yourself and your baby, and the idea of eating organic foods—those that are grown without chemicals—appeals to you. However, organic foods tend to be more expensive than conventionally raised food. Is it worth spending the extra money?

The American Dietetic Association (ADA) says no. There is no evidence that organic produce is better or safer than conventionally grown produce.

Other organizations disagree. For example, the Environmental Working Group (EWG) says that the U.S. government does not regulate pesticide use stringently enough and that Americans should choose organic produce whenever possible.

Pesticides and Fresh Produce

According to the nonprofit Environmental Working Group, these fresh fruits and vegetables are consistently the most—and least—contaminated by pesticides.

Highest levels of pesticides	Lowest levels of pesticides
Apples	Asparagus
Bell peppers	Avocados
Celery	Bananas
Cherries	Broccoli
Grapes	Cauliflower
Nectarines	Corn
Peaches	Kiwifruits
Pears	Mangoes
Potatoes	Onions
Red raspberries	Papayas
Spinach	Pineapple
Strawberries	Sweet peas

week 11

It's up to you to decide what you want and can afford to do. One option is to compromise and choose organic only when you're selecting the 12 fruits and veggies that, according to the EWG, have been shown to contain the most pesticide residue (see the "Pesticides and Fresh Produce" chart, page 97).

Whether you choose organic, conventionally grown, or some of each, what matters most is that you eat 2–4 servings of fruit and 3–5 servings of vegetables every day. Always wash produce—conventional or organic—before eating it.

Kegel exercises

As your uterus grows larger and the weight of the baby presses down on your pelvic floor muscles, they may weaken. That's not a good development because these muscles support the organs in the pelvis—the bladder, urethra, uterus, and rectum—and control urination. Kegel exercises to the rescue! Kegel exercises, which are named after the doctor who pioneered their use, strengthen pelvic floor muscles; this makes delivery slightly easier and helps prevent urinary incontinence. The exercises can also help make intercourse more enjoyable.

You can do Kegels anytime, anywhere. A good way to remember your Kegels is to do them at the same time each day or while you're doing a certain activity—riding the bus to and from work, for example. Here's how:

- Tighten the pelvic floor muscles. Do what you would do if you were in the middle of urinating and wanted to stop because you thought you heard the phone ringing. Or, even better, pretend you are in an elevator and you have to pass gas; hold the gas in and you will tighten your pelvic floor muscles from front to back.
- Hold the muscles tight and then release.
- There are several ways to do Kegels: You can hold the muscles tight for a count of four and then release for a count of four and repeat that for several minutes. Or you can hold the muscles tight for up to 10 seconds, release, and repeat 10 times several times a day.

Common Questions

Q. I was at my nephew's birthday party last week and just found out that one of the kids at the party had chicken pox. What should I do?

A. If you've already had chicken pox, or if you've had the varicella vaccine, you probably won't get it. Stay away from the infected person anyway, just in case. If you haven't had chicken pox, call your doctor immediately and let her know you've been exposed. You may be given varicella immunoglobulin, which can prevent you from developing chicken pox. Immunoglobulin works only if it's given within 96 hours of exposure, so time is critical. In pregnant women, chicken pox can cause pneumonia in addition to all those itchy pox.

Q. What about other illnesses? What do I do if I think I've been exposed to them?

A. Try as you might, it is impossible to live your life normally and avoid all contact with possibly contagious people (like the sneezing boy next door) and germs (like those inhabiting public restrooms). If you think you have been exposed to the following infectious illnesses, call your doctor right away:

Fifth disease. This oddly titled viral infection gets its name from being one of the five common childhood diseases that cause fever and a rash due to parvovirus. (The other four are measles, mumps, chicken pox, and rubella. Fifth disease is the least serious of the bunch.)

Primarily an infection of childhood, fifth disease may cause a rash or arthritis-like stiffness and joint pain. Or it may cause no symptoms at all. In rare cases fifth disease can cause severe fetal anemia that leads to miscarriage, fetal hydrops, or stillbirth.

Fifth disease is contagious before it shows any symptoms, so it's difficult to avoid. The best precaution is to wash your hands frequently, particularly after you've been with children.

Cytomegalovirus. Most adults have had this infection already, but because it produces few or no symptoms, they never knew they had it. If there are symptoms, they are similar to those of the common cold or flu: sore throat, fever, fatigue, and swollen glands.

Teachers, daycare providers, nurses, and parents of toddlers are at highest risk for cytomegalovirus. It is spread via body fluids, so if you change diapers, be sure to always wear gloves or wash your hands thoroughly afterward.

Unfortunately, if a woman catches cytomegalovirus for the first time during pregnancy, her fetus is at risk. The virus can cause birth defects such as blindness, mental retardation, and deafness. It is the most common cause of congenital-viral infection in the United States. If you've already had it and you become infected again, there's a much smaller chance that your baby will be severely harmed.

Lyme disease. This bacterial infection is spread by infected deer ticks. It causes a rash—usually a bull's-eye-shape rash—and if it's not treated in its early stage, it can go on to cause a wide variety of serious symptoms that affect the joints, heart, skin, and nervous system.

Pregnant women who get Lyme disease may receive ampicillin or a cephalosporin, both of which are safe during pregnancy. Little is known about the impact of Lyme disease on a fetus, although researchers suspect that in rare cases, Lyme disease acquired during pregnancy may be associated with stillbirth.

To prevent Lyme disease, check yourself, your pets, and other family members for ticks after spending time outdoors. If you find a deer tick, remove it: Use tweezers to grasp the head of the tick and pull it straight out. It takes 36–48 hours for a tick to transmit the bacteria, so do tick checks every 24 hours if you or your pets go outside in areas with tick infestation.

week 11

Week 12

Your Baby

The inside story

Your baby can swallow by now, and he might even get the hiccups! He's a whopping 3 inches long, and his head, which was half the size of his body last month, is now just a third as big as the rest of him. He's also less hunched over. His face is almost fully formed, and his nose, eyelids, and ears are almost completely developed. He's even got an upper lip.

Blood has started to pump through your baby's umbilical cord, carrying nutrients and oxygen from your body through the placenta to support your baby. The umbilical cord also works in reverse to rid your body of the baby's waste products now that his kidneys are excreting urine.

All of the major organ systems have finished forming by the end of your 1st trimester, so now they only need to grow. Your baby has opposable thumbs too, and his motions are more purposeful. In fact, some researchers say they can detect variations in personality even this early, such as whether your baby will be active or calm, a thumb sucker or not. Most of his motions right now are reflexes, but his muscles are starting to respond to his brain signals; he can kick and curl his toes. If you could prod your baby's hands right now, they would probably close because of reflex. He'll be holding your finger with a good, firm grip before too long.

Your Body

Sleep problems and solutions

Some women sleep like babies while they're pregnant. Others toss and turn. For still others, a good night's

---

Uterine fibroids

These noncancerous growths in the uterus seldom cause trouble during pregnancy. One in four women has them, but because the fibroids are so small, most of these women have no symptoms. When fibroids grow large, or when there are many of them, problems such as pain, changes in menstrual cycles, and infertility can occur.

If you have a history of fibroids and begin to feel unusual pain or pressure in your abdomen, call your doctor. In rare cases fibroids can cause miscarriage or other pregnancy complications.

sleep may come easily early in the pregnancy and then become more elusive during later months. Here are some ways to improve your sleep:

- Cut down on evening fluids. Frequent urination is a major sleep saboteur. Most pregnant women have to get up one, two, and even three times each night to urinate. You can reduce nighttime trips to the bathroom by drinking most of your fluids earlier in the day and limiting them after dinner.
- Keep heartburn at bay. Avoid spicy, fatty foods late in the day and eat lightly in the evening. Elevating the head of the bed or sleeping with an extra pillow may also help.
- Work out early. Exercise can help you sleep, but working out too close to bedtime might keep you awake.
- Practice sleeping on your side. It's best not to sleep on your back after week 24, because doing so can impede blood flow to major vessels and may make you feel nauseated.
- Cushion your expanding belly. As your pregnancy progresses, the weight of your growing baby may place uncomfortable pressure on certain parts of your body. Some women get comfort from the

Thyroid trouble

The thyroid is a butterfly-shape gland at the base of the neck. It produces hormones that manage your metabolism. Malfunctions of the thyroid are quite common in both pregnant and nonpregnant women.

Trouble occurs when your thyroid produces too many or too few thyroid hormones. Producing too little *(hypothyroid)* slows down your metabolism, leaving you feeling tired, sluggish, and sleepy. You may also have dry hair and skin or feel cold, depressed, constipated, or crampy. Producing too much *(hyperthyroid)* speeds up your metabolism, making you feel wound up and hyperactive. You may have heart palpitations, insomnia, breathlessness, heat intolerance, or increased bowel movements.

Because many of the symptoms of thyroid disease are interchangeable with the effects of pregnancy, diagnosis can be a challenge. However, it's important that thyroid disease in pregnancy be diagnosed because uncontrolled thyroid function can harm the fetus. Untreated hyperthyroidism may be associated with an increased risk of preterm delivery, severe preeclampsia, and miscarriage. Untreated hypothyroidism can lead to preeclampsia, placental abruption, low birthweight, and possibly low IQ in the infant.

The good news is that thyroid disease is relatively easy to treat. Underactive thyroid disease is treated with thyroid hormone replacement pills. Overactive thyroid disease is treated with medication that slows the thyroid down.

If you develop thyroid disease during pregnancy—or if you had it before you conceived—your doctor will do a blood test to measure the thyroid hormone levels every 6 to 8 weeks. Thyroid hormone levels tend to change in pregnancy, and medication will be adjusted as needed.

week 12

full-body pregnancy pillows that are sold in catalogs and baby stores. You can get similar full-body support by lining up several smaller pillows.

- Relax. If stress is keeping you awake, take a warm shower or bath before bed, practice breathing exercises, or ask your partner for a soothing massage.

Stuffy nose and nosebleeds

Pregnancy affects every inch of your body, even your nose. Pregnancy hormones can cause nasal congestion, nosebleeds, and stuffy nose in some women—although others breathe easily from conception to delivery. If your nose is giving you trouble, running a humidifier in your bedroom while you sleep may help. Saline spray may also help, but avoid decongestants and other over-the-counter medications. If your nose feels chapped, soothe it with a dab of petroleum jelly.

Your Self

Your lower risk of miscarriage

Good news! Your risk of miscarriage goes way down at the end of the 1st trimester. So if you haven't already

Preexisting high blood pressure

If you're among the 5 percent of women who had high blood pressure before you conceived, your pregnancy may be more complicated. Babies born to mothers with high blood pressure are at risk for being born prematurely or with a low birthweight. If you take care of yourself and have good prenatal care, however, you have an excellent chance of having a healthy baby. Here is what you need to know:

ACE inhibitors are a no-no. These high blood pressure medications are dangerous to your baby, particularly during the 2nd and 3rd trimesters. In the mother they can cause low blood pressure, severe kidney failure, and too much potassium; for the baby they can cause death. It's best to stop taking ACE inhibitors before you conceive. If you're on them now, immediately contact your doctor, who will switch you to a safer kind of drug. Don't stop taking your medication unless your doctor tells you to.

You are at risk for preeclampsia. One-fourth of women who have high blood pressure develop preeclampsia (also known as toxemia), usually after about 28 weeks of pregnancy. (See "Preeclampsia," page 253.)

You are at risk for placental abruption. Placental abruption, or separation of the placenta from the uterine wall, is dangerous for mother and baby. It can cause severe bleeding, usually after week 20. (See "Placental abruption," page 269.)

Your doctor will monitor you closely. Your blood pressure will be checked regularly, and your urine will be tested for protein. (One of the signs of preeclampsia is excess protein in the urine.) Some doctors ask their patients to monitor their blood pressure at home.

You can make a difference. Monitoring your weight gain, taking your medications religiously, and exercising will help cut your risk of complications.

shared the getting-bigger-by-the-day news with family, friends, and neighbors, now may be a good time.

"I'm pregnant, world!"

Many women share the news of their pregnancy around week 12, when miscarriage risk has gone down. If you're not quite ready to shout it from the rooftops, you can probably wait longer, because you won't start to show for a few more weeks. If this is your first pregnancy and you're of average height and weight, you can probably continue to hide your growing belly until week 20 or so.

Why wait? Well, once your friends, family, coworkers, and neighbors know you're pregnant, they'll want to talk about it and ask you an array of questions. Do you know if it's a boy or a girl? Are you going to quit work? What names do you have picked out? Have you had an amniocentesis? And so on. If you're not ready to answer all those questions, waiting a few weeks is the way to go.

Diet & Exercise

Pregnancy and posture

Growing a big belly and adding about 30 pounds to your frame can take a toll on your posture. Your enlarged belly can pull your body forward into a slump, tilting your pelvis backward and distorting the sway of your back. Poor posture can lead to pain in the neck, shoulders, low back, and hips.

Check your posture several times a day. Roll your shoulders back to open up your chest area. Align your shoulders with your hips. Pull your abdominal muscles in and tilt your pelvis forward, rather than toward the back of your body. Hold your head up, and if your chin juts forward, pull it back in toward your neck. Be gentle as you check your posture—you don't have to look like a marine.

It's good to snack

You may think of snacks as a nutritional no-no, but dietitians actually encourage pregnant women to eat three snacks along with their three meals each day. Eating six mini-meals instead of three large meals helps prevent heartburn and keeps blood sugar levels stable.

Snacking doesn't mean heading to the candy machine for a chocolate bar. Your three snacks a day—between breakfast and lunch, between lunch and dinner, and before bedtime (if it doesn't cause indigestion)—are three more opportunities for you to eat foods that are rich in vitamins, minerals, protein, fiber, and other nutrients. Here are some nutritious, delicious snacks that you can enjoy:
- Yogurt with granola and fresh fruit
- A frozen 100-percent-juice bar
- Low-fat cheese and whole wheat crackers
- Carrot sticks with low-fat ranch dressing for dipping
- Red, green, and yellow bell peppers with salsa for dipping
- Whole wheat bagel with 100-percent-fruit spread

week 12

- Apple slices with peanut butter
- Whole wheat waffle topped with fresh strawberries

Virgin party drinks

Just because you can't drink alcohol doesn't mean you have to walk around with a glass of tap water at your next party. Make your own nonalcoholic party drinks by blending fruits, fruit juices, or vegetable juices with mixers. These drinks do double duty, delighting your taste buds and providing important nutrition for you and your baby. Here are some simple ideas:

Virgin Mary. Combine low-salt vegetable juice with a squeeze of lemon juice, a shake of pepper, a dash of celery seed, and a splash of Worcestershire and/or Tabasco sauce. Serve over ice with a stalk of celery.

Party punch. Mix equal amounts of orange juice, pineapple juice, and seltzer. Garnish with a slice of orange or fresh pineapple.

Margarita. Combine orange juice, a splash of fresh lime juice, and a sprinkle of margarita mix.

Piña colada. Blend 1 part coconut cream with 3 parts pineapple juice and crushed ice.

Strawberry daiquiri. Blend fresh or frozen strawberries with a splash of lime juice and crushed ice.

Tahitian punch. Blend fresh strawberries, papaya, banana, and pineapple with orange juice and seltzer.

Mimosa. Combine equal amounts of orange juice and seltzer.

Common Questions

Q. What if I fall or am injured?

A. When it comes to accidents, you've got two strikes against you when you're pregnant: First, as your center of gravity shifts, you have less sense of balance and become less coordinated. Second, hormonal changes relax your ligaments, making them vulnerable to injury.

Use extra caution to make up for what you lack in grace. Ask for help when walking on ice or other slippery surfaces. Avoid high heels, clogs, mules, and any other shoes that compromise your stability. Take your time walking down stairs, getting out of the bathtub, and leaning over in the shower to shave your legs. Stay off ladders.

If you're injured, inform emergency health care providers that you're pregnant. If you cut yourself or get a puncture wound and haven't had a tetanus booster within the past 10 years, get one: Infection with the tetanus bacteria can be fatal to both mother and baby. Tetanus booster shots are safe during your pregnancy.

the.2nd trimester

2

Welcome to the "honeymoon" phase of pregnancy. You'll feel hungrier for food and hungrier for life. You'll stop feeling nauseous and start regaining your appetites and energy. With your new curves and only a modest belly, you may feel sexier than ever. You may also have a heightened sense of pleasure in the world around you as you revel in being a player in life's most essential creative cycle. The most exciting development in this phase will be feeling your baby move. At first, you'll notice a light, fluttering sensation, as if the inside of your belly is being stroked with a paintbrush. Soon, though, you'll get some solid kicks that your partner can feel too.

In this section

Week 13

Your Baby

The inside story

Your baby is ramping up his growth rate. Your baby's organs, now fully formed, will mature during this trimester in preparation for life after birth. You still supply his oxygen through your bloodstream, but your baby will exercise his lungs and work his chest muscles. His kidneys are getting some practice too, and the amniotic fluid now contains fetal urine. The placenta is working alongside your baby, producing hormones and red blood cells.

His skin is becoming more water-proof. His heartbeat will start slowing down, but it will be strong enough for you to hear during your prenatal visit. His brain is continuing to grow. In fact everything will start growing so fast this month that your baby will almost double in length by the end of the 2nd trimester. Grow, baby, grow!

Your Body

Dental care

Who wants to see the dentist when there are so many other, more exciting things to do during pregnancy? It may be a chore, but tending to your dental health is actually a baby-related activity. Your pregnancy will affect your teeth and gums, just as it's affecting the rest of your body. Looking out for your teeth during these hormone-flushed months will protect your health and your baby's health, not to mention your smile.

Yes, pregnancy affects even your mouth. You're eating more, and those pesky pregnancy hormones will cause your gum tissue to become swollen, softer, and more sensitive. This combination of factors will make you more susceptible to inflammation and bleeding of the gums, a condition known as pregnancy gingivitis. Half of all pregnant women experience this problem. Pregnancy gingivitis is caused by plaque, that sticky, colorless film that builds up on your teeth and causes tooth decay.

Brush and floss your teeth regularly throughout your pregnancy to keep plaque at bay. Use a soft-bristle or ultrasonic toothbrush to remove plaque buildup and reduce bleeding, and rinse out your mouth at least twice a day with an antiseptic mouthwash. In addition, keep your diet rich in foods that contain calcium and vitamin C.

The dangers of periodontal disease.
At your checkup your dentist can
determine whether you're at risk for
periodontal disease, a serious gum
infection that can destroy the fibers
and supporting bone holding your
teeth in place. Expectant moms with
periodontal disease may be seven
times more likely to have a baby
who's born too early and too small;
preterm births may be provoked by
the hormone prostaglandin, which is
found in oral bacteria and is responsible for inducing labor.

If your dentist diagnoses periodontal disease, she might recommend
that you have a common, nonsurgical
procedure called scaling and root
planing; this cleans plaque and tartar
from deep periodontal pockets and
smooths the root to remove bacterial
toxins. This procedure may cut your
chances of having a preterm birth and
alleviate gum swelling and tenderness. It's perfectly safe for you to
have a dental cleaning or a local anesthetic at this point in your pregnancy,
but tell your dentist about your
condition so that she can take any
necessary precautions.

**Your dental health affects your
baby's teeth.** Sometime between your
3rd and 6th months of pregnancy,
your baby's teeth will begin to
develop below the gums. It's crucial
for you to eat a diet that has sufficient
amounts of protein, calcium, phosphorus, and vitamins A, C, and D.
Why? To strengthen the baby's teeth.
Fluoride is also an important mineral
to add to your diet for your baby's

healthy tooth development. Practicing
good dental habits will help protect
your baby's teeth as well as your own.
Babies aren't born with the bacteria
that cause tooth decay, and studies
have shown that mothers are the most
likely source for transmitting plaque-
building bacteria to their children.

Your Self

Advice burnout

It's finally time to share your news,
and you do so joyfully. After all, it's
more rewarding to tell friends and
family about your pregnancy than it
would be to hoard your good news to
yourself, isn't it?

That's mostly true. Unfortunately,
the one thing you may not have anticipated when you started telling
friends and coworkers about your
pregnancy was the advice overload
that would come your way. Now that
your belly is showing, everyone wants
to manage your pregnancy.

Reaching out to you with advice is
a way for people to connect with you
and share your pregnancy, usually
because they're remembering their
own pregnancy experiences. Although
their intentions might be good, the
sheer volume of advice can leave you
feeling buried or insecure.

Unfortunately, a lot of the
pregnancy advice you get will be
based on tales, misinformation,
myths, or pregnancies different from
yours. You may be cautioned against
raising your arms lest you strangle the

baby, told that if you eat carrots your baby's eyesight will be perfect, or informed that you're having a boy because you're "carrying high." You'll be showered with homespun remedies and cultural superstitions and subjected to pressure by friends and family who advise you to have the pregnancies and childbirth experiences they had (or wish they'd had). Some of this advice can be hurtful, especially if it brings up a loaded issue. Your mother may disagree with your decision to return to work, for instance, or your friend might set out on a one-woman crusade to convince you to have an epidural or find out your baby's sex before delivery.

Whatever running commentary you get, bear in mind that it's probably delivered out of love for you and your unborn baby. That doesn't mean you need to take the advice. Whatever you're told, consider the source. You might want to smile politely and move on, or you can enlist an ally if someone is persistent in telling you to do things that conflict with your own ideas and preferences. Say, "My partner and I have decided that I should breastfeed," or "My doctor thinks another ultrasound will help clarify one of my prenatal tests." If someone is particularly meddlesome, she probably just wants to be involved. You might get her off your back by actually soliciting advice about something that matters less to you (like which maternity clothes you should buy) but still makes her feel included. And remember, if someone's

advice doesn't sound logical, it probably isn't. When in doubt, ask your provider for confirmation.

Sharing household chores

You unloaded the dishwasher, threw in a third load of laundry, and potted a few plants for the front porch. While you were working, your partner fiddled around with his computer. It's not your imagination: If you think you're doing more of the household chores even though you and your partner both work, you probably are. This won't necessarily change just because you have a baby. In fact if you're planning to stay home during a maternity leave or work less after the baby arrives, you can bet that your partner will expect you to do more around the house, not less. This is especially true if your partner is your husband. Researchers in the United States have shown that even when husbands and wives both work full-time outside the home, women take on more of the household chores. When couples have a child together, women also assume a greater share of childcare duties.

Now is the time to start divvying up the household responsibilities more fairly. If you're currently handling most of the cleaning and laundry, make a list of responsibilities and divide them up the same way that you might tackle a team project at work. Once your partner gets going on those chores, don't criticize his way of doing them. He may give up if you can't be flexible about standards.

You can take turns doing a certain chore (like cleaning the bathroom) and do it your way the next time. If your partner says, "I know you'd do a better job," or "I can't find the laundry soap," keep responding positively and offer encouragement. Don't step in and do the chore, or you'll be right back where you started.

If there is a certain chore that you both hate, like ironing or doing the bathrooms, have it done by someone else from time to time. It's worth the extra money to save your marriage, especially now that the two of you have a baby on the way and baby-related chores. If you successfully negotiate domestic tasks now, it will be a lot easier to renegotiate once the baby is born and your life is turned upside down.

Diet & Exercise

Understanding food labels

Reading food labels may not be as exciting as thumbing through the newest issue of your favorite magazine, but it can be an excellent guide for choosing foods. These parts of the food label will be most useful to you as you plan meals:

Calories. Counting every calorie you eat is unnecessary, but it's good to become aware of approximate calorie counts in foods to help you gauge whether to eat more or less.

Serving size. Servings are often smaller than you might expect. For example, the bowl of cereal you

normally pour may be closer to 2 servings than 1 serving.

Sugars. The sugars referred to on the food label include sugar found in the food, such as lactose in milk and fructose in fruits, and those added to the food, such as table sugar, corn syrup, and dextrose. Don't be fooled by a label that boasts "no added sugar." It may still contain a lot of natural sugar. For example, 100-percent apple juice has no added sugar, but because of its high natural-sugar content, it can cause blood sugar levels to skyrocket. No matter where the sugar comes from, your body processes it in the same way.

Fiber. Aim for 25–35 grams of fiber a day.

Vitamins. The label lists whatever vitamins are in that food, along with the "percent of daily value." Use this as a rough guide, because your vitamin requirements during pregnancy are higher. All vitamins are important, but vitamin A, any of the B vitamins (thiamin, riboflavin, niacin, B_6, folic acid, B_{12}, biotin, and B_5), and vitamins C and D are especially important.

Minerals. The food label lists whatever minerals are in that food, along with the "percent of daily value." Look for foods rich in calcium, zinc, and magnesium.

Sodium. You'll be shocked at how much sodium (salt) there is in the foods you eat. You expect to see a lot of sodium in a bag of pretzels or potato chips (approximately 210 to 250 mg per serving, depending on brand), but amazingly there's more sodium in a serving of raisin bran with a cup of skim milk (475 mg) than there is in pretzels. That doesn't mean you should have pretzels for breakfast instead of raisin bran in milk. It merely shows that checking food labels for sodium is enlightening.

You do not need to restrict sodium during pregnancy. If you had high blood pressure and swelling with a previous pregnancy, however, you may want to keep your intake at moderate levels.

Caffeine and alcohol

Drinking alcohol and consuming excessive amounts of caffeine are particularly dangerous during the 1st trimester, when your baby's organs are developing and the risk of miscarriage is higher. Once you've passed that supercritical time and are in your 2nd trimester, don't pop open a beer or go coffee crazy. Alcohol is still off limits, as it is throughout pregnancy. This is because the alcohol that you drink goes right through the placenta to your baby. Researchers don't know how much—or how little—alcohol it takes to harm a fetus, so the safest thing to do is to avoid it completely. As for caffeine, continue to limit yourself to about 300 mg of caffeine daily, or the amount in a cup or two of coffee. (See "The buzz about caffeine," page 43.)

Exercise

If you're lucky, you've been exercising all the way through your 1st trimester. Many women aren't so fortunate. Morning sickness and fatigue can keep them on the sidelines.

If you didn't exercise much during the 1st trimester, that's OK—you can start now (provided your doctor approves). Walking is a great fitness activity for all pregnant women, particularly those who are not athletic and who haven't followed an exercise regimen before conception. (See "New exercisers? Get walking," page 79.) If you jogged, ran, swam, or took aerobics classes before you got pregnant, you can ease back into those activities now; start slowly and gently if your body has been out of commission for a while. Listen to your body, and if you feel comfortable returning to your prepregnancy exercise levels, go ahead. You may find yourself breathless halfway through a workout that used to leave you feeling invigorated. That's because you're exercising for two!

Common Questions

Q. I was sick for almost my entire pregnancy three years ago, and labor was extremely painful. Will this pregnancy be like my first?

A. Not likely. It's very rare for any second pregnancy or birth to be a replay of the first. You may have been sick for your entire first pregnancy, yet find that you have very little nausea now. On the other hand, you may have been tired for just the first

8 weeks of that first pregnancy, but now—with a preschooler in tow, still begging to be carried—you may feel more exhausted for a much longer time.

Probably the most significant difference most women report between first and subsequent pregnancies is the ability to feel their babies moving much earlier. A first-time mom might notice her baby's fetal activity around 20 weeks; more experienced moms will feel those first butterfly movements as early as 16 weeks. That's not because second or third babies are stronger but because these moms now can distinguish between a baby's distinct motion and a gas bubble.

Your latest pregnancy is also likely to show sooner because your abdominal muscles may already be stretched. The good thing about this baby's lowered position is that you may not suffer the same heartburn you did during your last pregnancy; the downside is that you may find yourself making even more frequent trips to the bathroom this time around.

Your back may hurt more with this pregnancy if you can't get enough rest or if other children need to be carried or picked up. Teach older children to do more for themselves; for instance, your toddler can probably climb into her own car seat, and a preschooler can use a footstool to reach the sink. If an older child wants to sit on your lap, sit down first and let her climb up. You can also wear a maternity abdominal support garment to diminish backaches.

As for childbirth, well, there's probably nothing more unpredictable in nature than how a baby decides to make his appearance. Subsequent labors and births are generally easier and faster than the first because your body already knows what to do and your cervix is less rigid; the cervix will dilate and thin out faster when it's time for your baby to arrive.

Q. Can I paint the nursery?

A. As long as you're careful, yes. Most paints, including latex, don't contain harmful lead or mercury, so you can paint safely. The repetitive motion of using a roller or brush can be hard on your back, so ask your partner to tackle the task with you. As a precaution, open a window while you paint to let the fumes out. Avoid climbing a ladder or even a step stool; as your balance changes in pregnancy, you're at greater risk of falling. Stay away from oil-base paints that may contain solvents. Avoid using any paint removers or thinners because most of these are extremely toxic.

Week 14

Your Baby

The inside story

Your baby is almost fully formed now. Although she weighs just under 2 ounces, that will change rapidly in the weeks ahead. She'll soon be much longer than her current 3 or 4 inches. She now has a recognizable neck, and her head sits up a bit from her chest. Because her head has grown, her eyes are closer together over the bridge of her nose.

As her arms and legs continue to lengthen, she'll put them to good use. Your baby might move hundreds of times a day in her secure, thick-walled bedroom. A fine, downy hair called lanugo is growing over her body to protect her skin; it will stay there until it starts to disappear a few weeks before her birth. Your baby is also developing hair on her head, as well as eyelashes and the first hint of eyebrows. Her eyes are still firmly shut, however, and won't open until approximately 23 weeks.

By now your baby is also starting to produce hormones on her own. Her thyroid gland has matured, and her reproductive organs have accelerated their development. Boys are developing their prostate glands by week 14, and if your baby is a girl, her ovaries have descended. Blood is forming in your baby's bone marrow, and her lungs are working away, preparing for that big day when she takes her first breath of fresh air.

Your Body

Starting to pop

This is a momentous occasion: It's finally time to break out those elastic-waist pants! That tummy bulge is definitely there, as your uterus continues to expand to house your growing baby, the placenta, and increased amniotic fluid. To locate your uterus, lie on your back and feel about an inch below your belly button. It's safe to press down on your abdomen; you won't hurt yourself or your baby. Your body is a wonderfully safe place for your child, who is cushioned within the amniotic sac and the thick walls of your uterus.

At each prenatal visit, your provider will measure the height of your uterus by measuring from the fundus—or top of the uterus—to your pubic bone. Up to your 12th week of pregnancy, your fundus was even with, or below, your pubic bone. After that, it began rising in a regular progression and should continue to do so throughout your pregnancy. This is one indication that your baby is growing on schedule.

How big should you be? By 16 weeks your fundus should reach halfway between your pubic bone and navel. Between 20 and 40 weeks of pregnancy, the height of your fundus in centimeters should equal the age of your baby in weeks. (Practitioners always allow for a little extra growth, or a little less, because babies don't all grow at the same rate.)

Getting comfortable at night

Some of that advice overload you've been getting has probably included cautionary tales about never sleeping on your stomach or back for fear of injuring your baby. The truth is this: If a certain sleep position is bad for your baby or you, you'll know it because it will be so uncomfortable that your body will naturally shift.

Where do these cautions come from? Never sleeping on your stomach makes a certain amount of sense—after all there's a baby between you and the bed, and sleeping on your stomach may make you feel like you've rolled over onto a football. That position is probably more uncomfortable for you than it is for your baby, however, and the uterus is designed to protect your baby from harm.

As for never sleeping on your back, that rule stems from the fact that you have major blood vessels that lie to the right of your spine. Sleeping on

your back causes the weight of the uterus to press down on them and decrease blood circulation. When you compress one of these veins, known as the vena cava, less blood flow is returned to your heart. That can make your blood pressure drop enough to make you feel sweaty, dizzy, or even nauseous. But don't worry. Your body naturally protects you and your baby in this situation: By the time your uterus is heavy enough to compress the vein, you'll be so uncomfortable lying on your back that your body will flip over, even if you're asleep. So go ahead and sleep any way you like. If it makes you feel better, though, you can use pillows to wedge yourself onto your side; that will become your comfiest and most practical sleep position by the end of your pregnancy.

Heartburn causes and cures

That plate of cheese-drenched nachos with hot peppers never bothered you prepregnancy. In fact, your motto has always been "The spicier the better." But now you've got a devilish case of heartburn. As many as 50 percent of all women experience heartburn during their 2nd and 3rd trimesters, typically after meals or at bedtime. The feeling can range from uncomfortable to agonizing.

Also known as acid indigestion or reflux, heartburn causes a burning sensation behind the breastbone and, sometimes, a sour, bitter taste in the mouth. Why are you getting heartburn now? Because pregnancy hormones have slowed down your digestive process to help your baby draw extra nutrition and water from your body. Food moves more slowly through your intestines, and emptying time for your stomach is delayed. Progesterone, one of those pregnancy hormones, causes the muscle between your stomach and esophagus to relax. Together, all these changes offer more opportunity for stomach acids to churn and splash upward. Presto! You've got heartburn.

Heartburn has nothing to do with the health of your heart. It will probably go away after delivery, when your stomach has more room in your abdominal cavity.

To cool off your heartburn, try some of these tactics:

- Instead of eating three large meals, break your food intake into smaller portions (try six small meals) spread throughout the day.
- Avoid eating within 4 hours of your bedtime.
- When you eat acidic foods like oranges, tomatoes, or grapefruit, combine them with less acidic foods to reduce that evil fiery aftermath. For instance, eat tomatoes on your sandwich instead of in your salad and don't drink orange juice until you've had a bowl of cereal.
- Some women find that spicy foods, greasy foods, coffee, carbonated beverages, acidic foods, and chocolate exacerbate heartburn; others can eat those foods without incident but have different trigger

foods. Pay attention to what sets off your heartburn; then avoid it.
- Don't drink large quantities of fluids with meals, because drinking can cause you to swallow more air. These gulps of air may aggravate heartburn. If you feel thirsty, take small sips between bites of food.
- Skip drinks containing caffeine, because they help relax the muscle at the top of the stomach that holds in the acid.
- Chew gum after meals to increase saliva production; this will lessen your discomfort. Why? Saliva helps neutralize acid in the esophagus.
- Don't lie down or bend over right after you eat. Instead, sit up straight for at least an hour after you eat.
- Sleep with a few extra pillows so that you're in a more upright position at night.
- Generally an ordinary antacid like Tums or Mylanta can safely reduce the acidity of your stomach contents during pregnancy. Most over-the-counter antacids don't contain ingredients that can be absorbed, so they won't harm your baby. Check with your provider before using other medications such as cimetidine or ranitidine.

Your Self

Planning your maternity leave

Like most expectant working mothers, you may have to do some research on your employer's family leave policies, make a few financial and personal compromises, and carefully negotiate your maternity leave to get what you really want.

Talk to your supervisor first. Your planning will go better if you can bring your immediate supervisor on board as an ally. Plan to tell your supervisor about your pregnancy before you tell coworkers; most managers hate hearing things through the grapevine. Telling your supervisor early in your 2nd trimester will let her know that you're willing to work together to do what's best for the company. However, before you approach your boss with your news, talk with friends and colleagues outside of your company about maternity leave arrangements they've been able to negotiate. Decide on one that seems ideal for you and approach your manager with a specific course of action and an open mind.

Be proactive. Anticipate your manager's concerns and be ready to address them as you discuss your own needs. By asking your supervisor to help you form a plan that works best for you, your coworkers, and the company, you're showing company loyalty. As a result your supervisor will have faith that you're still focused on your job. Estimate when you would like to leave work, how long you expect to be gone, and what you think must be done before you go.

Put a priority on communication. Throughout your pregnancy continue to communicate with your supervisor about what steps you're taking to make this transition—and your absence from the job—easier on everyone involved. For instance, make a list of the duties you routinely perform each day; this will help your replacement fulfill your regular duties while you're out. In essence, you want to show that you're willing to manage your maternity leave the same way you do your job: with savvy, common sense, and knowledge of what's good for the company. Before leaving, create a folder and a computer file where your replacement can note changes that occur when you're gone. That way you can update yourself faster upon your return. Let your supervisor and other key coworkers know that they can contact you at home in an emergency.

Negotiating work leave

Most companies have two kinds of benefit policies: formal and informal. No matter what state or institutional policies your company has regarding maternity leave, you may be able to work out a better deal with your own manager. Here are some possible strategies for landing and paying for a longer maternity leave:

Ask for what you want, whether it's a longer unpaid leave or part-time work for a few months. Be prepared to meet your manager's objections with various solutions, and be flexible in return. For instance, your boss might let you take off a few more weeks after you deliver at a partial salary if you agree to do a project from home or come into the office for a few

Severe mood swings

Most women have mood swings during pregnancy—laughing hysterically at a friend's joke one minute, then swearing viciously at a driver who cuts them off on the highway the next—but sometimes those mood swings are too severe and can signal that you're affected by depression, anxiety, or anger that should be treated by a therapist. What if you weep for days on end or can't seem to get out of bed because everything feels too overwhelming? What if nothing you do, from exercise to talking, makes you feel better? If your day-to-day personality changes to the point where people close to you start commenting on your behavior and these disturbing emotions don't go away for long periods of time (as in weeks, not hours or days), you may have a serious problem.

Just like everyone else, pregnant women can become emotionally ill, especially toward the end of their pregnancies, when the double burden of physical discomfort and anxiety about childbirth seems like too much to handle. If you think you have any of the conditions described here, it's important to get help before your baby arrives.

Anxiety disorders. People with anxiety disorders avoid new situations. If you're saying no to dinner out—for fear of not knowing what to say to other people, for instance—you may be experiencing an anxiety disorder. This can be accompanied by panic attacks marked by a racing heart, night sweats, trembling, or difficulty breathing. Or you might find yourself obsessively worrying about things you can't possibly control, like terrorist attacks, global warming, or whether your child will have a life-threatening disease. If no amount of reassurance stops you from mulling over these dire possibilities, you may have an anxiety disorder.

Anger disorder. You may have an anger disorder if you yell at your partner or children more than usual or if you fantasize about hitting them or hurting other people. You may also have trouble keeping perspective about small things, like a child knocking over a plant. Your anger might build even after these incidents have passed.

Depression. Depression is marked by a lack of enjoyment in things that used to please you, like baking or spending time with your girlfriends. You constantly feel so tired that it's difficult to find the energy to do anything, so you sleep more than usual to avoid facing the world. You may feel such a huge amount of stress that you start forgetting things, and you prefer to be alone because it feels too much like work to interact with others.

hours each week. If you think you want to work only half-time for a few months after the baby is born, see if you can arrange a job-share position for that amount of time.

Use vacation time, personal days, or sick days to offset a portion of unpaid leave, if your company allows. Ask if you can borrow paid leave against future time off.

Adjust your tax withholding at work to reflect the extra deduction you'll claim for your new child. Don't wait until after the baby is born.

Investigate the laws. Several states mandate partial salary replacement for workers who are temporarily disabled for medical reasons, including pregnancy and childbirth. Find out if your company has a policy like that and if you qualify.

Cut back on any unnecessary expenses. Every time you whip out that credit card to purchase something major, ask yourself whether you'd rather have that new coat/rug/couch/car or more time at home with your baby.

Diet & Exercise

Weight gain so far

Your baby weighs just a couple of ounces now, so why have you gained 4 pounds—or more? Simple: Your body needs to make a whole lot of changes to support that tiny speck of a baby, and some of those changes mean extra weight for you. For example, the amount of blood pumping through your veins increases by 40 percent while you're pregnant and eventually contributes about 4 pounds to your weight. Also, your baby is surrounded by up to 2 pounds of amniotic fluid, and your breasts are getting larger and heavier as they prepare for breastfeeding.

If you're gaining too much weight, eat less and up your exercise. Don't go on a diet, though—if you starve yourself, you're starving your baby.

Sodium intake

Americans love salt and eat way too much of it: popcorn at the movies, pretzels at the ballpark, potato chips in front of the TV. Sodium intake should be limited to 2,400 mg a day, but the average American consumes 6,000–18,000 mg daily. Although there is no need to restrict your sodium intake during pregnancy, too much sodium can cause excess fluid retention, especially later in the 3rd trimester.

You don't have to eliminate all of the sodium in your diet, but cutting down is a good idea. Start by reading food labels. Foods that are high in salt include canned and dry soups, cured meats (ham, bacon, sausage), processed meats (hot dogs, deli meat), canned tomatoes, cheese, peanut butter, some breakfast cereals, packaged frozen dinners, fast food, seasoned rice, snack foods (potato chips, pretzels, tortilla chips), gravy, and flavor enhancers such as taco seasoning, cooking sherry, chili sauce, meat tenderizer, soy sauce, steak sauce, and Worcestershire sauce.

Once you start reading labels, you'll discover that there's salt in foods you never imagined would contain salt. For example, a serving of light Caesar salad dressing has 520 mg of sodium, and ½ cup of canned spaghetti sauce contains 580 mg of sodium.

Try these painless ways to decrease your sodium intake:
● Take the saltshaker off your table.
● In restaurants ask that your food be cooked without salt.

- Use lemon juice, herbs, and spices instead of salt to flavor food.
- Avoid MSG.
- Choose low-sodium versions of your favorite foods.
- When grilling meat, use low-sodium or salt-free marinades.

Proteins for vegetarians

If you're not a meat eater—or if you're temporarily nauseated at the mere thought of a hamburger—there are plenty of ways to get the protein you need during pregnancy without eating meat.

Some nonmeat sources of protein include dairy products (milk, cheese, yogurt), eggs, legumes (lentils, garbanzo beans, kidney beans, black beans, split peas), and nuts (peanuts, walnuts, cashews, pecans, and their butters). Protein-packed meals include a bowl of vegetarian chili, a cup of lentil soup, a peanut butter sandwich, or a bean burrito.

Watch for fat and cholesterol content when you choose nonmeat protein foods; meat-free doesn't automatically mean low-fat. Full-fat dairy products contain lots of saturated fat and calories; choose non-fat or low-fat dairy foods. Egg yolks are high in cholesterol, so limit yourself to four yolks per week. Nuts also pack a fair amount of fat. The fat in nuts is the heart-healthy monounsaturated kind, but it's still high in calories. When you eat nuts and nut butters, always measure serving sizes; they may be smaller than you realize. A serving of peanuts is 1 ounce, for example.

That's about the size of the small bags served on airplanes—you know, the bags you can eat 12 of during a cross-country flight.

Benefits of the buddy system

Staying motivated to exercise every day can be tough, especially when you would rather be lying on the couch than jogging on a trail. One great way to stay motivated is to exercise with a buddy who shares your desire to get moving regularly. Research shows that people who exercise with a buddy are more likely to stick to their fitness regimen, probably because it's harder to skip your workout when you know someone is waiting for you.

The best exercise buddy is one whose fitness level is about equal to yours. Why? Someone less fit will slow you down, while someone who's much more athletic than you may unknowingly cause you to push yourself too hard.

Common Questions

Q. I've been feeling really vulnerable lately. How can I take care of a baby if I'm barely able to get through the day without having somebody help me with something?

A. Think about it: Wouldn't it be stranger if you didn't feel vulnerable right now? Your body is going through more changes in 9 months than it went through during your entire adolescence, and pregnancy hormones are sending your emotions into a tailspin. Although the 2nd trimester is usually a period of calm as your hormone levels plateau and your energy returns, your metabolism is still on overdrive, preparing to support your baby's biggest growth period yet. In addition, there's all of this anxiety on the back burner: Is your baby going to be OK? Will you be a good mom? Will your partner still love you if you can't wear a bikini? Will you ever be able to keep the house clean with a toddler and a baby in residence?

What's more, your loved ones are all trying to do things for you that they never offered before. Many women are so accustomed to caring for others that when the time comes for them to be on the receiving end of someone else's attention and nurturing, their feelings of dependency may seem overwhelming. When your friends want to cook you dinner so that you can rest, you may long to wave them off and go trotting right back to work, denying that you need any help. You're used to being independent. But this is a time when it makes sense to accept whatever help is offered—gracefully—because your main job is to keep your body strong and rested for your baby's sake.

Q. I can't stop smoking, even though I know it's bad for my baby. Can you help?

A. If at first you don't succeed, then you owe it to your baby and yourself to try again. Smoking can harm your baby at any stage of pregnancy. Many studies have shown that pregnant moms who smoke are more likely to have babies with lower birthweights, cleft lips or cleft palates, asthma, learning disabilities, and behavioral problems. What's more, if you smoke after your baby is born, you increase the risk of SIDS (see "Common Questions," page 260).

This is a long way of saying that you should do everything possible to kick the cigarette habit. If you cannot quit entirely, then make a herculean effort to at least cut back on the number of cigarettes you smoke; this will reduce the health risks to you and your child. Here are some strategies to tap the next time you feel like smoking:

- Carry one of your baby's ultrasound pictures with you. Look at it every time you think about having a cigarette.
- Try aversion therapy. Every time you have heartburn or feel nauseous, say the word "cigarette" to yourself so that you start associating the word with a bad physical feeling.
- Tape your own scary warning to your cigarette packs: "Cigarettes will hurt my baby."
- Ask your partner to quit smoking or to refrain from smoking around you. That will reduce the temptation for you and lessen the effects of secondhand smoke on your baby.
- Figure out what prompts you to smoke and substitute an action. Do you smoke when you feel nervous and want to calm down? Then fiddle with a pencil or chew a piece of gum instead. Are you seeking stimulation? Try taking a short, brisk walk. The less you smoke, the healthier your baby will be.
- Hang out in places where smoking is prohibited, like movies and cafes.

- Ask your provider about using a nicotine patch, nicotine gum, or a medication to help you quit. Studies of how these methods affect pregnancy are still being conducted, so safety remains a concern.
- Your provider might also suggest alternative methods to reduce your craving for cigarettes, such as hypnosis or acupuncture.
- If all else fails, at least reduce the amount of poisons to which you're exposing yourself and your baby by smoking each cigarette only halfway down.

Q. This is embarrassing—my hemorrhoids are killing me! Is there any way to treat them safely?

A. Welcome to the sisterhood of mothers-to-be. Most women have hemorrhoids during pregnancy because their blood vessels are swollen with a higher blood volume than usual. Think of hemorrhoids as varicose veins in your rectal area that tend to be itchy or painful. The extra blood volume can cause hemorrhoids to plump up to the size of a marble, and your growing uterus exerts more pressure on the pelvic veins, increasing the swelling.

To ease your discomfort, try alternating ice packs with warm-water soaks. That doesn't mean you have to fill an entire bathtub every time; you can buy a small plastic tub (called a "sitz bath") at the drugstore. Fill it with warm water and position it over your toilet so that you can sit in the water several times a day. Some women get relief from witch hazel, which can be used to medicate a cold compress.

Using unscented, white toilet tissue can lessen irritation, and it might help to wet the tissue before you wipe your rectal area. You can also buy specially medicated moist towelettes to use instead of toilet tissue. If the pain or itching becomes intolerable, ask your practitioner to suggest a safe medicated suppository or topical anesthetic. You also might want to ask your provider about a fiber supplement or stool softener, because constipation and straining can aggravate hemorrhoid discomfort. Avoid sitting or standing for long stretches of time and lie on your left side while sleeping or watching TV to take some of the pressure off your rectal veins.

Your partner: His emotional journey

You've been grappling with the reality of pregnancy for many weeks now, filled with excitement, worn out by fatigue and morning sickness, supported by cheerleading friends and family members. But it may have taken until this trimester—when your pregnant belly is starting to pop out—to shock your partner into truly understanding that (soon!) there is a baby coming.

Your partner's emotional adjustment to your pregnancy will be similar to your own, marked by the same highs and lows that you've experienced in the past few months. For instance, many partners are so astounded by the physical changes brought on by pregnancy that they're alternately horrified and fascinated, especially when the baby's movements become visible. You may find that he has a newfound respect for you because of the many hardships you've endured so far.

Your blossoming body is no libido buster for your partner. In fact like most partners, yours may be excited by the changes in your pregnant body, even the seemingly unattractive changes such as bigger hips, dimpled thighs, and the new pregnancy posture you may adopt to balance your growing belly. Thanks to you (and the baby), your partner may start to form new ideas about what's beautiful and sexy in a woman.

However, if your partner has problems adjusting to the pregnancy, talk things out now, before baby's arrival makes your relationship even bumpier. It's possible that he's feeling left out, because so far the spotlight has been mainly on you. As your focus turns inward toward your new baby, he may be sadly anticipating that you'll be giving him the cold shoulder for the rest of your days together. Ease his fears by including him in the pregnancy. Make a point of enjoying activities together that are not all about the baby.

Your partner may also suddenly be seized by anxiety about how you're going to pony up the cost of raising a child. While you're feeling energetic enough to look at cribs and strollers and curtains in your 2nd trimester, your partner may fret about every expense and throw himself into work more than ever before. If you want your partner to be home more, ask him, because it won't be obvious to him that you need him there. If you want your partner to feel less insecure about money, work out a budget that details how you're going to cover expenses after the baby comes. This is especially important if either one of you is planning to take an unpaid work leave after the birth.

Your partner may also be worrying about how well he's going to handle the whole fatherhood thing, especially if he came from a family without a strong father figure or if he's never accrued any babysitting hours and hasn't a clue how to diaper a baby or how to hold one. Reassure him that you're in this thing together and that the two of you will work as a team to provide a loving home for this new life you're creating together.

Finally, give him time to bond with the baby. Tell him what a wonderful father he's going to be and why you think so. Encourage him to touch your belly and to talk or sing to your growing child. Before long he'll be looking forward to holding that baby in his arms as much as you are.

Week 15

Your Baby

The inside story

If you could see your baby right now, you'd laugh as she tests out her developing muscles by making lots of funny faces—squinting, frowning, even smiling in the womb. You'd be astonished by her paper-thin skin, through which a network of fine blood vessels runs like a series of miniature roads. She is developing lanugo, a fine, downy hair that covers her body and protects her skin. Lanugo begins to disappear before birth, but some babies—especially those born early—may still have a fine covering of it on their shoulders, backs, and foreheads as they come into the world. This hair usually disappears within a week or so after birth. Beneath her skin, your baby's skeleton is hardening, transforming from cartilage to bone as she continues to absorb calcium. Her bones will stay flexible, however, so that she can easily make the journey through your birth canal. They won't harden enough for her to stand until she's a toddler.

Her ears are nearly in position, and she can turn her head. She can make fists and point her toes too, though most of the time these movements are reflexive. Her hair has started to grow, and it may have a little color as the pigment cells of her hair follicles kick in. You'll need to decide soon whether you want to know the sex of your baby before you give birth; the external sex organs are nearly complete, so an ultrasound can reveal whether you're having a boy or a girl.

Your Body

Varicose veins

Oh, your aching legs. Half of all pregnant women develop varicose veins in their legs. These swollen, blue, ropelike veins aren't solely due to weight gain. They are evidence that your circulatory system is struggling to move 40 percent more blood through veins and arteries all over your body. Sometimes this extra blood increases the pressure on vein walls to the point where veins stretch and their valves don't close properly. Blood can ooze through those leaky valves and pool in your veins; this is what makes them become varicose—stretched out of shape and sometimes even twisted.

Extra risk factors for varicose veins include having a job that requires long periods of sitting or standing, having thin-walled veins or an injury, and gaining too much weight. Usually varicose veins will return to normal after your baby is born, but they can still be uncomfortable. Women who have them in their legs complain of heaviness, additional fatigue, pressure, and aching. Varicose veins can be permanent and tend to worsen with each pregnancy, so it's worth trying to prevent them or to ease the discomfort they cause.

Here are some tips for keeping your legs healthy during your pregnancy:

- When you rest, keep your legs elevated higher than your heart. That will help the blood return to the heart instead of pooling in your legs.
- When you sit down, avoid crossing your legs, because that reduces blood circulation.
- Avoid standing or sitting for long periods of time.
- Follow an exercise plan to improve your circulation. Walking half an hour every day can help a lot.
- If you can't exercise, sit in a rocking chair several times a day and use your legs to gently rock back and forth, encouraging blood flow.
- Invest in support stockings. Put them on before you get out of bed so blood doesn't have a chance to pool in your ankles. Sheer maternity pantyhose offer gradient compression, which means that the pressure of the stockings is greatest at the ankle and decreases higher up on the leg. These stockings will help support your legs and squeeze the blood upward from your legs back toward your heart.

Multiple marker screening test

The 2nd trimester signals a new round of prenatal testing. During one of your routine visits between 15 weeks and 20 weeks, your health care provider may offer to draw blood for a "multiple marker" screening test, also known as a quad marker screen. This screen indicates if the fetus is at risk of having a chromosomal abnormality; it identifies about 75 percent of babies with Down syndrome and 80 percent of infants with neural tube defects such as spina bifida.

Although it's never fun to have another needle in your arm, this screening test can help you decide whether to have an amniocentesis (see page 126), which is a more invasive test with a higher risk to your baby. After your blood is drawn, it will be sent to a laboratory and tested for four different biochemical markers: alpha-fetoprotein (AFP), human chorionic gonadotropin (hCG), unconjugated estriol (uE3), and inhibin-A.

The results of a multiple marker screen are typically available within seven working days, when your provider will receive either a "screen positive" or "screen negative" test result. If you test positive on this screen, you'll be offered an ultrasound and possibly an amniocentesis for a definitive diagnosis.

Amniocentesis

Often referred to as an "amnio," this test is usually done between 15 and 21 weeks. With an accuracy rate as high as 99 percent, an amniocentesis can detect Down syndrome, other chromosomal disorders, and genetic glitches, including Tay-Sachs disease, cystic fibrosis, and sickle-cell anemia. It's generally offered to women over 35 because that's the age at which the risk of chromosomal abnormalities is approximately equal to the risk of the procedure. However, new data show the risk of miscarriage after amniocentesis is much lower.

How it's done. This is one of those tests that's scary in principle, but in fact it doesn't hurt much and usually has few side effects. Some women fear an amniocentesis because it involves a larger-than-life needle inserted into the abdomen. They may worry about the pain of the needle or be concerned that the procedure might harm their baby or cause pregnancy complications. Still others are anxious about the small risk of miscarriage associated with amniocentesis. Most of the time, these fears are unfounded, and your provider will recommend an amniocentesis when the benefits of having the test outweigh the risks.

There are no restrictions on what you can eat or drink beforehand. You'll lie on your back on a table while the practitioner does an ultrasound to determine the position of the baby. Next she will clean off an area on your belly with antiseptic solution. Many doctors do not use anesthetic because the numbing medicine is sometimes worse than the quick, thin amniocentesis needle.

Your provider will insert a long, hollow needle through your abdomen into the uterus and amniotic sac to draw a sample of amniotic fluid. You probably won't feel anything other than the pinprick, followed by a tugging or pushing sensation of the actual amniocentesis needle. Your amniotic fluid contains free-floating fetal cells that can be grown in a laboratory; at the lab, technicians will extract chromosomes or genes from these cells and analyze them for various abnormalities. It generally takes about 2 weeks to get the results of this analysis. The amount of amniotic fluid that is removed is generally replenished within the next 24 hours.

Risks. Because the ultrasound allows the technician to see the position of your baby, the chances of your baby being harmed by the needle are minuscule. The main negative side effect of an amniocentesis is miscarriage, but that happens to fewer than 1 in 200 women who have this test. In addition, about 1 percent of women experience bleeding, cramping, or leaking fluid from the vagina after the procedure. These symptoms usually resolve on their own. Therefore, the overall risk of an amniocentesis to you and your baby is low.

When test results indicate a problem

It's possible that your multiple marker screening test (quad marker screen) may suggest an abnormality when your baby is actually healthy. (This is known as a "false positive.") If you get a positive result, you may want to talk with your provider or a genetic counselor before deciding on the next step. Depending on your age, your comfort level, and a host of other factors, you may choose to have an ultrasound, an amniocentesis, or both.

False positives. There are a number of reasons why a false positive occurs on a multiple marker test. You might be earlier or later in your pregnancy than you thought, you might be carrying twins, or you might have altered hormone levels but the baby is normal. Your practitioner may offer an amniocentesis to confirm results.

Handling problems. If the amniocentesis confirms chromosomal abnormality, you may want a second opinion before you make any decisions about whether to continue the pregnancy or terminate it.

It's a horrible shock to learn that your baby has a medical problem. You will need time to absorb the news and gather information about your baby's condition. You can't predict now what your reaction to an abnormal test result might be. With so many medical advances, there are treatments for many conditions. Ideally you will meet with a genetic counselor both before and after diagnostic testing to help you sort out emotional and practical issues. This counselor will neither encourage you to have the baby nor urge you to end the pregnancy; if you have a positive test result, she will merely help inform you so that you and your partner can make that decision. You may have to consider some tough questions. For instance, are you prepared to raise a child with a severe disability? Are you willing to face a stillborn birth? How treatable is your baby's disease, both now and in the future? If the prognosis for your baby's survival is poor, would you rather cherish the rest of the time you have to carry this child or terminate the pregnancy now?

To test or not to test? Some parents elect not to have any screening tests because they know they would never terminate a pregnancy. However, many parents opposed to abortion have screening tests anyway because the test results may help them prepare for a baby with special needs, arrange for medical intervention in utero or after delivery, or arrange for a special needs adoption.

Rh incompatibility

You will have a blood test early in your pregnancy to determine whether your blood has a protein factor called Rh. If it does, you are Rh-positive, which is true for about 85 percent of the U.S. population. If it does not, you are Rh-negative. If you are Rh-negative, it alerts the practitioner to a potential incompatibility between your blood and your baby's blood.

Having Rh-negative blood doesn't pose a problem during pregnancy unless the baby's father is Rh-positive. If that's the case, then there's a chance that your baby could be Rh-positive and that your blood and your baby's are incompatible. (If both you and your baby are Rh-negative, then all is well.)

During pregnancy, red blood cells from your baby can cross the placenta into your bloodstream. This isn't usually a problem in a first pregnancy, but if this is your second pregnancy with an Rh-positive baby, there's a chance that your red blood cells will recognize this different blood type and rise up in revolt, creating an immune response against your own baby because your Rh-negative blood won't tolerate Rh-positive blood cells. (This can also happen after a miscarriage or an abortion with an Rh-positive fetus.) Your practitioner will give you an injection of Rhogam, an Rh-immune globulin, to halt your body's production of antibodies that might attack your baby's blood. This is typically done in the 28th week of your pregnancy, with a follow-up dose within 72 hours after birth if in fact your baby's blood tests show that he's Rh-positive. You may also receive a Rhogam shot if you're Rh-negative and experience any bleeding or if you have a medical procedure during which blood could be transferred, like amniocentesis.

If you have this immune response and don't receive the shot of Rhogam, your blood cells may treat the Rh-positive cells of your baby like a virus or any other intruder and make antibodies against them. The antibodies can cross the placenta to reach your baby and destroy his circulating red blood cells, causing severe anemia in your unborn child. In a small percentage of cases this can result in your baby's death.

week 15

Your Self

The ups and downs of sex

Multiple orgasms, powerful sexual fantasies, and a feeling that you can't get enough of your partner—sex during your 2nd trimester may be better than ever, especially since you're no longer nauseous and your energy has returned. Your increased blood flow is making your vagina feel plumper and tighter and increasing your vaginal lubrication. Many women feel far more sensual as a result of hormone surges and increased sensitivity in the pelvic region. If you've had trouble climaxing during sex in the past, you may find it surprisingly easy now. You might even experience multiple orgasms for the first time. Your increased desire could translate into new sexual fantasies. Have fun with your new sensuality and give free rein to your imagination. Think of good sex now as a sort of savings account you can draw on (and remember) when private time is chiseled away after the baby is born.

For other women, sexual fantasies and acts may become troubling as it becomes tougher to ignore the fact that there's a third person—your baby—in bed with you. Many women (and their partners) have difficulty resolving the conflict between their ideals of a "good" mother and a sexy one. Avoiding sex during pregnancy is not a good solution to these issues; sex can be an important way to connect as a couple.

Relaxation techniques

Deadlines, traffic jams, and interpersonal conflicts with family members and friends are stressors you will have to deal with during pregnancy, just as you do during other times of life. While a little stress can actually be good for you, boosting your immune response and preparing it for possible infection or injury, chronic stress can wear you down. (See "Chronic stress," page 163.) If you're pregnant and stressed-out, your mind-set may affect your baby's development. One study of women in their 3rd trimesters showed that those with signs of stress, such as high blood pressure, were more apt to have babies with increased heart rates than non-stressed mothers were. Researchers are also investigating the link between stress and premature births. So for your baby's health as well as your own, teach yourself to relax.

Stress-reducing techniques slow down the body and still the mind. They include meditation, breathing exercises, guided imagery, and progressive muscle imagery. All of these techniques help you focus on the mind-body connection in ways that allow you to maintain a quieter, deeper perspective on events in your life and things beyond your control.

Try this quick and easy relaxation practice:
- Set aside 15 minutes and retreat to a private place where you will not be disturbed.
- Sit or lie down comfortably.
- Close your eyes, or rest your gaze

week 15

where you won't be distracted.

- Allow your awareness to rest in the center of your body as you take 10 relaxed, full breaths, counting backward from 10 to 1. Inhale deeply and slowly. Slow down your breathing if you feel light-headed.
- As you inhale, picture a calm, peaceful place. Imagine yourself taking breaths of air in that place. Visualize the place in detail, picturing your peaceful baby beside you, and allow your mind and body to relax as you visualize this scene.
- Stretch your arms and legs, take several more deep breaths, and then congratulate yourself on time well spent.

Mindful walk

If you're the sort of person who has trouble sitting still, you might find it more relaxing to take a "mindful walk" than to meditate. A mindful walk serves the same purpose as other relaxation techniques, centering you in the moment by helping you become more aware of your body and your surroundings.

To do a mindful walk, go outdoors and start walking at a slower-than-normal pace. Experience the sensations of walking one step at a time. As you walk focus on each of your senses individually. Smell the aroma of the grass and trees; notice the buildings you pass; listen to the birdsong and the sound of distant lawn mowers droning or snow crunching beneath your boots. Stay present in the moment. When other thoughts intrude, gently acknowledge them; then nudge yourself back to the present moment by refocusing on current sensations. After you finish your walk, carry that mindfulness with you for the rest of the day by noticing your body's reactions to new sounds, sights, smells, and textures.

Prepping siblings

For every question you may have about your new baby, your older child probably has 10. Will the new baby share my bedroom? Will he steal my toys? Will Mom and Dad love him more? Young siblings, especially, may worry that they're being replaced by a new baby. Many of those fears won't translate into behavior issues until after the baby is actually born. Before the baby's arrival, put yourself in your older children's shoes and try to imagine the arrival from their perspective. In general your children will accept the new baby better if they know they still have a central place in your lives and hearts.

Start talking. When you talk to your older children about the baby, ease their fears by reinforcing the fact that they're moving "up the ladder" by getting a bigger room, a bigger bed, or a later bedtime than the baby. Refer to your new baby as "your little brother" or "little sister" instead of "Mommy and Daddy's new baby." This will reinforce the idea that the baby belongs to the whole family.

Reduce anxiety. Take your older children on a tour of the hospital or birth center to relieve any concerns they may have about the unknown. They'll be more comfortable when they know where you'll be when you're not at home, what will happen, and when you'll come back. Be as definite as possible about these things. Many hospitals now offer introductory programs for older children; the staff will show them the nursery and a room like the one you'll be staying in.

Discuss plans for your absence. Line up childcare for your hospital stay and let your children know who will be with them while you're gone. Choose a childcare provider whom they know and like. Arrange for someone to keep your children updated on your progress during labor.

Prepare for siblings to meet. Buy a small gift for your older children to give to the baby, and buy gifts for them from the baby too. When your older children meet the baby, plan for the baby to be in a bassinet and not in your arms, and if they want to exchange presents first, let them. Let older siblings set the pace of their first meeting with their new brother or sister so they can interact in a way that makes them most comfortable.

Don't be surprised if your older children occasionally express resentment or even anger toward the impending arrival. Even the sweetest older sibling might say he already "hates" his new brother or sister. The reality is that your children will experience intense emotions about this change in your life, just as you will. The best thing you can do is listen,

tell them that their emotions are understandable, and let them know that they still matter to you. Brotherly and sisterly love will come with time.

Diet & Exercise

A craving for comfort foods

Some pregnant women find that they can't get enough comfort foods—meat loaf, macaroni and cheese, chicken soup, spaghetti and meatballs, mashed potatoes, homemade chocolate chip cookies. Maybe being pregnant reminds them of their own mothers and the foods they prepared. Or maybe pregnant women crave these foods because they provide security during an unsettling time. Whatever the reason, if you crave comfort foods, find ways to make them a healthful part of your pregnancy diet.

Smart substitutions are the key. For example, if you make meat loaf, use 93-percent lean ground beef or a mixture of beef and ground turkey or chicken breast. (If you use ground poultry, buy meat that is labeled as the ground breast of the bird. If your ground poultry contains dark meat from the legs or thighs, it can have more fat than very lean beef.) Mix in grated carrots, zucchini, or other vegetables and sprinkle some wheat germ into the mix too. Make macaroni and cheese with low-fat cheese, bake your meatballs instead of frying them, and prepare mashed potatoes with a drizzle of olive oil and a sprinkle of fresh

Parmesan cheese rather than a big pat of butter and a spoonful of salt.

If you can't modify recipes, take small servings. Eating one or two homemade chocolate chip cookies is fine, but bingeing on a dozen of them is a no-no, no matter how comforting it might feel in the short term.

Maintaining strenuous exercise

If you're a hard-core exerciser who can't imagine a week without a long-distance run or a challenging hike, you'll be relieved to know that you can continue doing the strenuous exercise that you did before getting pregnant, within reason. (Of course, get your doctor's approval.) Use good sense and remember these tips:

- Your balance changes during pregnancy, so take extra care with activities that require balance.
- Avoid exercising in hot weather. If you become overheated or dehydrated, you will be uncomfortable.
- Wear supportive shoes or, if you're hiking, boots.
- Wear a sports bra that gives your breasts ample support.
- Drink plenty of fluids during and after exercise.
- Take light snacks with you.
- After the 2nd trimester, avoid exercises that require you to lie on your back.
- Stop exercising and call your doctor if you experience calf pain or swelling, chest pain, decreased fetal movement, trouble breathing, dizziness, headache, leaking amniotic fluid, muscle weakness,

contractions, or vaginal bleeding.
- Avoid activities that are dangerous, including those that put you at high risk for falling or abdominal trauma: basketball, soccer, downhill skiing, horseback riding, in-line skating, ice hockey, vigorous racket sports, gymnastics, scuba diving, rock climbing, and waterskiing.

Common Questions

Q. I may have broken my arm, and my doctor wants to X-ray it. I'm afraid the X-ray will hurt my baby. Shouldn't I wait until after the baby is born?

A. There's no need to wait. The American College of Radiology reports that diagnostic X-rays rarely pose a threat to an unborn baby. There is little risk of tissue damage with any ionizing radiation under 5 rads, and most modern X-rays emit many fewer than 5 rads. In addition, current X-ray equipment can pinpoint specific areas, such as your arm. There's very little chance that your baby would be exposed to any radiation at all, especially when you wear a lead apron over your torso.

Magnetic resonance imaging (MRI) has also been deemed safe to use during pregnancy, but a CT scan (computerized tomography) may be less so. A CT scan uses multiple X-rays to examine the body and create its three-dimensional image, so there's more risk of radiation exposure for your baby. The amount of radiation exposure also depends on what area of the body is being investigated. It's best if the abdomen and pelvis are shielded.

Even then, you have to weigh the risks against the benefits of having such a diagnostic test. Chances are good that your baby would suffer little or no tissue damage.

Q. I'm having a lot of vaginal discharge, and it has a strange odor. Should I be worried?

A. Probably not. It's normal to have increased discharge and a different odor during pregnancy. If the discharge is white and watery-looking, or looks something like egg whites and has an acidic smell, things are fine. Wash the outer area more often if it bothers you and wear cotton or cotton-crotch panties to stay drier. Bring extra pairs to work if necessary. Resist the urge to wear pantyliners because they may cause a rashlike effect or irritation of the sensitive skin in your genital area. Expect these secretions to increase even more later on in your pregnancy.

If your vaginal discharge smells fishy or rotten and looks yellow, green, curdled, or cheesy, you may have an infection. The most likely culprit is a yeast infection (see "Yeast infections," page 58), but it could also be a bacterial infection like trichomoniasis or bacterial vaginosis (see "Increased vaginal discharge," pages 255-256). Bacterial infections should be treated with a pregnancy-safe medication, so see your provider. She will do a slide to look for yeast, trichomonas, or bacterial vaginosis and/or a culture looking for chlamydia or gonorrhea. Then she'll administer proper treatment.

Week 16

Your Baby

The inside story

As you end your 4th month, get ready for an exciting development: You may start feeling your baby move for the first time this week. There's a real person in there, and he's about to make himself known! Your baby is still small enough to fit in the palm of your hand, but barely. He's growing fast now, reaching more than 4 inches in length and weighing in at about 5 ounces. His transparent skin is tinged pink as it adds layers, and he can kick his tiny feet and make grasping motions with his hands. His eyes are becoming increasingly sensitive to light.

By now, all of your baby's muscles and bones are in place, and his nervous system is starting to exert control.

Your baby is attached to the placenta by his lifeline, the umbilical cord, and that's growing thicker and stronger as his needs increase. Blood is constantly pulsing through the cord, bringing nutrients to your baby and helping to remove toxins from the amniotic fluid, which fills his trachea each time he opens his mouth. The placenta has grown too, in order to accommodate the thousands of blood vessels that are working hard to exchange nutrients and oxygen between your body and your baby's.

Your Body

Your energy returns

The 16th week represents a true turning point: Even after a long day of work, you'll find yourself excited to go shopping for the baby's nursery or meet your girlfriends for dinner. This is when most women feel their energy return; their nausea has subsided and they are feeling fewer waves of fatigue. You'll certainly feel calmer and more in control of your emotions, now that those nasty hormone surges have leveled out. Even if you are struck down by the need to cry or yell, you'll cope with it more successfully now because you're feeling better physically.

Despite this welcome return to a more normal life, don't be surprised if you occasionally feel a twinge of loss too. If this is your first child, you may secretly still feel that you're not ready to be a mother, and you may look mournfully at that strapless black cocktail dress because you don't know when you'll wear it again (or if it will ever fit in quite the same way). If you already have children, you may find yourself trying to fit in everything you know you won't be able to do later.

Continue talking to your partner about all of the decisions you'll have to make, such as whether to feed your baby by breast or bottle, who will clean the house for the first six months after the baby comes, how long you can afford to take off from work, and who will take care of your baby while you're working or otherwise out of the house. With those important choices made, you'll be able to relax and enjoy the remaining months of your pregnancy.

Stretch marks

As your body grows to accommodate your baby, your skin must stretch. If you're like about half of all pregnant women, you may start to notice lines on your breasts and belly by the 2nd or 3rd trimester. These lines, which are called stretch marks, are actually tiny scars caused by the skin stretching out so fast that it tears beneath the surface layer. Women who have very fair or very dark skin are the most inclined to develop visible stretch marks.

Not all stretch marks will disappear after pregnancy, but most will fade. Other than maintaining a sensible weight gain and hoping for good genes, there's really not much you can do to prevent them, though some women swear by everything from expensive creams to vitamin E. If you don't like the sight of your stretch marks after your baby is born, you can have them safely lightened with laser treatments in a dermatologist's office.

Foot changes

Toss your favorite designer shoes into the back of your closet, if you haven't already, because they're not going to fit again for quite some time. Higher hormone levels may cause you to retain water, making your feet swell.

To prevent discomfort, raise your legs above your heart for 20 minutes several times a day. This will encourage blood to flow back away from your feet toward your heart. You can also improve circulation by sitting with one leg raised, rotating your ankle a dozen times in each direction, then switching legs and doing the same thing on the other side. Rotate your ankles in this way at least 10 times at each sitting. Then try writing the alphabet, one letter at a time, with each foot.

Sleep on your left side to relieve pressure on the vena cava (the largest vein returning blood to your heart). Excessive weight gain will make foot pain worse, so monitor your pregnancy pounds. Remember to prop up your feet above the level of your heart when you are watching television and even during the night. To relieve extreme discomfort, ice your feet and ankles for 20 minutes every hour; this will reduce swelling. By late pregnancy you will probably need to buy larger shoes to support your widening feet. Avoid buying any shoes that lace, though, because they'll be tough to tie during your last weeks!

week 16

Late miscarriage

Though they are rare, affecting only about 2 percent of pregnancies, late miscarriages do happen. Late miscarriages are defined as those that occur between 14 and 20 weeks. It is traumatic to lose a baby you've carried this far. You may have told people about the pregnancy, had reassuring prenatal testing, and already felt the baby moving. Many times it is possible to determine why it happened and predict the health of future pregnancies.

The symptoms of a late miscarriage are similar to those of an early miscarriage and usually include severe cramping and bleeding. You may also notice large clots of tissue passed with the blood. Contact your provider immediately if you have any of these symptoms. Although it may be too late to save your baby, your provider can take important steps to protect your health; for instance, you may be hospitalized to be sure that you don't hemorrhage. If your bleeding and cramps continue after the baby and placenta are expelled from your body, you might have a minor surgical procedure called a D&C (dilation and curettage) to remove any remaining pregnancy tissue in your uterus.

Following a late miscarriage, your provider will try to determine the cause of the miscarriage in order to prevent others in the future. For instance, if your cervix dilated too early and provoked preterm labor, your provider may be able to use cerclage (a technique that involves sewing the cervix shut) to prevent late miscarriage during your next pregnancy. Other times your doctor will gain information from the placenta, the autopsy, or laboratory tests. Even though you are grieving, at some point after your loss it is important for you and your partner to review what has happened in order to determine what, if anything, can be done differently with the next pregnancy.

These are some of the causes of miscarriage after the 1st trimester:

- Fetal structural problems like spina bifida and congenital heart defects.
- A maternal anatomical problem, such as a uterus divided in two.
- A problem with the placenta, such as placental abruption or abnormal implantation.
- An infection that kills the baby, such as parvovirus, cytomegalovirus or toxoplasmosis.
- An infection that causes a leak in the amniotic sac or preterm labor.
- An incompetent cervix, which is one that is too weak to hold the pregnancy.
- Antiphospholid antibodies syndrome (APS), which is the condition of having too many antiphospholid antibodies in your bloodstream. About 15 percent of women with recurrent miscarriages have these antibodies; this can cause blood clots in the placenta.

In addition to the medical issues, this is an upsetting experience emotionally. Take as much time as you need to process (see "Miscarriage," page 35). Many around you, including your doctor, a social worker, and your family, may provide support.

Severe heel pain can plague pregnant women and may be caused by fasciitis. Start by getting shoes with good heel support. A visit to a podiatrist may also be beneficial.

Changes in the vagina

As your blood flow continues to increase and your body's estrogen and progesterone levels soar, the tissues in your vaginal area may become pumped up into a permanent state of sexual arousal. The color of your engorged labia will change as well, from a pale pink and red to a bluish purple; this is another result of the blood rush to all parts of your body. On the labia, you may also notice new bluish veins, which increase if you stand or sit for a long time. Not to worry—these are just like the varicose veins in your legs.

Sometimes this new pressure on your genitals, along with increased vaginal lubrication, puts you in a state of constant desire during your 2nd trimester. You may find yourself wanting to make love with your partner or masturbate many more times a week than you ever have before. Most women don't find that this is a bad thing. However, some women find that their partners are taken aback by this new lustfulness, especially if they are accustomed to initiating sex. Your partner may also be put off or nervous if your genitals look and feel different. That's why, as your body continues to change, it is important for you both to lay your cards on the table and be honest about your ever-shifting physical and emotional needs.

Your Self

Questioning your identity

You may sometimes feel as though you've stepped into someone else's life. Your body is changing, and so are your thoughts about the world around you. Naturally you still have some days when things are almost the same as they were before pregnancy. Now that you feel better, you may get up and go to work, tend to older children, then make dinner and watch television. You do the laundry and go out to lunches with girlfriends. However, as your body continues to change, you're beginning to take stock too. What sort of mother will you be? Who are you becoming?

You won't really know the answers to those questions for a long time yet, but it's important to ask them. When you're pregnant, there's a revolution going on inside you. That revolution will be mind-bendingly dramatic whether you've had children already or not and whether your actual labor and delivery are calm or chaotic. No matter where you are in your life right now, things will be different when this pregnancy ends. How different?

You will most certainly have to reorder priorities. Right now your career may be what makes you feel most passionate, or your partner, or your hobbies. Whatever your focus is now, it will shift after your baby is born. Even if you leap right back into your job after a few weeks off, or you have an au pair or partner who spends more time at home with your baby than you do, things that seem so important to you now will suddenly take a backseat to your new adorable baby's care.

There will be practical shifts in your priorities. You'll make changes to when you leave work or come home, how you get the laundry and vacuuming done, and how you sneak time alone with your partner. After your baby is born, you'll be at the beck and call of a person who weighs hardly more than a bag of sugar, so it's worth thinking about how you'll make room in your life for that new attention grabber.

Now that you're in your 2nd trimester, your emotions are less erratic, but you may still be more emotional than before pregnancy—and you can expect to stay that way. Some mothers describe this change in perspective as going from living in a black and white world to a world of neon colors. You're probably already feeling some of this, tearing up at a news account of a lost child or smiling at babies in the mall. This greater empathy with the world—and your awareness of your place in it—will continue to grow as you make the transition to new motherhood.

Finally, you are starting to realize—perhaps with fear, or maybe with relief—that your life is not quite as much under your control as you'd hoped. You've carefully chosen your practitioner and your birth center, but you're starting to become more aware that pregnancy, labor, and delivery are not things that you can plan completely, no matter how methodical or organized you are. Pregnancy and parenthood remind people that they are not always drivers of their own destiny on this earth, but sometimes merely passengers along for the ride.

Diet & Exercise

Caution with herbal teas
Herbal teas have a reputation for being soothing, caffeine-free, and perfectly safe. However, a label that says "herbal" or "natural" is no guarantee of safety. Herbs have been poorly studied, so no one knows exactly how they act or whether they cause harm. Large amounts of certain herbal teas have been shown to cause uterine contractions and may increase the risk of miscarriage or preterm labor. It's best to steer clear of herbs and herbal teas during pregnancy, especially peppermint, red raspberry leaf, black or blue cohosh, ephedra, dong quai, feverfew, juniper, pennyroyal, Saint-John's-wort, rosemary, and thuja. If you have other favorites, ask your provider before using them.

Staying motivated to exercise
The benefits of exercise come not from occasional no-pain, no-gain workouts but from consistent daily effort. That requires motivation, which is sometimes hard to come by.

If you're having trouble staying motivated, try these steps:

Schedule your workout each day. Make an appointment with yourself, write it in your date book in pen, and treat it as seriously as you would a doctor's appointment.

Record your progress. Keep a log of how many minutes you exercise each day. You'll be pleasantly surprised to see how quickly the time adds up.

Start a streak. If you've exercised for 10 days straight, it's a lot easier to motivate yourself to walk again on the 11th day.

Mix it up. Avoid boredom by doing a variety of activities and exercise.

Make it a part of your social life. Instead of meeting a friend in a pastry shop, meet for a brisk walk.

Reward yourself. Set a goal and buy yourself a bouquet of flowers when you reach it.

Keep it fun. If you think of exercise as drudgery, you're unlikely to stay with it. Pick activities that are fun, and you'll enjoy exercise more.

Swimming and water exercise

If there's a perfect pregnancy exercise, it's got to be swimming. Swimming is a low-impact activity that works your muscles and your cardiovascular system without taxing your joints and ligaments. The risk of injury is low, you can't get overheated, and it provides a weightless feeling that's heavenly for someone who is carrying around all those extra pregnancy pounds. Unless your doctor tells you to stop exercising, you can continue swimming all the way through your pregnancy. When your prepregnancy bathing suit gets too tight, invest in a maternity bathing suit or borrow a larger-size swimsuit from a friend.

Remember to drink water before and after you swim. If it's a long workout, take short drink breaks. Like any other aerobic exercise, swimming increases your body's need for water. Be careful not to swallow pool water; it may contain bacteria.

Common Questions

Q. What happens if I develop a fever during my 2nd trimester?

A. With a charged-up metabolism and hormone changes, your body's going to naturally run hotter than usual. However, if your fever rises above 100 degrees, you'll be uncomfortable enough to want to do something about it. If you have cold or flu symptoms, your fever is probably related to the pesky virus that's making you sniff and cough. Fevers are much less likely to cause fetal damage in the 2nd trimester than in the 1st trimester, but you should still try to lower it with acetaminophen (the ingredient in Tylenol), which is safe at any stage of pregnancy. Tepid baths and cool air might help too. However, if you have a fever over 101 degrees with no cold or flu symptoms, make an appointment to see your provider. The fever could signal an infection that needs prompt medical attention.

Q. I had an unexpected miscarriage two days ago, and I can't stop crying. How do I grieve my loss?

A. No matter when you miscarry, it's never easy to accept that loss. A late miscarriage can be extremely difficult because you've grown attached to your child. Ask your health care provider to refer you to a therapist or a support group for people who have experienced miscarriage.

When a baby is miscarried before 24 weeks, there is no legal requirement to bury or cremate the baby, but some hospitals offer this service. You may decide to have a funeral for your baby, or you may prefer to grieve privately with your partner. Either way, it might help you grieve if you name your baby and gather mementos—such as an ultrasound photo, baby clothes, and photos taken of you during your pregnancy—and put them in a special box to look at from time to time. Some parents mark their loss by planting a tree or by making a donation to charity in their baby's name. After the initial shock, you will need time to grieve. Although the pain will decrease over time, you will always remember your baby.

Q. Help! I spotted a little blood after my husband and I made love last night, and now I'm terrified that I'm having a miscarriage.

A. If it was just a little blood and you have no cramping, there's no cause for concern. It's common for pregnant women to spot after intercourse in their 2nd and 3rd trimesters. The increased blood supply to the cervix and vaginal walls means that congested blood vessels are more likely to break during intercourse, especially at the tip of the cervix, where they come in contact with a man's penis during penetration. (See "Bleeding and spotting: What's normal and what's not," page 36.) Now that you're in your 2nd trimester, it might be time to try out some new positions that allow you to control the depth of your partner's penetration, like woman-on-top or side-by-side (see "Sex and your growing belly," page 170), to prevent this from happening.

Week 17

Your Baby

The inside story

Your baby is growing stronger by the day. You can feel that for yourself as those first timid flutters become more pronounced pokes from her busy little feet and hands. She can touch her own face, and she may be looking for her thumb to suck.

Your baby is now about 5 inches long—that's not quite as long as a ballpoint pen—and her body systems are in good working order. Her circulatory system and urinary tract are functioning, and she is inhaling and exhaling amniotic fluid as she learns to breathe.

Pink nipples are forming on her chest, and your baby has mammary glands even if she's a he. If your baby is a girl, her ovaries are busy developing tiny follicles. She will have 6 million eggs or so at this point in your pregnancy, but that number will fall to about 1 million by the time she is born.

If you could see your baby, she'd look long and lanky, with legs not much bigger around than your thumb. Soon she'll start developing a layer of fat that will keep her warm after birth. In fact, a newborn weighing about 8 pounds at birth will have more than 5 pounds of fat on her body.

Your Body

Dizziness

Are you feeling dizzy when you move from sitting to standing? That's normal. When you stand, it takes a little while for the blood that's been pooling in the lower part of your body to make its way back to the upper part of your body. You can reduce dizziness by getting up more slowly. However, if you are so dizzy that it feels like you might lose consciousness, tell your doctor.

Feeling your baby move

Get ready for one of the most exciting parts of pregnancy—feeling your baby move for the first time. Many women can't quite believe they're pregnant until the baby moves, even if they've heard a heartbeat or seen the baby on ultrasound. Your baby's movement is the reward for everything you've gone through so far.

Ordinarily women start to feel their babies move at about 20 weeks, although this varies. You may feel it as early as 16 weeks or as late as

week 17

23 weeks. If you've had a baby before, you're likely to notice the movement earlier because it's already a familiar sensation that you've experienced in a previous pregnancy.

At first the movement feels like a flutter. Then over the next couple of weeks, the faint flutter turns into stronger movements. At 20 weeks you may wonder if that funny feeling is the baby moving; by about 25 weeks you'll have no doubt that there's a living being inside you. By 30 weeks you'll become convinced that your baby has learned how to do somersaults. If you look down at your belly later in your pregnancy, you'll actually see your baby moving.

Your baby has been on the move since you were 6 weeks pregnant, but you didn't feel it because the baby was so small. By about 20 weeks, a baby is large enough to make itself felt to you.

If you're not noticing any fetal movement, it might be because you're not paying close enough attention. At first the feelings really are subtle. Take a few time-outs during the day to sit still in a quiet place and focus on what you feel. Sometimes it takes real concentration to feel the movement.

If you don't feel your baby moving by 22 or 23 weeks, call your doctor. A quick fetal heart check using your doctor's Doppler will be reassuring. You may simply have a mellow baby. Also the location of the placenta makes a difference. If the placenta is in front of the uterus, your baby's movements may be less noticeable. Weight plays a role too: Slender women usually feel fetal motion earlier than overweight women.

Sacroiliac back pain

Low-back pain is very common during pregnancy. Often the pain is centered at the sacroiliac joint, which is the place in the lower back where the sacrum bone joins with the hip. You have two of these joints, one on

Kidney stones

Kidney stones are hard masses that form in the kidney. They may be smaller than a poppy seed or as big as a marble. Pregnancy doesn't cause kidney stones to form, but pregnant women do sometimes develop them.

Often, kidney stones go unnoticed, passing out of the body in the urine. Trouble comes when they get stuck in one of the ureters, the tubes that connect the kidneys with the bladder. This causes tremendous pain in the back, side, or groin that may be accompanied by nausea, vomiting, or blood in the urine. The pain may come and go in waves.

If the kidney stone is small, doctors usually recommend taking acetaminophen to help with the pain and drinking large amounts of water to try to flush the stone out of the body. If the stone is too large to pass, stronger pain medication is sometimes used; rarely is a surgical procedure needed. Lithotripsy, a procedure that uses sound waves or lasers to break up kidney stones, is not safe for pregnant women.

Terminating a pregnancy

If you've received heartbreaking news following your amniocentesis or other diagnostic tests, you may elect to terminate your pregnancy. Some parents make this wrenching decision after learning that their child will be born with a severe disability or a condition that will cause the child to suffer through potentially painful treatments for a disease that is incurable.

Before 12 weeks of pregnancy, all but 1 percent of U.S. abortions are done by a vacuum suction technique (also called aspiration). By the 2nd trimester, however, most practitioners will use a dilation and extraction (D&E) technique to terminate your pregnancy. Other options include chemical installation and vaginal delivery. The technique used will depend on several factors, including your gestational age. Discuss these techniques with your provider.

Before making the decision to terminate your pregnancy, confirm the diagnosis and thoroughly discuss the possible extent of your child's disability. Your health care provider can help put you in touch with specialists who can provide specific information, including high-risk obstetricians, genetic counselors, therapists, pediatric surgeons, and developmental pediatricians. Perinatal social workers or therapists may also help prepare you for the onslaught of emotions that may accompany a pregnancy termination. After an abortion you can expect to feel weepy, angry, and exhausted, so having such support in place is essential for surviving this ordeal.

To find a genetic counselor, contact the National Society of Genetic Counselors, 233 Canterbury Drive, Wallingford, PA 19086; 610-872-7608; www.nsgc.org. Or contact the Society for Maternal-Fetal Medicine, 409 12th St. SW, Washington, DC 20024; 202-863-2476; www.smfm.org.

each side. If the tendons of the joint are pushed, pulled, or yanked too much in the wrong direction, they can become inflamed, causing pain around the hip bone and lower back.

Sacroiliac pain is common during pregnancy for several reasons. Because of its location, the sacroiliac joint receives pressure from the growing uterus; that pressure may irritate it. Also your growing belly may be pulling you forward as you walk or sit, changing your posture and putting unaccustomed pressure on the sacroili-ac joint. If you started pregnancy overweight or have gained excess weight since conceiving, you're at higher risk for sacroiliac pain.

Take acetaminophen for the pain. Apply ice, alternating with heat; limit each to 20 minutes and always end with ice. In some cases walking helps relieve the pain; in other cases, rest is best. Do what feels right for you. This condition usually fixes itself, but when it interferes with your life, call your doctor to discuss other treatment options.

Even more frequent urination

Like the uterus, the bladder is a muscular sac that expands as needed. When you're not pregnant, your bladder can hold up to a pint of urine. During pregnancy your uterus is the star of the show in the pelvic cavity, and as it grows, everything else gets squished, including your bladder. A squished bladder holds much less urine than a bladder that has room to expand—that's why, as your pregnancy progresses, you need to urinate more often. Your bladder will return to normal after delivery.

Frequent urination may indicate that you have a urinary tract infection (UTI). If you see blood—even a tint of pink—in your urine, if you run to empty your bladder and only empty drops, or if you feel burning while you urinate, call your doctor right away. A UTI can be cleared up easily with antibiotics. If left untreated, a UTI can cause a kidney infection that can lead to preterm labor.

Your Self

Maternity leave laws

Knowledge is power, and that's true when you're making preparations for your leave from work and, perhaps, your eventual return. Before making any final decisions on the length and conditions of your maternity leave, find out what you're entitled to by law.

The federal Family and Medical Leave Act (FMLA) entitles eligible employees to take up to 12 weeks of unpaid, job-protected maternity leave. This law applies to all businesses with 50 or more employees. It requires the employer to continue to offer you the same health insurance coverage at the same price that you would pay if you had remained at work. Your employer must also keep your job (or an equivalent position) open for you when you return. However, pay attention to the law's fine print. For example, you're eligible only if you have been at your job for 12 months or more. And if you don't return to work after your maternity leave, your company may ask you to reimburse it for the premiums it paid to maintain your health insurance coverage while you were on leave. The U.S. Department of Labor (www.dol.gov) or your company's human resources department can fill you in on all the details of the FMLA.

Although it is not mandated by law, some employers offer paid leave for all or part of your absence; others may allow you to collect short-term disability payments.

Making daycare decisions

If you're considering a daycare center or a home-based family daycare, spend a few hours observing the facility. Pay careful attention to the interactions between staff members and children. Ask about schedules, parent participation requirements, and staff qualifications. Take note of hygiene. Do the staff members wash

Single moms

There are many situations that lead women to be single moms. Some women are forced into this situation; other women have chosen to have a baby on their own. Whatever led you to be a single mother, it's important to remember that you're never alone. There are people and resources to help you out—and you'll need them. As any parent will tell you, babies are a lot of work and can be very expensive. That's why being prepared for your new life with a baby is especially important for single moms.

Even financially independent women can be shocked by the cost of having a child; baby clothes, formula, diapers, childcare, and a college plan add up fast. Make a budget now to see how your current income will work once the baby arrives. Include all that you spend right now; then add the things you'll need for the baby. It's often helpful to write down everything you spend money on for a week to see where your money really goes each month.

For the emotional ups and downs of pregnancy, find a community of other mothers, both pregnant and experienced, to help get you through the bad days and celebrate the good. There are many support groups for expecting mothers in most communities through churches, organizations, and hospitals. Ask your practitioner to help you find support groups especially for single mothers.

Find a friend, labor coach, or relative willing to attend childbirth classes and the delivery. If your baby's father is a friend, ask him if he'd be willing to be involved. If he's willing, work out an arrangement so that he can take part in his child's birth and care too. Ask the baby's father, or friends and relatives, to help out in the first few weeks after you have the baby. That can be an overwhelming time for new moms, especially while they're still recovering from delivery.

Your friends can be a great resource in providing care for your infant. You also can ask relatives to step in temporarily while you sort things out if infant care is too pricey. If you own your own home, consider getting a roommate to defray expenses. Another mother, who will understand a crying baby in the middle of the night, is ideal. An au pair can provide less-expensive childcare in exchange for room and board.

Finally, remember that single parenthood—just like parenting with a partner—offers as many rewards as it does stresses. You can raise a happy child—no doubt about it. After all, one good parent is better than two bad ones, and you and your baby will love one another and enrich each other's lives in ways that go far beyond measure.

their hands before and after changing diapers? Do they disinfect toys and eating surfaces? Ask about food: When your baby is old enough to eat solid food, will that be provided or will you bring it from home? Take along your checkbook: Even though your baby's birth is months away, you may be asked to put down a deposit to hold a space.

Check out all your childcare options before deciding what kind of care you're most comfortable with. Some mothers like the sense of community at a daycare center, for example, but others want their babies to be cared for in a home setting.

Diet & Exercise

Alternative exercises

At this point, training for a marathon is definitely not a good fitness option. Instead consider activities that allow you to build strength and increase your flexibility gently. Keep in mind that some of these activities include moves that require balancing, which can be a challenge during pregnancy. To avoid falling and injuring yourself during balance moves, hold on to a chair or wall for support.

Yoga. This ancient Indian system of breathing and exercise can help ease the discomforts of pregnancy and prepare your body for labor. Yoga postures, also known as asanas, gently stretch and strengthen the body, while controlled breathing and meditation relax and focus the mind.

There are several schools of yoga. Although they teach similar positions, they differ in their intensity; some incorporate strength and cardiovascular training as well. Hatha is a generic term for yoga; it is generally used to describe gentler kinds of yoga.

Stick with gentle yoga. Avoid Bikram (also known as hot yoga), which is practiced in a room heated to 105 degrees. It's not good for your body to get that hot. High-intensity power yoga classes are not appropriate for most pregnant women. In yoga, as in all exercises during pregnancy, don't strain while stretching—stretch only to the point where you feel a mild tension; then relax as you hold the stretch. Do not bounce or strain.

Tai chi. Originated in China around the 13th century, tai chi is a slow, graceful exercise that enhances relaxation skills, physical alignment, and mental focus while building leg strength, endurance, and stability.

Tai chi is a great exercise for pregnant women because it is a nonimpact activity with a low risk of injury. Because it focuses on posture, it helps prevent back pain by teaching you how to avoid arching your back to accommodate your growing belly. Tai chi also reduces stress and sharpens coordination.

Pilates. Named after its early-20th-century founder, Pilates (pronounced puh-LAH-teez) builds flexibility and strength through a series of controlled movements performed either on specially designed exercise equipment and supervised by a

Herniated disks

Pregnancy can put your back through the wringer. Extra weight and changes in posture can tax the vertebrae—the bones that make up the spine—and the disks, which are the gel-filled cushions between the vertebrae that act as shock absorbers. Injuries or sudden movements can cause a disk to bulge out between the bones. This is called a herniated disk; it's also referred to as a slipped disk. If the disk presses on a nerve, it can cause mild, moderate, or severe pain down the front, back, or side of one leg, sometimes accompanied by numbness or tingling.

If you herniate a disk, take acetaminophen. If the pain is very bad, your doctor might prescribe a stronger painkiller. Herniated disks may fix themselves over the course of a few weeks, usually with a combination of rest and pain relievers initially. When the pain first strikes, experiment with lying and standing positions to see what brings relief. If those don't work, try bed rest. Some people find relief from disk pain by doing a yoga pose called the cat or camel stretch. (See "Staying limber," page 173.) Do this stretch only with your doctor's OK. Working with a physical therapist can help improve your posture and strengthen the muscles that support the back. This may prevent the disk from herniating again in the future.

trained Pilates instructor or on an exercise mat. Pilates, traditionally used by dancers for injury rehabilitation, has become popular during the past few years. It's a favorite exercise of many celebrities who credit it for toning and strengthening their bodies.

Pilates is also a favorite of obstetricians because it focuses on strengthening the core abdominals and lower-back muscles.

Finding a class. Many health clubs, YWCAs, spas, community centers, hospitals, and HMOs offer these classes. Look for classes with an experienced instructor and, ideally, only 12 to 15 participants. The instructor should make you feel safe and should be sensitive and willing to listen to you; she should not be pushy or militant. If possible choose a class designed for pregnant women. If not, be sure to tell your instructor that you are pregnant; she can warn you if certain postures aren't suitable for a pregnant woman. While in class listen to your body and don't do anything that feels uncomfortable. If you are more comfortable exercising at home, there are many yoga, tai chi, and Pilates books, DVDs, and videos available to buy or rent. Choose ones that focus on pregnancy.

Common Questions

Q. Should I move to a bigger house to make more room for my growing family?

A. Don't call your real estate agent yet. Having a big house with plenty of room for children is nice, but it's not always the right solution. Here are some things to consider before putting up that "for sale" sign.

Emotional concerns. Expectant parents often overlook an important consideration: Moving can take you away from the emotional support system that you will desperately need after your baby is born. Here's what often happens: A couple lives and works in the city. The woman has friends at work and in her neighborhood or apartment complex. When the couple decides to start a family, they move out to the suburbs, and the woman quits her job to stay home full-time with her baby. The couple has a nice house, but the woman feels isolated because she's left all of her friends in the city. Being alone can be very depressing for a new mother who's home with an infant.

That said, if you can afford a new home that brings you closer to family and friends, moving might be a good idea.

Financial concerns. Buying a new house can also be a bad move if it leaves you financially strapped. Think twice before committing to mortgage payments that will leave you little money for the many necessities a baby requires. You'll be shocked at how fast the cost of diapers adds up. And if you buy a home with a mortgage that requires two salaries to pay, what will happen if one of you loses your job or wants to stay home with your baby? Being a new parent is stressful enough without adding financial problems to the mix.

Renovation issues. If you decide a new house is best for your situation, be careful not to take on more than you can handle as far as renovation goes. Ask yourself if you really have the time, energy, money, and patience to renovate a house while you are pregnant or have an infant. You might be better off buying a home that needs less work.

If you do renovate, keep in mind that homes built before 1978 may contain lead paint. Exposure to even small amounts of lead can be dangerous for your baby. If painted surfaces need sanding or scraping, stay out of the house until the dust is cleared away; you can get lead in your body by breathing lead-tainted dust, and that lead can cross the placenta and damage your baby's brain and nervous system. For more on lead paint, contact the Environmental Protection Agency (www.epa.gov).

Week 18

Your Baby

The inside story

If you had an ultrasound this week, you might see your baby sucking his thumb, or frowning as if to say, "You again?" His fingerprints are nearly complete, and his heart has formed completely so that you can see the heart's different structures on the ultrasound. Your baby's senses are rapidly maturing too. He has more taste buds than he needs. At long last he's able to use his ears. His inner ear bones and nerve endings from his ears to his brain have developed enough so that your baby might startle if he hears a loud noise. He can also sense sounds like your heartbeat and blood pumping through the umbilical cord. If there were light in your womb, he could detect that too.

Because your baby's visceral organs, such as his heart and liver, are growing fast, he's sitting more erect inside you to make room for them. He now has 200 bones, and they're continuing to harden; at birth he'll have about 300 bones, but some of those will fuse later, which is why the adult skeleton has only 206 bones in all.

Your baby is as big as the placenta, which is still his main source for nutrients and oxygen. The placenta is also a waste disposal system, rushing baby's waste into your bloodstream, where it will be filtered through your kidneys and liver.

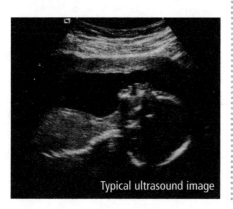
Typical ultrasound image

Your Body

Leg cramps

Sometimes the least serious ailments cause the most aggravation. Leg cramps are an example of this. These cramps usually occur in the lower leg, often at night. They can be quite painful and can interrupt your sleep. You may hear that leg cramps are caused by too little potassium or too much phosphorus in the diet, but those are myths. The truth is, doctors don't know what causes them, but it

week 18

probably has something to do with your circulation slowing down when you're at rest.

The best treatment for leg cramps is to stand barefoot on a cold tile floor and lift your toes up. This stretches the calf and often brings relief. Daily exercise also helps.

Rarely, leg pain is the sign of a blood clot. If your leg pain increases in intensity, and if your leg feels swollen and tender to the touch, call your doctor right away.

Breast lumps

Unfortunately, being pregnant doesn't protect you from breast cancer. Although it is less common in women of childbearing age than it is in older women, breast cancer does strike women in their 20s and 30s. Many of them find the cancer themselves in the form of a breast lump.

If you performed breast self-exams every month before pregnancy, keep doing it. If you have never examined your breasts, start now. If you find a lump, tell your doctor. Don't be too alarmed, however. Your breasts are busy getting ready for nursing, and they may develop lumps that are perfectly benign.

Your Self

Boosting your energy at work

It's three o'clock, and you're wiped out. You don't know how you're going to last another 2 hours at work. How can you energize yourself?

Don't go for a sugar infusion. Eating a candy bar may wake you up for a few minutes, but you'll crash later on.

Do eat a healthy snack that contains protein and complex carbohydrates, such as whole wheat crackers with peanut butter or a bowl of bran cereal with milk. Protein stimulates the brain's neurotransmitters, and complex carbohydrates release a slow, steady stream of energy that will carry you through the rest of the afternoon. Protein also takes longer to digest.

Don't pour a large cup of coffee. You're better off without the caffeine, particularly late in the day. Although caffeine remains in the body for 3–5 hours, it can keep some people awake for up to 12 hours.

Do go for a walk. Five minutes of brisk walking (outside or inside) will get your blood pumping.

Heart palpitations

Don't panic if your heart suddenly begins to pound. Heart palpitations are common in pregnancy because you have as much as 40 percent more blood, which is needed to bring adequate oxygen to your baby.

Your heart may be pounding because you're consuming too much caffeine. If so, cut down or eliminate caffeine from your diet. Occasionally palpitations can be a symptom of an overactive thyroid, so it's worth mentioning to your doctor during your next visit, especially if you have any of the other signs of thyroid disorder. (See "Thyroid trouble," page 101.) In very rare cases, palpitations accompanied by shortness of breath can be a sign of a cardiac arrhythmia, an abnormality of the heartbeat. Call your doctor right away if your heart pounds and you have trouble breathing.

Travel safety

The best way to avoid travel risks is to stay home, but what fun is that? (After all, a long weekend relaxing on the beach might be the best thing for you.) With a little extra planning, you can travel safely throughout your pregnancy. (See "Travel safety in mid-pregnancy," page 168.)

For plane, train, or automobile travel of more than a few hours, put support hose on. You can buy support stockings from any medical supply store. The thigh-high or maternity support hose will be more comfortable and effective than knee-highs.

Car travel. The most important rule is to wear your seat belt. A recent study of more than 440 pregnant women in car crashes showed that maternal mortality was six times higher when the woman was ejected from the automobile, and their unborn babies were five times as likely to die. Using a conventional lap belt alone has been shown to cause some injury to unborn babies, so wear a seat belt with a shoulder strap passed over the shoulder and across your chest between your breasts.

When you're on a long car trip, stop every 2 hours or so to stretch your legs and find a restroom. You don't want to rely on road food, so pack nutritious snacks and lots of water to keep you going. Break that 12-hour trip home to see family for the holidays into two days because at this stage of your pregnancy fatigue will be a major factor. Be sure your air conditioner is in good working order for summer trips because it's easy for you to feel overheated.

Air travel. You may have heard somewhere that air travel during early pregnancy is unsafe because of the link between exposure to solar radiation during pregnancy and childhood cancers. However, the American College of Obstetricians and Gynecologists states that the risk from casual air travel is negligible. For example, one round-trip, cross-country flight delivers only 6 percent of the solar radiation exposure that the National Council on Radiation Protection and Measurements deems safe for pregnant women.

You will, however, want to book flights early to get the best possible seat. Look for flights that aren't full so you can put up your feet on an empty seat; choose an aisle or bulkhead seat for more legroom; and stand up and stretch or walk around during long flights. Pack lightly, roll your luggage on wheels, and bring a carry-on bag with energy-boosting snacks and bottled water.

Gas expands with altitude, so avoid eating any bloat-producing foods before you fly. Sip water during the flight to fight dehydration, which can be aggravated by the dry air in the cabin. Pack a pair of thick socks too and wear them instead of shoes while

week 18

you're in the air. Your feet will likely swell whether you wear shoes or not, so choose comfortable footwear with expandable ties, adjustable straps, or elastic panels.

Travel abroad. Traveling outside the United States requires extra planning during pregnancy. Check that your destination has a modern medical facility and ask your provider for a copy of your health records to take with you. For a physician referral for international travel, contact International SOS Assistance (800-523-8930; www.internationalsos.com) or the International Association for Medical Assistance to Travelers (716-754-4883; www.iamat.org).

Find out your immunization status too, if you're leaving the country. Are your vaccines up to date for diseases that are common in the region? Avoid travel to any area where serious disease is a risk. If you have any questions about the health precautions that are currently being advised in a particular foreign country, call the Centers for Disease Control's International Travelers Hotline (404-332-4559; www.cdc.gov/travel/). Many immunizations are safe during pregnancy, while others are relatively safe only at certain times. Check with your doctor. In general, you must weigh the risks of having the vaccine against the risk of getting the disease it would protect you from. Certain vaccines, such as those for hepatitis A, hepatitis B, or tetanus, are considered safe even during early pregnancy.

This might also be a good time to contact your insurance company to find out what it covers if you're out of the country. Also consider buying traveler's insurance in case pregnancy complications arise and you can't use those plane tickets after all.

On-the-road rest stops

Yeast infections are often a problem for pregnant travelers, especially in hot, humid places. Wear lightweight, loose cotton clothing over cotton underwear and always change out of a wet bathing suit immediately after going for a swim.

Since clean restrooms aren't always available, and you'll be in and out of the bathroom more than you ever dreamed possible, plan plenty of stops. Carry a roll of toilet paper in your purse (take the cardboard tube out and flatten it first) and wear clothing that's easy to get in and out of. (No overalls or jumpsuits that take forever to unbutton or unbuckle.)

Always keep a granola bar or crackers in your purse for emergency provisions if you feel faint or dizzy on your trip.

Diet & Exercise

Meal-replacement drinks

You can't help noticing that the grocery store shelves are filled with energy drinks, which are sometimes called meal-replacement drinks. The truth is that these drinks don't make sense for the average pregnant woman. And they are no match for a real meal; some of them contain nearly as much sugar as soda.

It's fine to grab one occasionally if you don't have time to eat a meal, but don't rely on them. For a fast meal, you're better off reaching for a container of yogurt, a couple of slices of whole wheat bread, and an apple. Or make your own energy drink by blending skim milk or yogurt with soft fruit such as cantaloupe, peaches, strawberries, apricots, raspberries, or blueberries. Pour it into a thermos you can take in the car or to work.

Strength training

If you did strength training before conception and you're having a normal pregnancy, you can continue to lift weights. You may have to modify your routine though by switching to lighter weights and doing more repetitions. The training benefit will be nearly the same, and you will reduce your chance of joint injury. You should skip the abdominal strengtheners altogether.

The best way to do strength training during pregnancy is under the guidance of an experienced instructor. Sign up for a pregnancy fitness class or splurge on a session with a personal trainer who can advise you on how to lift weights safely.

Stretching abdominal muscles

You don't need to stretch your abdominal muscles; your baby is doing that for you. Avoid doing abdominal stretches during pregnancy because they can cause a widening of the gap that occurs between your rectus abdominis muscles during pregnancy. Save the abdominal stretching for after your baby is born.

Common Questions

Q. How can I find a good pediatrician for my baby?

A. Make a list of the doctors your friends recommend and then call their offices and ask for a meet-and-greet appointment. (Pick up on subtle clues by listening to how well the staff handles telephone calls. Are they polite? Do they keep you on hold forever?) Most pediatricians are willing to meet with expecting parents or talk with them by phone. You're going to be spending a lot of time with your baby's pediatrician, so it's important to choose someone you like and respect and who has an efficient office. Here are some questions to ask the office staff or the doctor:

- What days and hours are you available? (Some pediatricians offer weekend appointments for sick children.)
- How are middle-of-the-night emergencies handled?
- Is my health insurance accepted? If so, does the office bill my insurance company, or do I have to pay up front and be reimbursed?
- Is there someone on staff who can help instruct me on breastfeeding?
- To what hospitals do you admit patients?
- Are same-day appointments available?
- What are your thoughts on circumcising a baby?

week 18

Q. I have a stressful job, but I want to keep calm for the health of my baby. Any hints for stress busters at the office?

A. Pregnancy can be a time of anxiety, and a stressful job can make that even worse. Finding ways to relax is important because life is only going to get more stressful after your baby is born.

Throughout the day, make time for short relaxation sessions. These allow you to shift from shallow chest breathing—which is how you breathe when you're nervous—to deep, calming abdominal breathing. A mini-relaxation session lowers your heart rate and blood pressure; it helps your body back down from the anxiety response that it automatically adopts in a stressful situation. You can do a mini relaxation anytime, anywhere.

Here's how to do a mini relaxation: When you feel anxious, stop whatever you're doing and slowly take a deep breath. Slowly count: one, two, three, four. Pause. Then exhale: four, three, two, one. Repeat two or three times.

Do these mini relaxations throughout the day: when you're stuck in traffic, when you're angry at a coworker, or when you're racing to get things done.

Your partner: His reactions to your changing appearance

Your body is changing: You're gaining weight, your legs are swelling, and your face is puffy. It can be hard to feel sexy when you are changing into a larger, fleshier version of yourself. And if you don't feel attractive, you may be wondering how your partner feels about the new you.

Some men think their pregnant wives are sexier and more gorgeous than ever. But not all do. If your partner seems to be reacting negatively to your appearance—or if he is making critical comments about your size—talk with him about it. Let him know that his comments sting, even if he's just kidding.

Remind him that this is only temporary. After your baby is born, you will look more like yourself again. It may take you a while to lose the weight you've gained, but with determination (and his support), you can return to your prepregnancy weight. More important, remind him that you are going through all of these changes so that you can both become parents.

Be open with your partner about what you need. He may not realize his comments hurt you. By working together, you can go beyond appearance and build a deeper bond.

Week 19

Your Baby

The inside story

With all of those exhilarating new muscles and nerves to try out, your baby will probably stretch upon waking, though at this point she's still waking with her eyes closed. She probably weighs about 7 ounces now, and she could be as long as 8 inches. Her eyes and ears are finally in position. If you saw her on an ultrasound this week, you'd probably be able to tell whether she has her grandmother's nose or her father's chin. You might also discover whether your baby is a boy or a girl.

As your baby gets ready to be more in control of her own movements, her body is busy making myelin, a fatty substance that coats and insulates the nerves throughout her body so that electrical impulses can travel from her brain out to the tips of her toes and back again. She has as many nerve cells as an adult now.

That fatty coating on your baby's body is getting thicker. Her oil glands are now producing vernix caseosa, a greasy white coating designed to protect her delicate skin from the harsh amniotic fluid. The coating will mostly disappear by birth, but if your baby is born early, she might look like she's been dipped in yogurt. Because she is still developing fat on her body, her skin is loose-fitting and wrinkled, but that will change soon.

Your Body

Douching

Douching is never a good idea, but it's an even worse idea during pregnancy. The vagina maintains a delicate balance of good bacteria and bad bacteria. Flushing it with water or other fluids can irritate the vagina. Worse, it can change the balance of bacteria, which can cause infection in the vagina or bladder.

Feeling light-headed

No, you're not imagining it. When you move quickly from lying or sitting to standing, you may occasionally feel light-headed. Although it can be alarming to stand up and have to sit right back down because you feel a little dizzy, don't worry: Light-headedness is very common in pregnancy, particularly in tall women and women with hypoglycemia, or low blood sugar. Light-headedness has several causes: dehydration, hunger, and low blood sugar. Drink

week 19

Signs of trouble

Every woman worries about her baby and whether her pregnancy is progressing normally. The chances are very good that if you've made it this far, everything will be fine. That said, it's good to know the warning signs that something is going wrong. Watch for the following:

- **Bleeding from your vagina.** A tiny bit of spotting after intercourse, especially during the first 18 weeks, is probably nothing to worry about. More bleeding than that could be a sign of a miscarriage (in the 1st trimester), problems with the placenta (in the 2nd trimester), or premature labor.
- **Leakage of fluid from your vagina.** This is almost always a worrisome development, so call your doctor right away if you have fluid leaking from your vagina. It could be premature rupture of the membranes or an incompetent cervix.
- **Contractions that occur early in pregnancy** on a regular, measurable basis. Random, sporadic contractions are usually Braxton Hicks (see page 214); regular contractions may mean labor, particularly if you feel more than six in an hour.
- **Abdominal cramping or severe abdominal pain.** If you feel persistent, painful cramping in your abdomen, call the doctor—you could be in labor.
- **Severe nausea or vomiting.** How much you should worry about nausea and vomiting depends on what is causing them. If you've caught the stomach bug that everyone else in your family had—in other words, if you know why you're vomiting—you and your baby will be fine, even if you feel terrible. (If you are vomiting so much that you can't keep fluids down and are getting dehydrated, however, call your health care provider.) If you don't know why you're vomiting, give the doctor a call and let her determine whether it is worrisome.
- **Severe headaches, blurred vision, or extreme dizziness.** These are symptoms that always merit a call to the doctor because they could be a sign of pregnancy complications or nonpregnancy-related illness.

plenty of water and eat something every couple of hours to chase away hunger pangs and keep blood sugar stable. Avoid making any sudden moves; dangle your legs over the side of your bed before standing.

Boy or girl?

If you have an ultrasound around this time, the technician or doctor may be able to see whether your baby is a girl or a boy. Ultrasounds can be an effective way to determine the gender of your baby. Unlike amniocentesis, however, ultrasounds are not foolproof when it comes to showing whether your baby is a boy or a girl. Usually it's obvious if the baby is a boy because his scrotum and penis are discernible. Sometimes, though, the scrotum and penis aren't visible because of the position the baby is in, making a boy look like a girl. And sometimes the umbilical cord can slip between the legs of a girl and look like a penis, making a girl look like a boy. An ultrasound at this point is probably accurate, but don't paint the nursery pink or blue unless you have an amniocentesis.

Of course, just because modern science has the technology to determine whether you're carrying a son or daughter doesn't mean you have to find out. There's nothing wrong with waiting until delivery day to know your baby's gender.

Some parents-to-be ask to be told their baby's sex, but they keep the information to themselves. If that's your inclination, go ahead and save the secret. You don't owe it to the world to tell everything you know.

Your Self

Your maternity wardrobe

Do you need a little retail therapy? Head out for some new maternity clothes, if you haven't already. Maternity fashions have improved significantly in the last few years, and you'll likely be surprised at the cute tops, dresses, and jeans you'll find. Some women love making this switch from their old clothing to their new "Look at me, I'm going to be a mom!" outfits, but others dislike it. Both feelings are normal.

Undergarments. As you borrow or buy new clothes, don't overlook what goes underneath. You're probably busting out of your old bras by now. Invest in two new bras that fit your expanding breasts. Select ordinary bras in larger sizes, if they're comfortable, or choose nursing bras, which offer roominess and support now and when you're breastfeeding. Try on several before deciding which feels best. Nursing bras can be expensive, and you don't want to get home and realize they don't fit.

If you wear pantyhose, you'll probably start outgrowing your prepregnancy hose if you haven't already. Some women find that maternity pantyhose are comfortable because they expand to fit a growing belly without binding at the waist; others just go up to the next size in their own preferred prepregnancy style. Try both to see what works best for you.

Shoes. Your shoes may be feeling tight soon. While it doesn't happen to all women, many find that their feet increase a half or full size during pregnancy. If you discover that the shoes that fit perfectly a few weeks ago now feel tight, buy or borrow new shoes. The last thing you need during pregnancy is blisters caused by too-tight shoes.

Proper fit is especially important in your exercise shoes. When buying new shoes for walking or jogging, go to a good shoe store with knowledgeable salespeople and have your feet measured. Choose a walking shoe if you walk and a running shoe if you run; walking shoes and running shoes are built differently, and wearing a

week 19

running shoe to walk, or vice versa, can cause soreness in your legs and feet. Don't scrimp on exercise shoes. You want a style with plenty of cushioning because your feet are carrying more weight than they are accustomed to.

Diet & Exercise

Eating smart on the road

Double cheeseburgers, candy bars, thick chocolate milk shakes—it's a challenge to eat healthfully when you're on the road and fast-food restaurants and junk food vending machines beckon at every turn. Is it possible to put together a healthy meal under these conditions? The answer is yes. It takes some creativity, but you can find (relatively) nutritious meals while on the road.

After feeling the heat of public pressure, fast-food and other restaurants have added more-nutritious foods to their regular menus. Most now offer salads with grilled chicken and low-fat or non-fat dressing. Look for these foods:

Salads with low-fat or non-fat dressing. Leave off the croutons and go light on the shredded cheese. Topped with sliced grilled chicken, these salads make a good meal.

Grilled chicken sandwiches topped with lettuce and tomato. Be sure to ask for no sauce because the sauce can have more fat and calories than the rest of the sandwich. For a little extra zing, ask for a side of taco sauce,

salsa, or barbecue sauce and add it to the sandwich. Order the grilled chicken and not the "crispy" chicken, which is breaded and deep-fried.

Baked potatoes. Leave off the butter and top a potato with chili or with salsa. If you don't like the taste of your spuds without butter, use a small amount. It's still a better choice than french fries.

Orange juice. Most fast-food places have 100-percent orange juice. Choose the small or child-size serving. Larger sizes may have more calories than you need.

Plain hamburger or cheeseburger. A small burger or small cheeseburger is a good option. Pile on the lettuce, tomato, onions, pickles, catsup, or mustard, but avoid any special sauces or mayonnaise.

French fries. If you have to have them, ask for the smallest size. In some restaurants that's still too much, so ask for the size that's included in the child's meal. If the only available sizes are enormous, tremendous, and gargantuan, throw away what you don't need before you start to eat. A large-size order of fries can have up to 520 calories and 25 grams of fat.

Low-fat milk. Most fast-food places now carry milk, and usually it's the low-fat kind.

Breakfast sandwiches. Choose the kind that's served on an English muffin, rather than a biscuit or croissant. Go light on the cheese and select ham rather than bacon or sausage (ham has less fat).

Convenience stores. Many of these

stores sell cereal, orange juice, and milk, although you may have to buy a large box of cereal. Ask for a coffee cup and a plastic spoon. Other healthy choices include tomato juice, cheese and crackers, yogurt, raisins, and peanut butter and rye bread (whole wheat bread in a convenience store may be too much to ask). Check the selections of heat-and-eat foods: You may find a vegetarian burrito or soup that you can warm up in the microwave oven.

Whenever possible pack food from home to take with you on the road. That way you'll always have a healthy meal or snack on hand. And remember to drink plenty of water while you're on the road; it's a great way to prevent constipation.

Give yourself small indulgences

Now that you've read the lecture on healthy eating, it's time to talk about indulgences. Pregnancy shouldn't be 9 months of food prison. Of course you can indulge in treats like ice cream, cake, chocolate, potato chips, and tortilla chips once in a while. When you do, really make it count by eating mindfully. If you sit in front of the TV eating chip after chip, you barely notice that you're eating, and before you know it, you've mowed through the whole bag. But if you measure out a serving of chips and, without the TV to distract you, pay attention to the crunch and the taste and the delicious saltiness of each chip, you'll appreciate them more. Chances are, you'll derive more

enjoyment from one serving of a treat eaten thoughtfully than several servings carelessly wolfed down.

Make your indulgences special—so you'll enjoy them more and need them less. If you're going to have a small piece of chocolate, splurge on the good stuff. Head to the gourmet store to buy a truffle. If you're craving cheese, bring home your favorite cheddar or Monterey Jack, rather than finishing up the cold, leftover pieces of grilled cheese sandwich from your 2-year-old's lunch plate.

Common Questions

Q. Why are my nipples already secreting fluid?

A. Your breasts are setting themselves up to become milk factories. The number of milk ducts is increasing, the milk glands are preparing for milk production, and the nipples are beginning to protrude more, making them easier for a baby to suck. During pregnancy some women notice a thin, yellowish liquid coming from their nipples. This is colostrum, which is the first fluid a nursing baby receives from the breasts. Colostrum, which contains nutrients and health-protecting antibodies, is produced for a day or two after delivery, followed by milk.

It's perfectly normal to leak colostrum during pregnancy—and it's also perfectly normal not to. Colostrum secretion during pregnancy says nothing about your breasts or ability to breastfeed successfully.

week 19

Q. Can I still pick up my 2-year-old now that I'm pregnant?

A. Lifting anything up to 35 pounds should be fine, even if it's a squirming pre-schooler. To avoid straining your back, always practice good lifting techniques. Bend at the knees, not at the waist, to lower yourself. Use your leg muscles when lifting and hold the object (or child) as close to your body as possible to put most of the strain on your arm muscles, not your back. Keep your back straight as you lift and carry. Switch your load from one side to the other every 10 minutes or so to avoid overusing one side of your back.

Week 20

Your Baby

The inside story

Your baby is really making himself known now, popping you with his feet or fists whenever he feels like turning or twisting around, which may seem to happen more at night than any other time of day. At this time, he still has plenty of room to perform somersaults. (Lucky you!)

At nearly 10 inches long, your baby is looking more human by the day. Specific areas in his brain are developing for each of his five senses, and his skin is now developing its various layers. Hair and nail growth continue too. An ultrasound might show him swallowing amniotic fluid, an action that helps his digestive system develop. Some researchers speculate that the amniotic fluid contributes nutrients to your developing baby.

Although your baby's lungs are still not quite developed enough for him to survive outside your body, you'll hear his heartbeat as a powerful whooshing sound during prenatal visits. It'll sound like a tiny racehorse coming home to the finish line.

Your Body

Your expanding uterus

Think of your uterus as a stretchy rubber balloon that expands on an as-needed basis. This muscular organ is located above the bladder and in front of the rectum. It is held in place by strong ligaments, and it is remarkably elastic, stretching to about 500 times its prepregnancy size. It grows in weight too, from a couple of ounces to more than 2 pounds. When your pregnancy is over, the uterus returns to its original size.

Round-ligament pain

If you didn't know your body houses something called round ligaments, you will soon. Basically, these ligaments are attached from the sides of the pelvis to the uterus. When the uterus grows, the ligaments must stretch with it. Round-ligament pain is common between weeks 16 and 20. It may feel like a dull ache in the lower abdomen (on one side or both), or it may feel like a sharp, shooting pain that travels down into your groin.

It is a normal, albeit sometimes annoying, part of pregnancy. Most women find relief by resting with their feet up and occasionally taking

week 20

High-risk pregnancies

Most pregnancies are considered "low-risk," which describes healthy pregnancies that proceed in a routine way; this is one time in your life when being ordinary is good. Pregnancies are considered "high-risk" if either the mother or baby has a health concern or another issue that makes the pregnancy or delivery riskier than an ordinary pregnancy.

Who is high-risk? A pregnancy is high-risk if the mother had a preexisting medical disorder such as diabetes or lupus; if she develops a complication during pregnancy such as early preeclampsia or placenta previa; if the baby is believed to have a birth defect or other problem; if the mother is obese; or if there is more than one baby. In some cases, women who have conceived through in vitro fertilization or other assisted reproduction techniques are considered to be high-risk during pregnancy. Some doctors consider any pregnancy in a mother over age 40 to be high-risk. Not all doctors subscribe to this belief, however. Some feel that maternal health and fitness matter more than age. With these doctors, if you are a healthy, fit 42-year-old, your pregnancy will be considered lower-risk than the pregnancy of an unhealthy, unfit woman who is much younger.

Precautions. If your pregnancy is high-risk, you may be monitored differently, with more frequent doctor visits or tests, depending on the reason for concern. In some cases, your doctor may recommend that you stop exercising, change your diet, or decrease your activity for the remainder of your pregnancy in order to reduce the risk of harm to you or your baby.

Your doctor may refer you to a high-risk obstetrician, or you may choose to see one on your own. High-risk obstetricians (also called perinatologists) are specialists who are trained to manage the complications that a high-risk pregnancy can bring. Your doctor may also recommend that you give birth in a hospital, such as a university-affiliated teaching hospital or a hospital with a neonatal intensive care unit that is fully equipped to provide state-of-the-art care for you and your baby.

Where you live enters into these decisions. You have more choices of specialists and hospitals if you live in New York City or Boston than you would have in a small town that is hundreds of miles from a major city. Again, the nature of your complication may determine your course of action. If you're having twins and everything seems normal, you and your doctor may feel comfortable having you give birth in a community hospital. However, if you're having triplets and you started the pregnancy with uncontrolled high blood pressure, it makes sense to see a perinatologist and deliver in a hospital that is well prepared for potentially difficult deliveries.

acetaminophen. Roll over carefully, and soak in a warm tub if it's really bad. This pain usually disappears by week 21.

Heightened sense of smell

Now that you're well into your 2nd trimester, your extra-sensitive sense of smell may return to normal. Or it may last until delivery. Not all women develop a heightened sense of smell during pregnancy. If you have, don't worry: Your nose will come back to its senses sooner or later.

Your Self

Chronic stress

Scientists don't know for sure whether high levels of chronic stress harm your baby or put your pregnancy at risk. However, there is some reason to believe that stress might impact your baby. According to the March of Dimes, very high levels of stress can contribute to preterm birth or low birthweight in full-term babies. What qualifies as "very high levels of stress"? Like beauty, stress is in the eye of the beholder. What puts stress on one person can often invigorate another.

Your body's reaction. When something that you perceive as distressing happens, your body undergoes a very real and very dramatic physical response. It's called the "fight or flight" response, because it physically prepares you to either confront a danger or escape from it.

Here's an example: You're lounging by a pool, when suddenly a toddler falls in. Nearly every system of your body becomes immediately prepared to deal with the stressful situation. Your heart begins to pump like crazy, rushing blood to your muscles. Your breathing becomes shallow and rapid. Stress hormones pour into your bloodstream. Your immune system and digestive system temporarily shut down, and your brain switches into a state of hyperalertness. You now have the power you need to jump up, run to the pool, plunge into the water, and save the child from drowning.

After you place the child into the arms of his frightened mother, you return to your lounge chair, and over time your body's systems return to their normal, non-stressed state.

If you are chronically stressed, however, your body remains in a constant state of alert. Your "fight or flight" reaction occurs over and over, and your systems never have a chance to return to normal. Your heart rate, breathing rate, and muscle tension stay elevated. Your body overflows with stress hormones. Your immune system remains suppressed, compromising your ability to fight disease. Constant surges in blood pressure and cholesterol production damage your blood vessels.

Protecting your baby. While scientists search for answers, pregnant women can try to avoid stressful situations and stressful people whenever possible. Getting enough sleep, eating well, exercising regularly,

week 20

spending time with supportive friends and family, doing yoga, and practicing meditation or other relaxation exercises can also help you reduce feelings of stress and bring your body from a state of emergency to a state of calmness. (See "Alternative exercises," page 146.)

Dealing with nosy relatives

One of the healthiest habits you can develop during pregnancy is the ability to say "No." It comes in handy when you have a newborn too. "No, you can't hold the baby because you have a cold." "No, I can't help out with the church picnic four weeks after giving birth." "No, the baby's head is not a funny shape." You get the idea.

Practice saying no to any relatives or in-laws—or neighbors, for that matter—who ask you questions that you'd rather not answer. It's perfectly fine to say, "No, I haven't decided whether I'll go back to my job." "No, we haven't chosen a name for the baby." "No, you can't put your hands all over my belly."

You have a right to decide what information to share and what to withhold. And you don't owe people a long explanation about why you're saying no. Take the baby's name, for instance: If you want to tell everyone what name you've chosen, that's fine. But you don't have to; nor do you have to answer questions about medical test results, health problems, your baby's gender, or how much weight you've gained.

Cramping after orgasm

Don't blame it on your partner. If you feel cramps in your uterus after having an orgasm, rest assured that this is a normal occurrence. It has no negative impact on your baby or you.

If cramping continues for more than a few minutes or comes and goes on a consistent basis—for example, every 6 minutes—call your doctor because what you're feeling may be premature labor. Although a small amount of spotting after orgasm in early pregnancy (before week 18) is probably nothing to worry about, spotting later in pregnancy, and substantial bleeding after an orgasm or at any other time, is a cause for concern and merits an immediate call to your prenatal provider.

Diet & Exercise

When heartburn persists

Heartburn can become more and more of a problem as your pregnancy progresses. Antacids are thought to be safe during pregnancy, although sodium bicarbonate should be avoided because of its high sodium content. If your heartburn persists despite diet, sleep modifications, and antacids, your doctor may recommend other medications.

B vitamins are your best friend

There are eight B vitamins, and they're usually referred to as the B family. Folic acid is the B family's superstar because it helps prevent

Foods high in B vitamins	
Vitamin	Food
Thiamin (B1)	Some lean meats including pork and liver, wheat germ, cereals, whole grains, enriched breads, tortillas, dried beans
Riboflavin (B2)	Milk, yogurt, eggs, enriched breads, cereals, meats, poultry
Niacin	Turkey, fish, nuts, peas, dried beans (especially black-eyed peas)
Pantothenic Acid (B5)	Salmon, chicken, yogurt, sweet potatoes, milk, corn, eggs, kidney beans
Pyridoxine (B6)	Chicken, pork, peanut butter, black beans, soybeans
Folic acid	Navy beans, wheat bran, whole grains, leafy greens such as spinach, legumes, orange juice, asparagus, broccoli
Vitamin B12	Beef, salmon, eggs, dairy products
Biotin	Egg yolk, legumes, nuts, peanuts

neural tube defects. But the other seven are critical too: They help the body properly use energy and nutrients, among other jobs. The best way to consume any nutrient is in food. Use the food guide, above, to make sure the B family is well represented in your body.

Common Questions

Q. How can I handle the emotions that come with a high-risk pregnancy?

A. How you cope depends on the nature of the risk. Here are some suggestions:
- **Educate yourself.** The more you know about the complication, how to reduce your risk, and what lifestyle changes you should make, the better. The March

of Dimes is a great place to start. Visit its website (www.marchofdimes.com) or check your phone book for a chapter near you.
- **Ask questions.** This is the time to jot down your questions and get the answers from your doctor. If you are sent to a specialist (high-risk obstetrician, neonatologist, or pediatric surgeon), make the most of the visit by asking for information. There are no "silly" questions.
- **Ask for help.** Turn to family, friends, neighbors, your church, or whoever else can help you with rides to doctor's appointments and hospitals, household chores, caring for your other children, and stopping by with meals. People want to help, but they can't if they don't know what you need.
- **Join a support group.** In-person and online support groups are a great way

to get information and feel less alone.
- **See a social worker or therapist.** It sometimes helps to talk things out with a professional if you find yourself feeling depressed or unable to cope.

Q. My ultrasound shows that I'm pregnant with more than one baby. What now?

A. Don't run out and buy a double stroller just yet, especially if the ultrasound was performed very early in your pregnancy. Here's why:

6-week ultrasound. Even though your ultrasound shows twins, it's still early in your pregnancy, and there is a chance that the pregnancy will "self-reduce." In other words, one fetus (or more) will die, either because of a genetic abnormality or because most of the nutrition is going to another fetus. The fact is that far more multiples are conceived than are actually born.

Because multiples frequently self-reduce during the first couple of months of pregnancy—before many women have an ultrasound—women who have conceived multiples and lost one may never know that there was more than one baby to start with. If your first ultrasound is at 20 weeks, you may see one baby and never know there was a second or third.

12-week ultrasound. If an ultrasound shows multiples at 12 weeks, there's a higher chance that all will survive, but you're not out of the woods yet. You really can't count on twins or triplets until you get past 18 weeks. After that benchmark, the chance of both or all of the babies surviving is much greater.

Next steps. Having more than one baby can be a shock, particularly if you have no multiples in your family, did not conceive through assisted reproduction, or are a younger mother. (The older you are, the higher your chance of multiples.) Multiples can add complications to your pregnancy. For example, multiples are more likely to be born early. The thought of having two or three babies can be overwhelming; the reality of caring for all of them at once is two or three times more overwhelming.

Your doctor will advise you on health-related specifics such as how much weight you should gain and how to tailor your nutrition and exercise regimen to accommodate multiples. As for emotional support, most women benefit from talking with mothers who have successfully delivered and are raising multiples. Seek out friends and acquaintances who have had multiples and ask them to share their experiences. You may also want to join a "mother of multiples" club in your community, if there is one.

Your partner: How he can interact with baby

Those poor dads. With all the action happening in the mother's belly, Dad can feel pretty left out. You can draw him out of the shadows and into your baby's life by including him in some of these ways:

Invite him to accompany you to medical appointments. Give him a book on fatherhood to occupy him while you're sitting in the doctor's waiting room.

Ask for his input on decisions such as which crib to buy and what color to paint the nursery. Even if he'll happily leave those choices up to you, he may like being asked.

Give him the lead role in your pregnancy. He shouldn't have to play second fiddle to your mother, your sister, or your best friend.

Talk with him about his own father. Ask him how he thinks his parenting style will differ from his father's.

Encourage him to rub your belly. Some partners hold back from doing this. Welcome him by placing his hands on your belly.

Set aside "kick time" for him. Many babies are at their most active when you lie down at the end of the day. Schedule a half hour or so before bedtime for the two of you to lie in bed together feeling the baby kick—you from the inside, your partner from the outside.

Invite him to talk and sing to your baby. Research shows that babies are born recognizing familiar voices.

Give him jobs to do. For example, ask him to burn a CD with music you might want to listen to during labor.

Week 21

Your Baby

The inside story

Congratulations! You're officially halfway through your pregnancy! Your baby is halfway to her birth size too, measuring an amazing 9 or 10 inches long and growing fast. It seems like she hardly ever sleeps now that she's big enough to be felt, though in reality a baby kicks only several times per hour, then sleeps for a period of time, awakens, and kicks some more. Because she still has room to move in your uterus, you'll feel the kicks in random places. At this point, it's tough to tell a foot from a fist.

As she continues to plump out, your baby will start to look like a little doll, complete with eyebrows. She's now completely covered with that white, pasty layer of vernix caseosa. Most of that substance will probably disappear before birth, except in certain places like the creases of her neck and behind her knees. Up until this point, her liver and spleen have produced nearly all of her blood cells. The liver will keep doing that until after her birth, and now her bone marrow's getting up to speed, churning out red blood cells as well.

Your baby's brain is growing as fast as the rest of her, and it will keep growing rapidly for several more years. Meanwhile, meconium is forming in her bowels—that's a blackish green, sticky substance that originates in your baby's digestive tract—and it will probably be passed through with your baby's first stool.

As your baby's senses develop, she's becoming increasingly aware of your eating and sleeping habits and of light and noise levels outside your body.

Your Body

Travel safety in mid-pregnancy

Head for the hills or the beach or the big city! This is the best time in your pregnancy to take a trip. Miscarriage isn't much of a risk now, your morning sickness has probably ended, and you're still small enough to get around easily. Use these travel tips to make the most of your last vacation (at least for a while) without night feedings, diaper bags, or a babysitter:

- Move around. The riskiest thing about travel during pregnancy is the possibility of getting a blood clot, and travel often requires long hours of sitting in a planc, bus, train, or car, which increases that risk. Get up and walk around every hour or so. Avoid crossing your legs, and if you have varicose veins or swelling problems, consider wearing support hose.

- Take your most comfortable shoes and clothing. Support hose are especially important if you're going to be sitting in cars, planes, or trains for long periods of time.
- Head off dehydration by drinking extra fluids (choose water rather than caffeinated beverages, which can contribute to dehydration), breathing steam from a cup of hot water, and using an over-the-counter saline nasal spray.
- Most airlines allow pregnant women to travel until the 36th week of pregnancy, though expectant mothers at risk for premature labor or who have placental abnormalities should avoid flying.
- Forget those multicity tours. Opt for a single destination and a pace that allows you to get off your feet in the middle of each day.
- Choose a cool climate over a hot one, now that your metabolism is in high gear, or at least be sure your hotel has air-conditioning and you can stay out of the sun.
- Beat jet lag by avoiding new time zones or start switching time zones before you leave. Switch to local time when you arrive.
- Take your good habits with you. Pack your prenatal vitamins and stick to a healthy eating plan. Continue to exercise daily.
- Lift luggage carefully: Stand

alongside your suitcase, bend at your knees, grasp the handle, and straighten up. Better yet, have your partner or the bellboy carry it.

- If you have a problem with swollen ankles, wear loose-fitting shoes. Rotate your ankles and elevate your feet to improve circulation.
- Get the name of a local obstetrician and carry it with you. Also carry your medical records and insurance card.
- Check with your health insurer to find out if you're covered for health problems that occur while you're traveling and determine whether you need your insurer's approval before receiving care.
- Pick a safe destination. Now is not the time to travel to countries with unsafe drinking water, high rates of infectious diseases, or civil unrest. If you must travel to a foreign country where vaccinations are recommended by the Centers for Disease Control, check with your health care provider to weigh the risk of every vaccination against the risk of getting the disease at this point in your pregnancy.
- Don't drink the water or swim in it if you're in a country where water standards are questionable. If you're in a region where the water poses hazards, don't eat raw or unpeeled fruits and vegetables.
- When you drive, wear a lap belt and shoulder harness. The lap belt should strap beneath your abdomen, and the shoulder belt should be snug without cutting

week 21

into your shoulder or neck.

- Bring extra pillows and socks no matter how you travel. They'll come in handy for comforting your back and feet.

Your Self

Sex and your growing belly

Even when you and your partner both have the energy and desire to make love, there's a major hurdle now—a very round hurdle. If this is your first child, there may be a learning curve to go along with your body's new curves as you face the challenge of combining parenthood with a great sex life. You'll need a sense of humor, an appreciation of the absurd, and a lot of tender, frank conversation.

Good positions. Don't ever assume that your partner knows what you want, and always be clear about what feels good—and what doesn't—during lovemaking. The missionary position is probably out now. Your partner can't really hurt the baby by lying on top of you, but he'll probably feel like he's lying on a watermelon, and you might gasp for air. Ask your partner to hold himself up on his arms to take the pressure off or sit on top of him to better control speed and penetration during intercourse. Your plumper vaginal tissues will probably cause lovemaking to be more pleasurable for both of you, and this position makes it easier for you to orgasm.

You can also try a rear-entry position, as long as your partner is careful about how deep and fast he penetrates you. Get up on your hands and knees and, for extra support, hold on to the headboard or stack pillows beneath your upper body.

Another comfortable position for late-pregnancy lovemaking is the back-to-front style. From behind you, your partner can slide his penis in and caress your genitals at the same time while he moves in and out and reaches around you to gently stroke your breasts.

Concerns about the baby. Now that your belly is so prominent, your partner may be afraid that he's going to hurt you or the baby. Reassure him that if a certain position is uncomfortable for you, you'll tell him. Remind him that the baby is well protected inside your thick uterine walls and that there's no chance of infection because of the mucus plug blocking your cervix.

Getting comfortable with your body. If this is your first child, you may feel shy about showing off your body, even in front of your partner. That may cause you to avoid sex or any type of intimacy. Instead of shying away from the topic, talk with your partner. He may surprise you by saying how great and sexy you look to him. Men aren't always good at saying what they're thinking. So while you may be thinking he's turned off by your growing belly or bigger thighs, you're probably off the mark.

Even if you don't go through a phase of feeling lustier this trimester, revel in body-to-body contact with

Psychiatric disorders and medications

Depression, anxiety, and other psychiatric disorders are common in women of reproductive age. If you're living with one of these disorders and taking a medication to control it, you may be wondering if you need to stop taking that drug to have a healthy baby. There is no simple "yes" or "no" answer.

Antidepressants. Depression affects up to 25 percent of adults in the United States each year, and women are twice as likely as men to experience it. The onset of major depression tends to occur during the childbearing years, and pregnancy appears to neither promote nor protect against it. Based on years of using antidepressants, physicians may give the green light to pregnant women to use tricyclic antidepressants (Elavil, Norpramin, Pamelor, and others) and SSRIs (selective serotonin reuptake inhibitors) like Prozac and Zoloft. Other medications may be less appealing because they can harm the baby's development.

Mood stabilizers. Lithium, valproic acid (Depakoate), and carbamazepine (Tegretol) are common treatments for bipolar disorder. Unfortunately, all of these drugs are linked to a higher risk of miscarriage and birth defects. For instance, valproic acid and carbamazepine have both been associated with a tenfold increase in neural tube defects if taken during the 1st trimester.

Antipsychotics. There are three basic groups of antipsychotics: high-potency agents, low-potency agents like Thorazine (chlorpromazine), and newer drugs like Risperdal (risperidone), Clozaril (clozapine), and Zyprexa (olanzapine). Each of these drugs has been linked to various fetal effects if taken during the 1st trimester.

If you have a psychiatric disorder, it is important to discuss it with your provider. Psychiatric symptoms can hamper your pregnancy if they affect your emotional state, your ability to take care of yourself, and your potential to engage in harmful behavior. You and your provider can weigh the risks and benefits of using specific medication during pregnancy. For instance, how well did you function without it before you were pregnant? Do you have a history of psychiatric hospitalizations or suicide attempts? Are you likely to have self-destructive thoughts if you stop taking this drug? Is there another effective medication that's safer to take during pregnancy? Discuss your concerns with your practitioner and mental health provider.

your partner while you watch a movie or lie near the fireplace, holding hands and talking about the future of your growing family. Time together as a couple is what's important.

Setting rules for relatives

Now that your pregnancy is out in the open, everyone's getting involved. Your mother-in-law has suggested that she come and stay for a week to take care of you and the new baby. Your sister wants to videotape the birth. Your own mother decides she should move in with you a month before the baby comes, "just in case."

Learning to set boundaries with family members is a crucial step toward your own development as a mother; it is also essential for the health of your relationship with your partner. Together, you and your partner need to decide whether you want to invite people to participate in the birth and to help out afterward. Is it important for you and your partner to be alone in the delivery room, or would you both feel more comfortable if another woman were there too? Do you want time alone to bond with the baby, or do you want help with older children and housework?

Decide what photographic or video record you want of your labor and delivery. Some practitioners or facilities prohibit cameras in the delivery room, so it's important to know that beforehand. You may also prefer to keep your baby's birth a private experience rather than having someone videotape those intense hours.

Each of these boundaries is unique for every couple. The important thing is that they're your decisions and nobody else's.

Diet & Exercise

Peanuts and allergies

Peanut butter is an ideal food for pregnancy. It contains fiber, vitamin E, folate, and heart-healthy monounsaturated fat. Studies have shown that eating peanuts and peanut butter can help lower cholesterol and blood sugar. Peanuts also help with weight control because they have a strong satiety value, meaning they keep hunger at bay longer than many other foods, particularly those that are high in carbohydrates. When you're planning meals and snacks, keep in mind that peanut butter is high in calories: Two tablespoons, which is the amount most people use on a sandwich, have 190 calories.

If you're allergic. About 2 percent to 2.5 percent of all adults (and many children) suffer from food allergies. Allergies to peanuts are the most common food allergies (followed by shellfish, eggs, wheat, soy, dairy products, and tree nuts). If you're allergic, you should stay away from peanut products at all times, including during pregnancy. Food allergies can show up as rashes, swelling of the skin, nasal congestion, nausea and diarrhea, or anaphylactic shock, which is life-threatening.

If you're not allergic. Will eating peanuts during pregnancy increase the risk of your child having a peanut allergy? There is no clear answer to this question. However, there is evidence that the protein from peanuts ingested by mothers is secreted into breast milk; researchers suspect that if peanut protein goes into breast milk, it probably can cross the placenta too. It makes sense for women who have a close relative with a peanut allergy to avoid eating peanuts during pregnancy and while nursing because their children may have a greater-than-average chance of developing a peanut allergy.

Zinc

This mineral helps the body build and repair cells and is essential during pregnancy. If you eat animal foods, you're probably getting plenty of zinc. It's found in milk, meat, cheese, eggs, and yogurt, and there's probably some in your prenatal vitamin too.

If you are a vegan—a vegetarian who eats no animal foods at all, including eggs and dairy—you'll benefit from seeking out plant foods that contain zinc. These include whole grains (breads, cereals, and the grains themselves), legumes, tofu, and nuts. Taking an extra zinc supplement is necessary only if your doctor advises it.

Vitamin B₁₂

Vitamin B_{12}, also known as cobalamin, is another essential pregnancy nutrient found mainly in animal foods. A diet low in B_{12} can contribute to anemia, so vegans' diets should include plant foods that contain B_{12}, such as fortified breakfast cereals.

Staying limber

During pregnancy, you ask your muscles to do more than ever before. They usually rise to the occasion, but sometimes they get a bit stiff. The following stretches will help your hardworking muscles stay limber. When you stretch, remember to hold the position until you feel a gentle stretch, never a sharp pull. Be sure to breathe while you stretch. Move fluidly and gently—never bounce. If any stretch feels uncomfortable, don't do it. The best time to stretch is after exercise, when your muscles are warm and most flexible.

Cat/camel back stretch. *To set up:* Get on your hands and knees on the floor. Hands should be shoulder width apart and directly under your shoulders. Knees should be hip width apart and directly under your hips.

The move: Slowly begin to tuck your chin in toward your chest while gently arching your back, tilting your pelvis back, and pulling your abdominal muscles toward the ceiling. Stay in that position for 20 seconds. You should feel a stretch in your back. Then slowly and gently bring your head up, tilt your pelvis forward, and relax your abdominal muscles. Stay in that position for 20 seconds. Repeat both stretches 2 or 3 times.

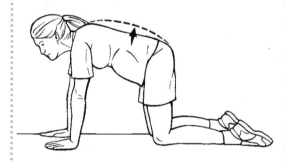

Calf and thigh stretch. *To set up:* Stand about 3 feet from a wall. *The move:* Keep your back leg straight with heel on the floor and turned slightly outward. Step in toward the wall with your front foot, bending your knee. Your front foot should be about halfway between your back foot and the wall. Place the palms of your hands on the wall, lined up with your shoulders, elbows bent. Lean into the wall until you feel a stretch in the calf and thigh of your back leg; keep your back heel on the ground. Hold for 20 seconds. Then stretch the other leg. Repeat the stretch 2 or 3 times for each leg.

Arm and chest stretch. *To set up:* Stand about a foot from a wall, feet shoulder width apart, knees slightly bent. The wall should be on your right side. Place your right arm against the wall beside you with the palm of your hand placed firmly on the wall, thumb pointing up.

The move: Gently turn away from the wall. You should feel a stretch in your arm and chest. Hold for 20 seconds, repeat with the other arm, and repeat 2 or 3 times on each side.

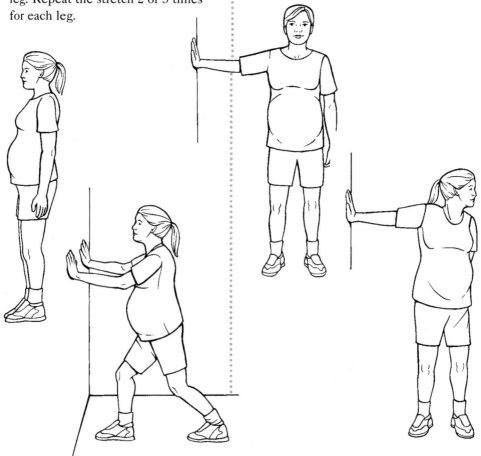

Two-part arm/shoulder stretch. *To set up:* Stand with your feet shoulde width apart, knees slightly bent, arms by your sides.

The move: With palms facing each other, slowly raise your arms in front of your body and over your head. Your arms should stay parallel to each other, and your elbows should not be bent. When your arms are straight up, reach for the sky. Hold the stretch for 10–20 seconds and then slowly return your arms to starting position. Now, beginning with your arms at your sides, lift your arms straight out from the sides of your body, palms facing the floor. When your arms are straight out from your shoulders, gently pull them back, keeping them straight with palms facing the floor. Hold 10–20 seconds; then slowly return to starting position. Repeat 2 or 3 times.

Quadriceps stretch. *To set up:* Stand with a table or chair in front of you. Hold on to it with your right hand to keep your balance.

The move: Keeping your right leg planted firmly on the ground, bend your left leg back toward your buttocks while you reach your left hand back to hold your foot. (The palm of your hand will be on the laces of your shoes.) Keeping your left knee pointing toward the ground, pull your left foot gently toward your buttocks. You should feel a gentle stretch in the

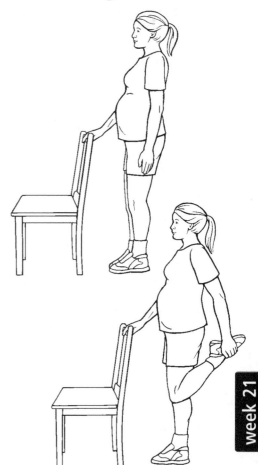

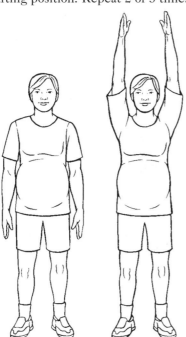

front of your thigh. Hold for 10–20 seconds and then return to starting position. Switch sides and repeat the stretch. Stretch both legs 2 or 3 times.

Common Questions

Q. My belly button is suddenly sticking out and feels very sore. It's annoying! Why is this happening?

A. During pregnancy, your uterus pushes so hard against your abdomen that your navel is forced to pop out. After the baby is born, your belly button will go back to being an "innie," if that's what you had before, or it will at least flatten out. Meanwhile, your navel is getting pressure from the inside and coming into unexpected and uncomfortable contact with your clothing, so wear soft, loose, breathable shirts and try not to lean against anything with your stomach.

Q. My baby is kicking so hard that it hurts! Can my baby damage my body?

A. Your little gymnast is reveling in those new muscles now that he has some control over them. He doesn't have a ball to play with; he's got to entertain himself somehow. No matter how great the pain, it's very unlikely that his kickboxing could do any damage to you beyond a bruised rib. The pain may feel especially weird and intense if this is your first pregnancy, but it's not dangerous.

To get your baby to punch a little less, try eating different foods and tracking what causes him to bounce around. You can also tell your tiny stepdancer a story, sing a song, or rub your belly to distract and soothe her; or shift positions so that the kicks aren't always in one (increasingly tender) place.

Q. I want to quit my job for the first year after my baby is born. My husband is in agreement, but now I'm nervous about problems I'll face getting back into the job market. What can I do?

A. Your concerns are not at all unrealistic. However, you can have the best of both worlds and enjoy more time with your baby without severing your connection to work.

For starters, keep up that computer savvy and become proficient in whatever new software is being used in your field. Depending on what kind of job you have, you may want to consider taking a class that gives you more knowledge or teaches you a new skill. Many classes are taught online now, which is a great option for stay-at-home moms.

You can also continue attending conferences and trade shows while you're on maternity leave. And you can subscribe to magazines and newspapers that will help you keep up with business developments and industry trends at home and abroad. You might seek out per diem or consulting work with either your old employer or new ones. If you can't find paid consulting work, consider volunteering as a way of exploring a job change or keeping your skills up-to-date.

Your partner: His anxiety over baby bills

While you're worrying about swollen ankles, kicks in unexpected places, and how you'll weather childbirth, your partner may be focused on finances. He may suddenly fret about losing his job, worry that he can't cover the bills while you take unpaid maternity leave, or feel frantic about paying for college. This sudden breadwinning zeal is a normal rite of passage for most dads-to-be, though you may feel somewhat abandoned if your partner is suddenly working longer hours when you're feeling needy.

It may help calm your partner down if the two of you put all your financial cards on the table to see what sort of hand you have. Do you have a plan for retirement? Are your credit cards paid up? Have you thought about how you're going to pay for diapers, baby equipment, formula, and out-of-pocket expenses for visits to the pediatrician?

Financial planning isn't the most romantic activity in the world, but it's a great way to take stress out of your relationship now, before the baby arrives. Yes, there's sticker shock involved. Who knew they could charge that much for a package of diapers you're just going to throw away? And the thought of college bills might send you both running for the smelling salts. However, you don't have to pay for 21 years of family life all at once. Begin by making a list of things you really can't live without and a list of things you'd rather not do without. Then track your spending, month by month, to see if you can start living according to a budget. See a financial planner together if the two of you are having a tough time deciding on priorities.

Week 22

Your Baby

The inside story

It's time to pull out your favorite children's book! This week, your baby can hear you more clearly because the bones of his inner ear are developed enough to detect vibrations. Some studies suggest that your baby will feed more vigorously if you read to him in utero, so why not try it? It's fun and it's a great way to connect with your baby.

Your baby will be busy exploring other sensations too, stroking his face as he gets to know himself. His fingernails have grown long enough to cover his fingertips by now, and his liver is capable of removing destroyed red blood cells (bilirubin) from his blood. (Babies who haven't yet developed the ability to do this are sometimes jaundiced and may look yellow at birth; this is easily treated with light.)

Your baby's heartbeat is so powerful now that you may be able to hear it with just a stethoscope. He continues to practice swallowing, gulping down amniotic fluid not for nourishment but because he's opening and closing his mouth to work his jaw muscles and tongue. Since everything you eat crosses through the placenta, your meals season the amniotic fluid he's swallowing. Your baby's taste buds are now developed enough to taste different flavors. In fact, ultrasounds of babies may even show them grimacing after their mothers have eaten garlic or spicy food. These different tastes prepare your baby to prefer your own uniquely flavored breast milk.

Your Body

Once a cesarean delivery, always a cesarean?

Just when doctors think this question has been answered for good, new research emerges to turn the medical community on its ear again.

Medical history. In the 1960s, the cesarean delivery rate was 6.6 percent. By 1978, that rate had skyrocketed to 15 percent. More than 98 percent of women who'd had one cesarean continued having the procedure with each new baby to protect against the higher risk of uterine rupture faced by women whose uteruses were scarred by prior surgery.

There were a number of reasons why the cesarean rate continued to climb: Moms and babies got bigger; multiple gestations increased in number; and breech babies were rarely delivered vaginally.

In 1988 the American College of Obstetricians and Gynecologists (ACOG) began discouraging routine repeat cesareans, saying that the risks of this elective surgery—which include infection and increased complications for both mom and baby—outweighed the benefits. The rationale for this advice? Despite the fact that more babies were being born by cesarean, about the same percentage died or were born brain-damaged or with other problems. This philosophy coincided with a new movement toward natural childbirth as the best choice for most mothers and babies.

For the next few years—roughly from 1988 through 1996—VBAC (vaginal birth after cesarean) was very common, until large studies revealed that a small percentage (less than 1 percent) of women with a prior low-transverse scar could rupture that scar in labor. Those studies also showed that only a small percentage of those women had catastrophic outcomes for the mother and/or baby. In response the ACOG recommended that VBAC be conducted in the safest possible environment for mom and baby. This means there should be a surgical team immediately available to do a cesarean delivery and an individual skilled to attend the baby.

What's right for you? Are you a good candidate for a VBAC, or should you schedule a repeat cesarean delivery?

First, you must know what kind of uterine scar you have. You are not a candidate for a vaginal delivery after a cesarean delivery if you had a high vertical incision on your uterus. Always ask your prenatal provider what type of scar you have because the scar you see on your skin may not be a reflection of the scar on your uterus. Like all of your medical decisions during pregnancy, this is one where it pays to be informed about your provider's philosophy and birth facility.

It might seem simpler to elect a cesarean and be done with it. After all, you can pick a convenient date and have pain medication, and that's what the guidelines suggest, right? Well, it's not that easy. A cesarean delivery is safer now than ever before, yet it's still a major surgery. Operative complications might include a risk of injury to other organs, blood clots in the legs or lungs, infection, excessive blood loss, and complications from anesthesia. In addition, healthy babies born by cesarean are more apt to need admission to intensive care units for various reasons, and moms who give birth by cesarean may have more challenges breastfeeding.

A VBAC does pose a greater risk than a vaginal birth for a woman who has never had a cesarean, but that risk is small if you're a healthy woman with an uncomplicated pregnancy. The risk of uterine rupture at the site of your previous cesarean scar rises slightly if you have your labor induced. When prostaglandins (med-

Blood clots and DVT

Superficial venous changes—like the threadlike purple or red lines you might see developing just beneath your skin during pregnancy—aren't serious. Most fade away after childbirth, or you can have them safely removed by a dermatologist. You may also notice varicose veins at this point in your pregnancy. These are the result of extra blood pooling in your veins, usually in your legs (see "Varicose veins," page 124). Although they can be unsightly and uncomfortable, you usually won't have to treat them with anything other than added rest, putting your feet up, and wearing support stockings.

However, occasionally venous changes can pose a problem during pregnancy. Pregnant women are seven times more likely to develop blood clots in the deeper veins, a condition known as deep vein thrombosis (DVT). Perhaps the most serious consequence of untreated DVT is a pulmonary embolism, caused when a bit of the blood clot breaks off and makes its way into your lungs.

Your blood usually clots for a good reason: to stop bleeding and help your body heal after an injury. DVT occurs when your body signals the clotting process to begin at the wrong time or in the wrong place. Most people who get these blood clots are older; however, pregnant women are at risk for them because uterine pressure slows down their circulation and pregnant women's blood has more factors circulating in it that cause clotting. In addition, you might not be as mobile as you were before you were pregnant, and immobility is another risk factor for DVT. You may also be more at risk for DVT if your family members had blood clots, if you're obese, if you have a serious infection, or if you have had a traumatic accident or a cesarean delivery.

Fortunately, the symptoms of DVT are pretty obvious. Your leg or groin area will be cool and pale, but the area where the blood clot forms will swell and become red and hot. It may be painful to walk, and it might hurt if you flex your toes toward your knee. Call your practitioner immediately if you have these symptoms so that you can have a diagnostic ultrasound and get treatment. Treatment usually includes hospitalization and heparin, a pregnancy-safe medication that thins your blood. You'll most likely keep taking this blood thinner throughout your pregnancy and for a period of time after the baby is born.

ications used to prepare the cervix for delivery) are used, there's a higher risk of a uterine rupture, in which case you'll need an emergency cesarean. However, Pitocin (it's like oxytocin, which your body produces naturally) is sometimes used to strengthen contractions; it doesn't increase the risk of uterine rupture.

Even though the risk is low, many practitioners won't support a VBAC delivery without easy access to good emergency care both by a physician and anesthetist.

Still, about 60–70 percent of women who get support and care during a VBAC have successful, uncomplicated vaginal births. So it's worth seriously considering a vaginal birth if you've had a previous cesarean. You're a good candidate if the following is true:

- Your previous cesarean delivery was performed with a low transverse incision.
- Your pelvis is adequate, and you have no other uterine scars or previous uterine rupture.
- You are giving birth in a place where you have rapid access to an emergency cesarean if labor fails.
- Your labor has begun spontaneously and you are already dilated when you arrive at the birth center or hospital.

Say good-bye, waistline

By your 6th month, you can't hide that basketball-size bump under your shirt. Your uterus has swollen to an inch or so above your belly button, and you're much more conscious of it as you reach into high cupboards or bend over to tie your shoes. At this point your uterus probably measures about 9 inches; your health care provider will measure it during each prenatal visit to be sure that your baby is developing normally.

You may start to worry about falling now that you're feeling a little clumsy and your uterus has grown above your pelvic bone, making it harder to see where you're going. Be assured: Between the amniotic fluid and those thick, muscular walls, your uterus is a safe haven. You'd have to be seriously injured for anything to happen to your baby. Still, you may find yourself

adopting that protective stance of expectant moms everywhere, always standing with your hands folded over your belly, or even patting it from time to time as you talk to your baby or try to distract him from kicking you in all the wrong spots.

Aches and pains

You may hear some friends vow that they "just loved" being pregnant. But they're not telling the whole truth and nothing but the truth. Every pregnancy is accompanied by some discomfort, and you shouldn't feel like a wimp if you notice some aches and pains as you grow your baby. Here are the most common aches and pains that strike during the 2nd and 3rd trimesters with suggestions for heading off the ouch:

Hip bone and pubic bone aches. Your cartilage will get looser and stretchier in your hips and pelvic region as your body gets ready to open up and send your baby into the world. These aches should subside on their own after birth.

Backaches. They're almost inevitable because the ligaments in your back are relaxing just as your abdominal muscles are stretching around your uterus. About half of all pregnant women complain of back pain as their pregnancies progress. To minimize discomfort, lift heavy objects with your legs, keeping your back straight. Strive for an erect posture rather than the swaybacked stance that too often accompanies pregnancy. Keep exercising too so that your muscles will stay strong to support that extra weight around your middle.

Headaches. That increased blood flow is good for your baby, but it can be bad for your head. You may need to eat every few hours to keep your blood sugar up. Take steps to draw blood away from your forehead and back down toward your legs by putting an ice pack on your forehead for 20 minutes or laying a hot-water bottle across your feet. You might also ask your partner to let you lean back into his hands while he supports your head at the base of your skull. Or press on the ridges below your eyebrows and the middle of your cheekbones. Get lots of fresh air too.

Urine leaks

Get ready for little "oops" moments that are one of the least glamorous aspects of pregnancy: a slight loss of bladder control. You may experience occasional urine leaks, usually when you're sneezing or laughing, or find there's a steady drip that you can't turn off.

What causes urine leaks in pregnancy? The bladder is basically a balloon that stores urine. When you urinate, your bladder muscles tighten to squeeze out the urine—and then to shut off the flow. The added weight and pressure of your uterus on the bladder can weaken your muscles so that some urine leaks out. The best way to prevent this, both before and after pregnancy, is to do Kegel exercises (see "Kegel exercises," page 98) to keep your bladder muscles strong. If this doesn't help, and you're leaking enough to soak through your underwear, talk to your provider to be sure it is just urine and not amniotic fluid. The problem should resolve itself after your baby is born. If it doesn't, don't despair. Your provider has many ways to resolve this.

Your Self

Protecting your career

You're naturally starting to wonder how you're going to juggle work, a newborn, and any other children you might already have. This is a good time to think quietly and rationally, while you still can, about how to manage your career.

Don't be afraid to explore your wildest fantasies of the perfect work-family-fun life. This will involve asking some tough questions and perhaps facing potentially heated arguments with your partner and friends. Beware: Working-mother guilt is a nasty little beast that can pop its head up in unexpected places. Ironically, stay-at-home moms often feel guilty too. Because they're not earning money they're feeling pressure from parents who paid for their college educations, or they resent giving up their own dreams of a rewarding career.

Whatever your decision, you should know that 50 years of research on working moms and their children has shown that a mother's choice to work or stay at home doesn't influence how her children will turn out (unless her job makes her miserable). Happy, stable families and good childcare are the most important predictors of your child's future success.

You can't know now how you'll feel about working outside the home after your baby is born. You may be washed over by feelings of intense longing for him once your maternity leave is over, or you may feel so confident in your daycare provider that you eagerly hit the ground running, briefcase in hand. Either way, it will help you maintain perspective on the whole issue of working moms if you ask yourself these questions now—and perhaps again and again through the years as your child reaches different ages and stages:

- Can you comfortably live on just one salary?
- What would be the long-term effects on your Social Security, health benefits, and other retirement plans if you quit your job?
- Would you put raises and promotions at risk by quitting? If so, how much do you care?
- Are you thinking of a career change anyway?
- How does your partner feel about how much you work (or don't)?
- How would you feel about yourself if you were pushing a stroller and picking up toys instead of walking to board meetings and having business lunches out?
- Does your job allow for flextime, job sharing, telecommuting, or any

other part-time options so that you can stay home more hours each week without completely giving up your career?
- Could you take a longer maternity leave and head back to the office when your baby is a little older?
- Are you satisfied with your daycare options?
- Could you and your partner each work part-time?
- How stressful is your career? How successful are you at leaving that stress in the office instead of bringing it home?
- And the big one: Do you love what you do at work and feel good at the end of the day?

Nighttime waking

Ah, welcome to parenthood, where day and night often feel the same. Now that you're in your 2nd trimester, your belly is bigger, the baby is popping you a good one every time you lie down, and you feel like you have to urinate every 20 minutes. That adds up to a lot of night wakings. You're in good company: It's a rare pregnant woman who sleeps through the night, leading some folks to conclude that this is nature's way of training a mother for her hectic life with a newborn.

Insomnia and night wakings won't hurt your baby, but you might have trouble getting through the day if you're up half the night. Here are some strategies for coping:

Chill out. Your body temperature is higher now that you're pregnant, so it may help you sleep better if you lower the thermostat in the bedroom.

Keep a food journal. If your baby reacts to spicy or sugary foods by becoming more active, don't eat them at dinner. Otherwise, your baby's dancing shoes are likely to wake you up at night.

Use a humidifier. By this point in your pregnancy, your husband's snores probably can't outdo yours. Humidifying the room will reduce pregnancy congestion and snoring.

Stack those pillows. Getting comfortable is the hardest thing about going to bed in the second half of your pregnancy, so use pillows to support whatever position works.

Drink a warm cup of milk with honey or eat a small turkey sandwich before bed or when you're having trouble getting back to sleep after waking up. Milk and turkey contain L-tryptophan, a sleep-inducing amino acid.

Reduce heartburn. Sleep in a slightly upright position, either on a stack of pillows or in a recliner.

Revel in the quiet. If you wake up and have trouble falling back to sleep, practice some deep breathing with your hands cupped over your belly and imagine your baby sleeping inside you.

Sing a lullaby. Your baby can hear you now, so if you sing him to sleep, you may find yourself feeling drowsy too. It's a great way for your baby to get to know your voice.

Diet & Exercise

Staying safe outdoors

Before you head out the door to walk (or jog or run), be sure you have got all of these safety points checked off:

- Carry a cell phone programmed with emergency numbers. The chances are remote that you'll need it, but it's good to have just in case.
- Carry identification.
- Watch your footing. Because pregnancy affects your balance, you may trip more easily on an uneven path or sidewalk.
- If you trip and fall and feel you may have hurt yourself, don't try to hobble home. Call someone to pick you up or, if you think you may be badly hurt, call an ambulance. If you hit your belly, call your health care provider.
- Whenever possible walk on sidewalks, paths, and trails rather than roads.
- Stay hydrated. Drink water before (8 ounces), during (8 ounces for every 15–20 minutes of exercise), and after (8–16 ounces) your walk.
- Stay cool by dressing in layers. Check the temperature before you go out and dress as if it's 10 degrees cooler. Take off (or add) layers as you warm up and cool down.
- If you must walk on a road, walk on the left side, facing traffic.
- Use caution with a personal stereo. Listening to music or a radio program while you walk can help the time fly by, but it can also limit

your ability to hear what's going on around you. Keep the volume low or put the headset over one ear only so you can still hear what's happening in your environment. Even if you're on a safe sidewalk, bicyclists or runners may come up from behind and startle you if you can't hear them.

• Choose safe routes. Now is not the time to be exploring desolate parks or unknown neighborhoods.

At-your-desk neck stretch

If you sit at a desk for long periods of time, or if all of the tension in your body seems to collect in your neck, you know what it's like to have stiff, tight neck muscles. Stretching neck muscles can make them feel better, but it's important to stretch correctly.

Many people do the 360-degree neck roll, but experts say bending the neck back as if to look at the ceiling can be dangerous for some people, including those with osteoporosis, arthritis, or a history of neck injuries.

Here are two ways to stretch your neck muscles safely. Start each by sitting in a straight-back chair, face forward, hands in your lap, feet flat on the floor. Repeat each stretch several times a day:

• Slowly tilt head to the right, bringing ear toward shoulder as far as it will go without pain. (Don't pull your shoulder up to meet the ear.) Hold 3–6 seconds. You should feel the stretch on the left side of your neck. Return to the starting position. Repeat on the left side.

Relax and then repeat 2–3 times.
• Slowly bend head forward, bringing chin toward chest as far as possible without pain. Slowly roll chin to the right, bringing cheek to shoulder as far as possible without pain. (Don't pull shoulder up to meet the cheek.) Hold 3–6 seconds. You should feel the stretch on the left side of your neck. Roll chin back to starting position and stop. Repeat on the left side. Relax and then repeat 2–3 times.

Common Questions

Q. Since I'm older, my boyfriend and I decided to get pregnant before my wedding, which is next spring. He seemed really happy at first, but now he's acting weird, almost as if he's jealous of the baby. Is this normal?

A. Definitely. You're probably getting all sorts of pampering at work, from your friends, and even from strangers, while your partner is left out in the cold. It's not his fault or yours. Although our culture encourages men to be more involved in pregnancy and childbirth, there's really not much for your boyfriend to do at this point other than worry—about you and the baby, money, and his own increased responsibilities after marriage and fatherhood land squarely on his shoulders. He probably doesn't want to talk about that because he knows he's supposed to be supportive. In addition, you're probably doing just what you should be doing, which is bonding with your unborn baby by talking to her or mulling over names and nursery colors. Your attention is no longer devoted exclusively to your boyfriend, and you can't blame him for feeling displaced and perhaps even resentful of this new love in your life.

To make your boyfriend feel more secure, pick your head up from your belly and notice him. Pay attention to what he's doing and ask what's happening at his job and how he's feeling about all that's going on. Make a special date to see a movie he's been looking forward to and eat at his favorite Thai restaurant. Buy him a new tie, leave a sexy note in his drawer, or surprise him with a picnic in the backyard on Sunday afternoon. It may seem as if it will take more energy than you have at the moment to focus on both your boyfriend and your baby, but this is good training for your life as a family, so why not get started?

Q. I'm in my 6th month of pregnancy, and everyone at work seems to be coming down with the flu. Is it safe to get a flu shot?

A. Step right up. There is no evidence that a flu shot is harmful to an unborn baby. The Centers for Disease Control recommends that all pregnant women get a flu vaccine. At the beginning of the flu season (October–March) some health care providers may hesitate to send women in their 1st trimester of pregnancy for flu shots, but there is no need to worry. The benefits of getting a flu shot far outweigh the risk of contracting influenza. Women in their 2nd and 3rd trimesters may be more susceptible to respiratory diseases because their immune systems are altered during pregnancy. The last thing you need now—just when things are starting to calm down and you have more energy—is a week in bed with the flu.

Week 23

Your Baby

The inside story

This week your baby is so busy that it feels like she's walking around in your belly. And guess what? That's exactly what she's doing, pushing her feet against the uterine wall in preparation for taking those first steps alone.

At this point, your baby is about 11 inches long and weighs just over 1 pound. She is developed enough to have a chance of surviving outside of your body with intensive care. Her nostrils are unsealed, and she's capable of muscular breathing, but her lungs need a little more time to mature.

Her other organs are almost in full gear. Her pancreas can now produce insulin and makes more if she's exposed to high levels of blood sugar in your body. Her brain is still growing rapidly inside her skull, which has four plates that aren't completely closed to allow for that brain growth. Even after birth, these skull plates won't be completely joined, because the human brain triples in size during the first year of life.

Your baby's lips are more distinct, and her eyes may flutter open occasionally, though she won't really open them fully until the 7th month. She has more pigment in her skin this week, and more fat is accumulating beneath it.

Your Body

Anemia and fatigue

If you've listened to friends who are new mothers, you know that you should have tons of energy during your 2nd trimester. But suddenly you're feeling tired every minute, and you can hardly focus on the tasks at hand. What's going on?

Expectant women need twice as much iron as they did before they were pregnant, and one of the main causes of fatigue after the 20th week is an iron deficiency that results in anemia. Iron deficiency anemia is the most common type of anemia throughout the world. It can be caused by an inadequate consumption of red meat and other foods high in iron and vitamin B_{12}. If you suspect that you're anemic, ask your provider to test your blood for iron deficiency.

If your iron stores are low, your red blood cells aren't getting enough iron to support your muscles and your baby. Many women experience this during the 2nd trimester because their babies are growing rapidly and absorbing extra iron from their blood. If left untreated, you suffer the risk of increased stress on your heart due to inadequate hemoglobin and low oxygen saturation in your blood, less resistance to infection, and a lower tolerance to heavy blood loss or surgical intervention during your delivery. If you are really anemic, your baby's health may suffer too.

Luckily it's easy enough to fix. Your provider will probably suggest an iron supplement. Once you add more iron, you may have more constipation. Increase your fluids and stay active.

Forgetfulness

The car keys have mysteriously disappeared for the third time this week. You stop at the grocery store for milk and come home with everything but, and you can't concentrate on the most mundane tasks at work. One of the most frequent complaints among pregnant women is that they "just space out." You aren't losing your mind, just the ability to focus.

It's usually temporary, but it's definitely a given with most pregnancies that you'll be in a bit of a fog. This is partly a result of hormones (are you tired of that word yet?) that are

Lupus

Just a quarter-century ago, women with lupus were advised not to have children. Lupus is a disease involving flukes in the immune system that cause the connective tissue and organs to become inflamed. Although an expectant mother with lupus still faces greater health risks and a possibly greater likelihood of stillbirth or premature delivery than pregnant women without the disease, advanced medical care has made it possible for most women with lupus to safely have babies.

At this point in your pregnancy you have probably discussed your situation with your health care provider. Your provider is ideally an obstetrician experienced in high-risk pregnancies, and you should plan to deliver your baby at a hospital that can manage not only your care but your baby's specialized needs should he have them.

Although some women have more lupus flares during pregnancy, others do not. Some flares may be mild enough to treat with small doses of corticosteroids or by increasing other medications that you are already taking. You have a greater risk of developing preeclampsia, especially if your lupus has affected your kidneys; your provider will monitor you for sudden increases in blood pressure or spilling protein in your urine, because this condition can be serious.

What most pregnant women with lupus worry about is not their own health, but their baby's. While it's true that you face a higher risk of premature birth or a stillbirth, babies born to moms with lupus are actually no more likely to suffer birth defects than babies born to mothers who don't have the disease. A small number of them will have neonatal lupus, which is usually a temporary rash and abnormal blood count; it usually disappears by the time your baby is 6 months old and rarely shows up again.

keeping your baby-making machinery humming. But it's also because you're turning your attention inward, imagining your baby asleep or feeling the happy patter of little feet on your belly or wondering again whether to name him after your father.

Organization can help. Make extra copies of your car, office, and house keys and give them to friends or carry them somewhere other than your ever-disappearing key ring. Carry a small notebook or electronic organizer in your purse and make a habit of checking it frequently. And edit down your to-do list to a manageable size. After all, learning to be content while getting less accomplished is one more step in preparing for your busy life as a new mother.

Your Self

Pampering your soul

You're about to enter your final trimester—yikes! Don't be surprised if your stress level ratchets up a notch. There's still so much to do, from finishing up projects at work to stocking the nursery. And you may be feeling a new level of anxiety about delivery and new motherhood.

This is the perfect time to invest in beauty treatments for your soul. Find ways to unwind whether you're the sort of person who relaxes best from the outside in—exercising your body first to slow down your mind—or whether your path to inner peace is to focus inward and stay in the moment.

Breathing. If you're planning on going to childbirth class, you'll probably learn breathing exercises designed to ease labor pain. But this focused, controlled breathing isn't just for labor. Buy an audio book or take a class that teaches you deep breathing techniques you can do for short periods every day. You might also want to try transcendental meditation, which usually requires sitting upright, adopting a passive attitude, and chanting a simple word or phrase like "om" for at least 15 minutes a day. This is a technique that first came to the attention of the American medical community in the late 1960s, when researchers showed that meditation could reduce blood pressure. It's a common relaxation technique today.

Body work. If you're the sort of person who needs external stimulation to relax, consider hands-on treatments like massage and acupressure. Experienced practitioners can help your muscles relax and calm your nervous system with just the right touch. A massage therapist experienced in working with pregnant women will have a table with a cutout that accommodates your abdomen or pillows to support you in a comfortable reclining position. She will also know not to massage your uterus in a way that might stimulate contractions.

Music. You can also take a step beyond just listening to music through sound or music therapy. This technique depends on sound waves of different frequencies to elicit slower breathing rates.

Diet & Exercise

Taming junk food cravings

It's tough to break a junk food habit, particularly when you find yourself craving such things as potato chips, cookies, fast-food burgers, and chocolate. Trying to cut unhealthy foods out of your diet completely won't work; you'll get frustrated and give up after a day or two. Instead, use the chart below to make some smart substitutions that will satisfy your urges without adding too many extra calories.

Vegetarian diets

A vegetarian diet is fine for pregnancy, as long as you're careful to get all the nutrition you and your baby need.

Protein. Protein is essential during pregnancy. If you are a lacto-ovo vegetarian (you avoid meat, fish, and poultry but do eat eggs and dairy

If you crave ...	Try this instead:
Potato chips	Pretzels, which have much less fat.
A fast-food double cheeseburger	A small hamburger.
French fries	At home, make baked fries. In restaurants, choose the smallest order, eat 10 fries, and throw the rest away.
Cola	Club soda with a splash of fruit juice; or if you really love that cola taste, mix 1 part cola with 1 part club soda.
Chocolate chip cookies	A low-fat chocolate chip granola bar.
Large movie theater popcorn with butter	Smallest tub without butter, or even better, air-popped popcorn brought from home.
A large chocolate bar	A small chocolate truffle, mini chocolate bar, or 1 tablespoon of chocolate chips.
Pizza-parlor pizza slathered with pepperoni and mozzarella cheese	Home-baked pizza made with supermarket dough, fresh Parmesan cheese, and fresh chopped vegetables.
Ice cream	Sherbet, low-fat frozen yogurt, non-fat ice cream, or frozen 100-percent-juice bars (Check packages for calorie counts—some are nearly as high as ice cream's.)

products) or a lacto-vegetarian (you avoid meat, fish, poultry, and eggs but do eat dairy products), you can easily get the 60 grams a day recommended for a pregnant woman. In addition to dairy foods and eggs, plant foods such as beans, soy, nut butters, and whole grain bread contain protein. Even a vegan (someone who eats no animal products at all) can easily satisfy the daily protein requirement with smart food choices.

Calcium. This crucial pregnancy nutrient can come from dairy products and plant foods. Vegans and others who don't eat dairy can add calcium to their diet by eating plenty of dark leafy greens such as turnip and mustard greens, broccoli, bok choy, tahini, almonds, tofu processed with calcium, kidney beans, navy beans, garbanzo beans, calcium-fortified orange juice, and calcium-fortified soymilk.

Vitamin D. Your body needs vitamin D to absorb calcium. If you drink milk, you're getting vitamin D; if you avoid milk, you may need a vitamin D supplement. Talk with your doctor about this.

Zinc. Zinc is found in cheese, eggs, and yogurt, so only vegetarians who avoid these foods need to be concerned about getting enough. Whole grains, nuts, seeds, and legumes contain zinc.

Vitamin B$_{12}$. Vitamin B$_{12}$ is a nutrient that can be difficult for vegans to get enough of because it is found mainly in animal foods. Fortified breakfast cereals and supplements are the best way for vegetarians to get enough B$_{12}$. If you're a vegan, tell your doctor—an extra B$_{12}$ supplement might make sense for you. B$_{12}$ is a fat-soluble vitamin, which means your body stores it for future use. It's important to get enough B$_{12}$ during pregnancy so that if you breastfeed you'll have enough stored B$_{12}$ available to nourish your baby.

Common Questions

Q. I've had to get several ultrasounds, and I'm worried that they're hurting my baby. Are multiple ultrasounds safe?

A. Scientists have made many attempts to establish a connection between ultrasound exposure and every possible consequence to babies in utero, from leukemia to learning disabilities. No harmful effect has been established.

Of course, that doesn't mean that your provider should be making ultrasound a routine part of every prenatal visit. Each time a scan is suggested, ask the reason for it. The most common, valid reasons for having an ultrasound include dating your pregnancy, diagnosing unsuspected physical abnormalities, determining problems with the placenta or the baby's position, assessing whether you're carrying twins or more, and monitoring growth. If you have the scan, tell your provider and the technician exactly what information you want to be told and what you'd rather have them hold back (for example, the sex of your baby).

If an abnormality does show up when you get an ultrasound, discuss it with your provider. You can always request a second opinion from a specialist.

It's also important to have your ultrasounds done in licensed facilities. If you're in doubt about your hospital or birth center's ultrasound equipment and technician training, contact the American Institute of Ultrasound in Medicine for a referral to a licensed facility (301-498-4100; www.aium.org).

Q. There's a new place in the mall where you can get keepsake ultrasounds. I'd love to have an ultrasound photo album showing every week of my baby's development. Are these ultrasounds safe?

A. These so-called keepsake ultrasounds may be safe in some places, but there is absolutely no reason to get one. An ultrasound is a medical diagnostic test and should always be performed by licensed technicians on approved equipment.

The long-term effects of repeated exposures to ultrasound are not well enough known to give a blanket approval to every establishment that wants to sell pictures of babies in utero. Many parents have the erroneous idea that these keepsake videos and pictures are good diagnostic tools, when in fact they're not typically performed by doctors or trained sonographers. The American Institute of Ultrasound in Medicine and the FDA have therefore discouraged this practice. If you want a peek at your developing baby, ask your health care provider for pictures when you go for your regular ultrasound.

Week 24

Your Baby

The inside story

This week heralds one of the most important thresholds in pregnancy: Your baby is considered "viable." That means that he now weighs well over 1 pound and has a better than 50 percent chance of surviving with intensive care if you deliver prematurely. This is due in large part to the final development of airway passages and air sacs in his lungs.

During the remaining weeks of pregnancy, your baby will gain about 6–7 pounds. His ears are now extremely sensitive to sounds outside the womb, and he can recognize your voice. In fact, research shows us that babies have their earliest language lessons in the womb; after birth, they suck more vigorously if they hear tape recordings of people speaking in their native tongue than they do if they hear people speaking a foreign language. There is no evidence that babies prefer the voices of their fathers, grandmothers, or siblings, but they definitely recognize their mothers' voices and prefer them once they're born.

Through ultrasound scientists have learned that even unborn babies love to play. Yours will continue to pedal around on the uterine walls, and he'll try to grab everything around him with his increasingly strong grip. His favorite toy—well, his only toy, really—is the umbilical cord, which he might yank or swing or pull on for entertainment. Don't worry, though. This thick bundle of blood vessels is remarkably strong, and the force of blood rushing through it keeps the cord extended and prevents kinking.

Your Body

Freckles, moles, and more

Your hormones are at work again now that it's the end of your 2nd trimester. This time they're causing pigment changes in your skin. Your nipples are getting darker, as are your freckles. You may have a dark line of skin dividing your growing belly in half. This common complexion change is called "linea nigra" and is the result of darkening skin pigment during pregnancy; it usually fades or disappears completely over a few months after your baby is born. Other more bothersome changes may occur. (See "Common Skin Problems in Pregnancy," page 194.) If your skin starts to trouble you, ask your doctor

Common Skin Problems in Pregnancy

Problem	What it is/effects	Solutions
Dark spots on the skin	Approximately 90 percent of pregnant women find dark spots on their skin. This condition is called hyperpigmentation, and it results from excess production of melanin, a natural substance that gives color to the hair, skin, and eyes. These spots can appear anywhere on the body, but they most often occur on the breasts, nipples, genital skin, and inner thighs.	The spots usually disappear after you give birth.
Mask of pregnancy	In 70 percent of pregnant women, skin darkens in a masklike pattern on the face.	It might be unsettling to see this new face in the mirror, but this is a benign condition that should fade after your baby is born. Ask your doctor about a pregnancy-safe cosmetic to conceal it in the meantime. Stay out of the sun, because sun exposure tends to make it worse.
Growing moles	Freckles and moles often get bigger and darker during pregnancy. Usually it's nothing to worry about.	Point out moles to your obstetrician if they change shape or tend to bleed; it may be a sign of skin cancer. Your doctor will likely refer you to a dermatologist for a closer look.
Acne	You may experience flare-up of pimples on the face, trunk, and back	Reduce flare-ups by washing your face several times a day and avoiding heavy makeup. (See "Complexion problems," page 33.)
Red bumps	One of the most benign, common skin changes in mid- to late pregnancy is also the most annoying. It's called pruritic urticarial papules and plaques (PUPP), a fancy name for an itchy, bumpy red rash that you might get first on your belly. It can spread down your thighs, onto your bottom, or upward to your breasts. There's no known cause for PUPP, though some researchers think it might have something to do with how much your skin stretches, because women who gain a lot of weight in pregnancy are most apt to get it. Although the itching can drive you nuts, PUPP carries no serious health risks.	It will disappear after delivery. Your provider will probably tell you to treat it with oral Benadryl to reduce discomfort.

Problem	What it is/effects	Solutions
Stretch marks	Among the most despised of pregnancy side effects are stretch marks, those pinkish-purplish-reddish bands that can appear on the abdomen, breasts, hips, buttocks, or thighs. Approximately 90 percent of women develop stretch marks, according to the American Academy of Dermatologists. The marks usually appear toward the end of pregnancy, when your skin is stretching to accommodate your growing baby.	There's not much you can do about these, other than monitor your weight gain; some experts believe that rapid weight gain is the biggest culprit. Various creams and lotions are sold to help prevent stretch marks from developing or getting worse, but the jury is out on whether they work. Stretch marks generally pale to nearly invisible lines within a year after your baby is born. (See "Stretch marks," page 135).
Preexisting skin conditions	If you had eczema, psoriasis, atopic dermatitis, or other skin diseases before conceiving, they may worsen during pregnancy.	Talk with your doctor or dermatologist about how to manage these conditions if they flare up.
Skin tags	These little flaps of skin can appear on various parts of a woman's body throughout pregnancy. They form wherever your skin rubs against something, like the band on your bra.	If they don't recede after pregnancy, they can be easily removed.
Too much hair	You probably don't mind having a little extra hair on your head, but your face and chest are a different story! Changes in the endocrine system during pregnancy can sometimes cause the growth of unwanted body hair.	If this happens to you, it's safe to use chemical hair-bleach and hair-removal products, but check with your doctor to be sure. Rest assured that your body hair will return to its normal prepregnancy amounts a few months after your baby is born.

about skin treatments that are safe during pregnancy. The medications that worked for you prepregnancy may cause birth defects.

Sciatica

As your baby grows bigger, you may notice that she's lying on your sciatic nerve. Ouch! This nerve is the largest and longest one in your body. About the width of your thumb, the nerve originates at the lower end of your spinal cord. It splits there to run down through your pelvic area, through each buttock and thigh, and along each leg to each foot. Sciatica is the name for any pain associated with the sciatic nerve.

Some people describe sciatica as an intense pain that radiates from one buttock down the back of that leg. Others feel it more in their hips. Descriptions of sciatica include tingling, burning, prickling, or stabbing pain that may be there all the time or come and go. In any case, sciatica can make you truly miserable, especially if you happen to be on a long road trip or working in an office where it's difficult to get up and move around.

Chances are your sciatica will lessen or go away completely after you have your baby. For some women the pain will subside during pregnancy as the baby grows and moves off the nerve.

Meanwhile, to treat the sciatica, ice the area several times a day as soon as

Bleeding gums

One morning you're brushing your teeth and find that you're spitting blood when you rinse your mouth. That's a sign of gingivitis, or inflamed and bleeding gums, which affects up to 75 percent of all women during pregnancy.

During pregnancy, you're more apt to get gingivitis, which is caused by plaque, because your gums, like other tissues, swell in response to your new hormone levels, and your immune system may be less resistant.

Some studies show that pregnant women who have gum infections are at greater risk for having a premature or low birthweight baby. Head off gingivitis by brushing your teeth regularly with a soft toothbrush, flossing several times a day, chewing sugarless gum when you can't brush after a meal, and using an antiseptic mouthwash. Add a visit to the dentist as part of your prenatal care. Your hygienist can examine you for gum inflammation or infection, and a thorough cleaning to remove any plaque buildup can probably see you through the rest of your pregnancy. (See "Dental care," page 108.)

You may also have bleeding gums if you have a pregnancy tumor known as a pyogenic granuloma. That's a scary name for something that's no big deal: tiny, fleshy nodules that appear on your gums and may bleed easily. They generally disappear on their own after childbirth; you can have them removed before your due date if they bother you too much.

the pain hits. After a couple of days, apply a hot-water bottle. Some women get relief from warm baths. It's also safe to take acetaminophen, and you can talk to your provider about acupuncture. Stretching exercises that focus on the lower back, buttock, and hamstring muscles can reduce discomfort, as can swimming or walking.

When diarrhea strikes

At some point in your pregnancy, you may have diarrhea. Generally, it is brought on by gastrointestinal bacteria that you either picked up from someone else or contracted by eating spoiled food. These cases rarely last more than 72 hours.

Although it's a lousy way to spend a Sunday, you're better off letting diarrhea run its course than trying to stop it. It may worry you if the food you eat passes right through your body. However, missing out on nutrition for a couple of days isn't going to hurt you or your baby. The most important thing is to keep replenishing your fluids with clear liquids such as water, chicken broth, or juices.

If you have a severe or prolonged case of diarrhea, diarrhea accompanied by a fever, or stools that look bloody or contain mucus, contact your health care provider. Your provider may check you for other infections and parasites, especially if you've been around people with other serious illnesses or if you've traveled someplace (such as a foreign country)

where the water isn't considered potable. If you are very dehydrated, you may be treated with an IV, and your doctor may suggest an antidiarrheal medication.

Your Self

Keeping your focus at work

As your body grows larger, you may feel as if your cubicle is closing in on you. If you're dreading going to work each day, think about what you can do to make yourself more comfortable. Try these ideas to stay alert and focused throughout the day:

- If you're sleepy or overheated, take a brisk walk during your mid-morning coffee break, again at lunch, and in the afternoon before you go home. This is especially important if you work in a factory, kitchen, or other place where temperature extremes are the norm. You own body's thermostat is set higher during pregnancy, so keeping cool is essential.
- If you suffer from headaches at work, press a cold, damp paper towel to your forehead. If you can, turn off the light in your office for a few minutes and rest your eyes.
- You may be plagued with all sorts of aches and pains as your pregnancy progresses. If there's a particular complaint that seems associated with your job—neck strain, shoulder strain, or sciatica, for instance—investigate the ergonomics of your desk and chair.

Should you raise your chair? Bring in a footstool? Work part of the time standing up if you're always sitting down on the job, or vice versa. Good posture is critical for a healthy back, so invest in a maternity support garment if you're starting to have trouble keeping your posture in line. Dump all nonessentials out of your handbag too; this will help reduce strain on your neck and shoulders.

- Eat lunch somewhere other than huddled over your computer terminal and stock up on healthy snacks so you can avoid running downstairs to the junk food vending machine every hour.
- If your workplace has a refrigerator, store reusable cold packs there to use on aching muscles. When driving is part of your job, allow extra time so that you can stop and use a restroom or stretch your legs.

Feathering your nest

Some expectant moms never feel the urge to decorate the nursery, touch baby sweaters at the department store, or test the mechanics of that bright blue stroller a friend has donated to you. But many women use their 2nd- and early 3rd-trimester energy bursts to start feathering their baby's home with all sorts of new gear and clothing.

Although your baby doesn't need much more than diapers, a safe place to sleep, and you, it's still fun to shop—but you knew that already, didn't you? Getting your home ready for a baby represents a novel adventure for any first-time mom and a nostalgic wander down memory lane for experienced mothers. Always include your partner in your buying decisions or he'll start worrying all over again about the cost of this baby.

Where to begin? With a list, of course. There may be some items that you'd rather borrow than buy. If you haven't done so already, check your own closets and the attics of your friends to see what you can find for free. Next, look at what's left on the list and decide which items are absolutely necessary. An infant seat, a crib, and a changing table are good places to start. Then cruise the stores and virtual aisles of the Internet to compare prices on the big-ticket items. Don't let zealous salespeople persuade you to buy anything yet; at this stage, focus on comparison shopping and talk to friends and family about the items they found most useful. (For instance, most people will tell you that a Diaper Genie is nice for disposing diapers, but an infant swing is a better investment if your baby is fussy; so if you can buy only one thing, make it that.) And if a friend wants to throw a baby shower, accept the offer! Even if this is your second or third child, it's always nice to start with a few brand-new things to welcome the new family member.

In addition to buying things for your baby, you may feel a different sort of nesting instinct kick in—namely, the urge to get down on your hands and knees and scrub the floor, repaper the dining room, or clean out every closet. While it's fine to indulge yourself in some of this mania, bear in mind that you can get hurt doing heavier chores now that you're heavier and clumsier yourself; you might be better off investing your energy in a walk. After all, your baby isn't going to care one bit whether you've gotten that last tea stain off the kitchen counter.

Diet & Exercise

The right weight gain

In week 24, the recommended weight gain to date for an ordinary pregnancy in a normal-weight woman is about 14–16 pounds. If you've gained a lot more than that, review what you're eating and how much exercise you're getting. Now is not the time to go on a diet. However, cutting out junk food and increasing your intake of fruits and vegetables makes sense.

Also, if you've slacked off on your exercise regimen, now is a good time to get moving again. Buy a pedometer and start walking. Studies show that women who wear pedometers walk 1 mile per day more than those who don't wear these devices.

If you've gained a lot of weight, forgive yourself and then focus on what you can do from this point onward. Resolve to eat smarter and exercise to keep your weight gain on track for the rest of your pregnancy.

Maternity workout wear

Not so long ago, expectant mothers who liked to exercise had to squeeze into their non-maternity workout wear or buy larger-size workout wear that was too loose in some places and too tight in others. Today, several companies sell exercise clothing created specifically for a pregnant woman's figure.

Exercise clothes should fit without being restrictive, and they should keep you cool. Spandex-type fabrics fit comfortably and wick moisture away from the skin. Some women choose a one-piece unitard; others prefer shorts and a top. Either way, always wear a supportive exercise bra, especially during your 3rd trimester.

Common Questions

Q. How early can my baby be born without dying or having severe birth defects?

A. Only 10 years ago, a fetus wasn't considered viable until 28 weeks, but now more than half of all babies born at 24 weeks can survive. However, there are still serious risks associated with premature birth, including neurological impairments and death, and premature children are 50 percent more likely to need special education classes.

Among premature babies, those born between 35 and 37 weeks have the best chance of being healthy because they generally have mature lungs and don't need a tube to breathe. They may have trouble sucking or swallowing, and they may have jaundice. However, these babies can be treated immediately and often can go right home with you.

Babies born between 32 and 35 weeks may take a little longer to learn to control their body temperature, and some will need help breathing. Special techniques may be used to help these babies eat because sucking and swallowing may be a difficult task. Most of these children go on to develop normally; however, preemies of this age may be more likely to contract infections because of their immature immune systems.

Babies born between 27 and 32 weeks will probably weigh no more than 4 pounds. At least 80 percent of these babies develop normally, but many will need help breathing temporarily, even if their mothers were given steroids to help their babies' lungs mature faster. These babies are also more at risk than full-term infants for infection, feeding difficulties, vision problems, and gastrointestinal illnesses.

Babies born between 24 and 27 weeks have a higher death rate, but many survive. Not surprisingly these children suffer the most complications, and as many as 60 percent will need special help in school.

Always remember that every baby is different. Your premature baby may be 10 times feistier than another woman's baby born just as early.

Q. I called my doctor this morning because I was having cramps. I was afraid I was in labor already, even though there are weeks and weeks to go before my due date. She said I should come in for a fetal fibronectin test. I'm nervous. Does the test hurt? What will it tell me?

A. A lot of things can cause cramping during pregnancy that may be mistaken for preterm labor (see "False labor," page 255). The fetal fibronectin test is one way that your provider can decide whether this is true labor and whether you're in danger of delivering your baby immediately.

This test certainly won't hurt; the procedure is basically identical to a Pap smear. Your practitioner will swab your vaginal and cervical secretions and send the samples to a laboratory. A technician will then evaluate the secretions for any evidence of fetal fibronectin, a protein found in amniotic fluid.

The presence of fibronectin can indicate an increased risk of delivering your baby too early. If you test positive, your practitioner may ask you to decrease your activity or possibly to stay in the hospital. She may also prescribe medication to stop the contractions, or she may give you steroids to help your baby's lungs mature faster.

If the test is negative, your cramping is probably not a sign of preterm labor, and you are much less likely to be at risk of going into labor in the immediate future.

the.3rd trimester

③ *You're in the home stretch! You're no doubt excited, even giddy, at the thought of meeting your baby. Will your child have her father's red hair? Your love of the outdoors? You can hardly wait to find out. As your pregnancy draws to an end, your wait may be peppered by mood swings as dramatic as those of your 1st trimester. Fatigue is partly to blame. You may have trouble sleeping through the night because of your size—and because nighttime seems to be playtime for baby, whose movements feel like those of a gold-medal gymnast. Fortunately there are lots of exciting ways to pass these last weeks, from taking childbirth classes to choosing a crib.*

In this section

Week 25

Your Baby

The inside story

Your baby has definite alert and resting periods now. She's still much skinnier than she'll be at birth, but she continues to fill out. By the end of this week she'll probably weigh about 1½ pounds.

Her eyes are open now, perhaps even blinking and closing when she sleeps. The nerves around her mouth are becoming sensitive as she prepares to be able to suckle and nourish her own body after birth.

For now, though, you're still nourishing your unborn child via the umbilical cord; your blood carries nutrients to your baby through the cord, which consists of a single vein and two arteries. The umbilical cord is protected against your baby's gymnastics by Wharton's jelly—a gelatinous goo that keeps the umbilical cord from twisting and knotting as your baby continues to test her muscles and find things to occupy her waking time.

As your baby grows, so does her brain. Deeper grooves and furrows are developing in her cerebral cortex, which is going to be Command Central for many important functions including her ability to see, hear, smell, speak, and walk. Already her brain controls her rhythmic breathing, digestion, and body temperature; these three activities are essential in order for your baby to be able to live outside your body.

Your Body

Bigger and bigger breasts

Are you surprised at how big your breasts have grown? Breasts grow even larger during the 3rd trimester. You may even find that when you sit down your breasts rest on your belly. It's not a wonderful feeling, but at least it's for a good cause: Your breasts are preparing to produce milk that can later nourish your baby.

Although your belly will become smaller right after your baby comes out, your breasts will not. In fact 24 hours to 48 hours after delivery, they will grow even larger as they fill with milk. (It's a process also known as "letting down" or "having your milk come in.") Nursing or expressing the milk reduces their size until the next breastfeeding session, when they fill up with milk again. Your breasts will return to their prepregnancy size after you wean your baby.

week 25

Breathlessness

You may feel even more short of breath in the 3rd trimester. Why? As your baby grows larger and takes up more and more of the space inside your abdomen, other organs are squeezed and pushed aside. Your lungs don't have the room they need to expand with a full breath. Your diaphragm can't offer much help because it is compressed too. (This doesn't cause any permanent damage; after your baby is born, your organs will slip right back into their prepregnancy position.)

Don't worry. As always, Mother Nature has provided for your baby. Although you may feel as if you're getting less air, high levels of progesterone help you take deeper breaths and get more oxygen into your blood. And because your blood volume is higher during pregnancy, more oxygen passes back and forth across the placenta as you inhale and exhale.

Easing symptoms. If you become winded during the day, slow down for a few minutes. Your breath should return. Make an effort to sit up straight during the day to give your lungs more breathing room. You can also consciously breathe in a way that raises your rib cage; check that your ribs push out against your hands as you inhale deeply. At night you may feel as if you're hyperventilating. You can ease that sensation by sleeping with your head raised on more than one pillow. If your breathlessness is accompanied by chest pains, call your doctor right away.

Luckily most women get relief from this breathlessness before childbirth. When your baby's head drops into your birth canal—about 2 or 3 weeks before delivery—you'll have more room for your diaphragm and breathe more easily.

Asthma sufferers. Women with asthma sometimes find that their symptoms worsen during the 3rd trimester. If your asthma gets worse, talk with your doctor. Many asthma medicines are considered safe during pregnancy. (See "Asthma," page 85.) Doctors usually prefer to prescribe inhaled medications because they have a more localized effect and work well; if you discover that your chest feels tight, however, tell your doctor.

Other breathing problems

It might be tempting to dismiss any 3rd-trimester breathlessness as normal, but if you experience shortness of breath that's sudden, severe, or associated with chest pain or a faster pulse, get medical help immediately. This could mean that a blood clot has settled in your lungs; it's a rare but dangerous occurrence among pregnant women, especially those with blood clots in their legs.

Be aware, too, that breathing problems can be caused by pneumonia. Usually accompanied by fever, chest pain, and cough, pneumonia is the third-leading cause of death among pregnant women. Pneumonia can be viral or bacterial; with either one, potential complications can include respiratory failure,

Preterm labor and delivery

An ordinary pregnancy lasts 37 to 42 weeks, with 40 weeks being the average. Most babies arrive near their due date, give or take a week or two. However, about 12 percent of babies in the United States are born before the 37th week. This is known as preterm birth.

Risks to the baby. Babies do a lot of developing during the last trimester of pregnancy, and if they're born early, they face an uphill battle. Preterm birth is the leading cause of death among newborns. Those who survive are more likely than full-term babies to have lifelong health problems such as developmental delays, hearing loss, blindness, chronic lung disease, and cerebral palsy. About 25 percent of very premature infants (those born before 32 weeks' gestation) suffer significant, long-term impairment of brain development.

Your likelihood of a preterm birth. Researchers have identified some of the risk factors for premature births. A woman is more likely to have a premature baby if she:

- Has had a previous premature delivery.
- Is pregnant with more than one baby.
- Suffers from a chronic illness such as diabetes or hypertension.
- Was very overweight or underweight before pregnancy.
- Smokes cigarettes.
- Is African-American.
- Has had an infection such as bacterial vaginosis, a urinary tract infection, or sexually transmitted infections during pregnancy.
- Is under age 17 or over age 35.
- Has experienced severe chronic stress or anxiety during pregnancy.
- Became pregnant with the help of infertility treatments.
- Has particular or certain abnormalities in her cervix or uterus.
- Has experienced domestic violence during pregnancy.

Prevention. If you are at increased risk for preterm birth because you had a previous preterm birth, your doctor may recommend weekly progesterone injections known as 17P. In recent studies, administering weekly progesterone injections beginning at weeks 16–20 to women with a history of preterm birth reduced the chance of another preterm birth by as much as 33 percent. This medication is not for all women; talk to your doctor.

Warning signs. In some cases medical treatment can delay preterm labor and give a baby more time to grow before being born. Treatment works best when it is administered early, so watch for these signs of early labor. Even if you are experiencing only one of the following symptoms, call your doctor right away. It's better to be overcautious than to take the chance of letting premature labor continue without medical care:

- Contractions every 10 minutes or less.
- Fluid or blood coming from your vagina.
- A sense of pressure in the pelvis that feels as if your baby is pushing down.
- A low, dull backache or cramps that feel like menstrual cramps.
- A change in vaginal discharge from creamy white to thin and mucousy.

When you call the doctor, he or she will ask about your symptoms and your gestational age. (Remember to report the weeks.) He or she may ask you to come into the office or go to the hospital to be monitored and to have a cervical exam to see if your cervix is dilating. If you are having contractions with cervical change, then you are having preterm labor.

Medical interventions. If you have symptoms of premature labor, your doctor may order a fetal fibronectin (fFN) test, which measures the level of a certain protein in your cervical-vaginal secretions. A negative fFN test is a highly reliable predictor that delivery will not occur within the next two weeks. A positive fFN test is not nearly as reliable; you may deliver early, but then again you may not. There are no tests that accurately predict which women with preterm labor will have a preterm birth. Many times it is a nerve-racking wait-and-see situation.

Some doctors recommend bed rest to prevent preterm labor, although research does not show that bed rest actually helps to stave off premature labor. Despite the scarcity of solid evidence, however, most doctors are cautious and advise bed rest for preterm labor.

Although doctors can't stop preterm labor, they can administer tocolytics, a class of medications that can often slow down labor for two to three days. Although that might not sound like much time, it can make a difference: Even a few extra days in the uterus can increase a preterm baby's chance of healthy survival, especially at extremely early gestational ages (24–26 weeks). If you are at 24–34 weeks' gestation, you will probably be given corticosteroids, a medication that increases the amount of surfactant in the baby's lungs. Surfactant allows the baby to breathe easier and spend less time after birth on a ventilator. The baby needs to stay in utero for at least 48 hours after you receive corticosteroids to receive the drug's maximum benefit. If your water has broken, you may receive antibiotics to prevent group B strep infection (see "Common Questions," page 306) and prolong in utero time.

Medical care after delivery. After birth a preterm baby goes to the neonatal intensive care unit (NICU), which contains medical equipment that helps the baby breathe, stay warm, take in nourishment, and receive care for health problems. In the NICU, a baby receives treatment from a neonatologist, a pediatrician who is specially trained to help premature babies. A preterm baby may spend anywhere from a few days to a few months in the NICU, depending on how early the baby was born and what health problems exist.

Choosing the right hospital. If you are at increased risk for preterm delivery, investigate your hospital's NICU. Hospitals are given designations that indicate the level of neonatal care they provide. A level 1 hospital has no neonatal intensive care unit; a level 3 hospital offers the most advanced care, with state-of-the-art equipment and the most highly trained staff. If your hospital is level 1, you may want to consider going to a different hospital. Also remember that half of all preterm births occur in women who are not at high risk. If you're not at high risk and plan to use a level 1 hospital, ask your obstetrician what will happen if you have preterm labor. If there is time to safely transport you with baby in utero to a level 3 hospital, that is the ideal situation.

week 25

premature delivery, or infections that can harm your unborn baby.

Rib pain

If it feels like your rib cage is getting larger, you're right: It's expanding to make room for your lungs, which need extra oxygen, and for your baby, who may decide to stretch out and push his feet up under your ribs. Some women will feel pain in the upper right corner of their abdomen over the last few ribs. This may be caused by inflammation of cartilage attached to the ribs.

Shifting positions may lessen your discomfort because it may cause your baby to move into a new position too. During the day, sit in a straight-back chair with a pillow behind your lower back to help relieve the pressure and make breathing easier. A warm bath or a heating pad may also help.

There is some relief in sight: Your ribs may feel less stretched during the last few weeks of pregnancy, when your baby moves down into position for birth.

Multiplying multiples

Multiple births seem to dominate the news and celebrity magazines. That's not surprising. During the past 25 years or so, the number of twin births in the United States has increased 65 percent, and the number of higher-order multiples (triplets or more) has increased by more than 400 percent, according to the National Center for Health Statistics. Approximately three of every 100 babies born in the United States are multiples.

Why the increase? Part of the reason is that women in the United States are waiting longer to have babies. As a woman ages, her chance of having multiples goes up. Assisted reproduction techniques (ART) such as in vitro fertilization also contribute to the rise in multiples. About half of the births that result from ART are multiples.

Your likelihood of multiples. Multiples are more likely to be born to mothers who have them in their family. According to recent studies, maternal height and weight come into play too. Women in the top 25th percentile of height and those with a body mass index of 30 or greater (which is considered obese) are more likely than thinner, shorter women to have multiples.

Twins are most common. The vast majority of multiple births are twins; they account for about 95 percent of multiple births. Twins can be identical or fraternal. Identical twins, which account for one-third of twin sets, occur when one fertilized egg splits early in pregnancy and develops into two fetuses. With fraternal twins, each fetus develops from a separate egg and sperm. Identical twins share one placenta and amniotic sac; fraternal twins each have their own placenta and amniotic sac.

The chance of having identical twins versus fraternal twins is not linked to age, family history, or anything else that scientists have uncovered so far. Having identical twins is believed to be an unpredictable, random event.

Detecting multiples. In your mother's day, a woman discovered she was having multiples in the delivery room, when the doctor pulled out one baby and realized that the party wasn't over yet. Now ultrasounds show multiples as early as 6 weeks into pregnancy and can detect more than 95 percent of multiples by the beginning of the 2nd trimester. If you don't have an ultrasound, or if you have one later in your pregnancy, your doctor may suspect multiples after hearing more than one heartbeat. Multiples are also a possibility if you are gaining a lot of weight, if your uterus is much larger than your gestational age would suggest, or if you have severe morning sickness. Multiples may be in your future if you have abnormal results on the multiple marker screening test, also known as the quad marker screen; this blood test is done between weeks 15 and 20.

Risks and precautions. Women who are pregnant with multiples see their doctors more often. Their pregnancies are usually considered high-risk because they have a greater chance of miscarrying one or more of the fetuses. They're also at higher risk for premature labor, gestational diabetes, preeclampsia, iron deficiency anemia, and intrauterine growth restriction, which indicates that a fetus is growing poorly. Multiples usually arrive early: 60 percent of twins, 90 percent of

triplets, and virtually all multiples greater than triplets are born preterm. Here's a quick rule: On average, singletons arrive at 40 weeks, twins at 36 weeks, triplets at 32 weeks, and quadruplets at 28 weeks.

Multiples are often born by cesarean delivery because premature babies are less likely to be vertex (in the head-down position). Almost all high-order multiples (three babies or more) are delivered by cesarean. Many twins may be delivered vaginally, especially if baby A (the baby that is presenting) is head down and baby B is smaller or the same size as baby A.

Your Self

Enjoying your new figure

Some women love the physical feeling of being pregnant and relish their expanding figure. Others struggle as they watch the disappearance of the waist they worked so hard to keep trim and the expansion of the bottom that was wide enough to begin with, thank you very much.

If your full figure depresses you, keep your eye on the prize, so to speak: You're growing larger in order to bring a new life into the world. That said, you may still feel frustrated when you reach the point of weighing more than your partner or when you take up two seats on the commuter train instead of one. Harness those feelings and use them to fuel your resolve when you're tempted to binge

week 25

on a stack of chocolate chip cookies or skip your workout. And remember, the change in your body is temporary.

Spider veins

Have you noticed any thin red lines on your breasts? Those are called spider veins. They are capillaries that can appear just about anywhere on your body, although they're most commonly found on the breasts. Because of an increased need for oxygen, your body manufactures as much as 40 percent more blood during pregnancy. All this extra blood can plump up blood vessels and make them more visible beneath the skin. Spider veins are more visible in women with fair skin.

Diet & Exercise

When it's twins—or more

If the stork will be bringing you more than one baby, you may be encouraged to head to the refrigerator a few extra times each day. Your doctor will likely advise you to consume more calories and gain more weight than you would if you were having just one baby. Ordinarily, women who start their pregnancy at normal weight are advised to gain 35–45 pounds with twins and 50–60 pounds with triplets.

To gain those additional pounds, you'll need to consume an extra 450–500 calories a day (rather than 300) and more if you are very active. Bulk up your diet with nutritious foods: fruits and vegetables, lean protein, whole grains, nuts, beans, and non-fat dairy foods. Talk with your doctor about whether you need extra vitamin supplements beyond your prenatal vitamin.

If your multiples pregnancy is proceeding without complications, your doctor will probably allow you to exercise moderately. If complications arise, your doctor may recommend that you stop exercising, particularly during the second half of pregnancy.

When exercise is a no-no

If your doctor instructs you to stop exercising, you may wonder if your pregnancy will still be healthy. When doctors make decisions about whether a pregnant woman should exercise, they compare the risks with the benefits. For a woman with an uncomplicated pregnancy, exercise is a healthy choice because the benefits outweigh any possible risks. However, if you begin your pregnancy with certain health problems or develop them along the way, your doctor may decide that exercise could complicate your pregnancy. In that situation the healthier choice for you is not to exercise because the risks of exercise outweigh the benefits.

Pregnancy massage

One of the nicest gifts you can give yourself is a pregnancy massage. As your belly grows larger, the muscles in your shoulders and back have to work harder to keep you upright. Overworked muscles can tighten, and massage is a wonderful way to loosen them up.

Massage therapists who specialize in pregnancy massage have tables with fold-down panels that allow a pregnant woman to lie facedown with her belly supported but not squashed. You may also have a chair massage; the massage therapist will work on your shoulders and back as you sit in a chair and lean forward, resting your head on a padded surface.

Common Questions

Q. Can I train for labor?

A. Giving birth is a bit like running a marathon: The better prepared you are physically, the easier it is to make it to the finish line. Studies show that women who are in good physical shape before delivery have shorter labors and need fewer interventions such as forceps delivery, vacuum delivery, and cesarean delivery. According to their own reports, fit women feel emotionally better prepared for labor than women who are less fit.

Fitness makes a difference in several ways. Ample aerobic capacity helps you endure the physical demands of labor and delivery. Good flexibility makes it easier for you to labor in different positions. Strong muscles come in handy when it's time to push the baby out. Having an athlete's mind-set can help too: Some women athletes say the experience of competing in sports prepares them for the rigors of labor. You don't have to be a jock though: Even daily walking counts and will make a difference in your fitness.

Physical fitness doesn't guarantee a short, easy labor. Other factors play a part. For example, a woman who is well rested before delivery will have more stamina than one who is exhausted.

If you have been exercising throughout your pregnancy, keep at it, provided your doctor approves. If you've been sedentary so far, talk with your doctor about whether you can begin a gentle walking program or take a prenatal exercise class.

Q. Should I have a delivery and birth plan?

A. Many women have strong feelings about how they would like to deliver their baby. In order to ensure that their wishes are respected during labor, some choose to draw up a birth plan. A birth plan can include details about your preferences regarding some of the following:

- Labor environment (for example, soft music or dim lights)
- Who will be present during your labor and delivery (doula, midwife, partner, relatives)
- Medical or nursing students observing or participating in your delivery
- Mobility during labor
- Routine IVs
- Fetal monitoring
- Pain medication
- Episiotomy
- Cutting the umbilical cord
- Breastfeeding immediately after birth
- Keeping the baby in your room with you

Share your birth plan with your doctor, midwife, and/or doula. More important than the written plan, however, are the conversations you have with your nurse and delivery provider. Many women fear that they won't be able to articulate their needs in labor. If you speak up, you can get your point across, even between frequent contractions. Your partner or other trusted person who will be with you in labor can help you communicate.

Be prepared for the possibility that your preferences may change during labor, particularly if this is your first baby. Women who swear that they would never, ever consider using pain medication sometimes find themselves begging for it, and those who think they need medication may find they can get along fine without it.

Whether you have a birth plan or a mental image of ideal childbirth, a ready-for-everything attitude comes in handy during labor and delivery. It's reasonable to plan what you want ahead of time, but it's also important to be flexible.

Week 26

Your Baby

The inside story

You loved feeling those delightful first kicks. Now, however, you're more likely to say "ouch" as your baby's length passes the 14-inch mark and his weight climbs to nearly 2 pounds. In fact his movements are so strong that your partner should be able to feel them easily. Your partner might even hear your baby's heartbeat if he puts his head on your belly. Your baby is probably still in the breech position (head up) at this point because your pear-shape uterus offers him more legroom that way.

Although he's still wrinkly, your baby is now at 25 percent of his expected birthweight, and he's going to really pile on the ounces in the next couple of months. His spine is getting stronger, and if he were born now, he would have an 80 percent chance of survival. He's now capable of inhaling, exhaling, and even crying. That lanugo hair that grew all over his body is rapidly disappearing, and it will probably be completely gone by the end of the 7th month except for some fuzz on his back and shoulders. Your baby's eyes are becoming more sensitive; if you were to shine a light on your belly, he would notice.

Your Body

The best sleep positions

Finding a comfortable sleep position can be a challenge when you have a belly the size of a beach ball. Sleeping on your stomach is out because it's simply not comfortable. Lying on your back for too long might make you feel nauseated because your uterus presses on a large blood vessel called the inferior vena cava. Your best option? Side-sleeping.

Lie on your side—preferably your left side—because major blood

---

Fetal heart arrhythmia

An arrhythmia is an irregular heartbeat. Doctors sometimes discover that a baby has an irregular heartbeat, on an ultrasound, with a Doppler (a device that amplifies the sound of a baby's heartbeat), or with a stethoscope. It sounds as if the heart is sometimes skipping a beat. This is usually nothing to worry about; babies tend to outgrow their prenatal arrhythmias and have healthy hearts at birth.

vessels lie to the right of your spine, and sleeping on your left side allows blood to flow freely through these vessels. Insert a pillow between your legs and, if it helps, a pillow under your belly. Some women find that specially designed pregnancy body pillows help them slumber soundly, although with you and the body pillow in the bed, there may not be much room left for your partner.

If you wake up and realize you're lying on your back, it's all right; flip over to your left side and go back to sleep. Being on your back may be why you awoke—if your circulation is being compromised by your sleep position, you will start to feel uncomfortable, and your body will automatically switch positions, whether you awaken or not.

Braxton Hicks contractions

Think of Braxton Hicks contractions as fire drills: They are not a sign that labor is imminent; they are a way for your body to prepare for labor. These mild, cramplike contractions—which feel like a squeezing or tightening of the uterus—begin during the second half of pregnancy. They occur irregularly and usually last for 30 seconds to 2 minutes. Braxton Hicks contractions are named for the doctor who first described them.

Braxton Hicks contractions differ from woman to woman and from pregnancy to pregnancy. Some women have them several times a day; others don't seem to have them at all. They may occur more often after exercise or intercourse. They tend to feel more intense and happen more often as pregnancy progresses.

It's important not to confuse Braxton Hicks contractions with real labor contractions. Braxton Hicks contractions do not occur in a regular pattern, whereas real contractions do. If contractions occur regularly—every 10 minutes or more than 6 per hour—you may be in labor. Call your doctor right away.

Uncomfortable intercourse

You and your partner may start to find that your old, familiar lovemaking positions don't fit your new, curvier figure. However, you don't need the flexibility of a gymnast in order to maintain a love life during pregnancy.

Try experimenting with different positions. Consider making love side by side (either facing each other or with your partner facing your back); with you on top, leaning forward and supporting yourself with your hands and arms so he doesn't penetrate too deeply; or with him on top with his arms outstretched to hold himself up so he doesn't crush your belly. Unless your doctor advises against it or your partner has herpes, oral sex is another option, if you're both comfortable with it.

Your Self

The naming game

Choosing a name for your bundle of joy can be one of the most enjoyable—and, surprisingly, most stressful—parts of pregnancy. Here are a few suggestions to take some of the bumps out of the decision:

- Talk with your partner about his expectations regarding baby names. Is there a family name he'd like to pass on? Does he have any ethnic or religious traditions that he'd like to honor? Share your ideas too.
- Before discussing specific names, talk about the categories of names you and your partner both like: Traditional names? One-of-a-kind names? Names that start with a certain letter?
- Take advantage of the many books and websites that list thousands of baby names and their meanings.
- Be prepared for the possibility that you and your partner have completely different approaches to name-choosing. You might like to snuggle up with a book of 10,000 baby names; your partner may prefer a more free-form strategy, such as listing the names of his best high school buddies. There's no right or wrong way to go through this process. If each person is patient with the other's approach, you'll agree on a name eventually.
- Be open-minded. Avoid saying no automatically when your partner suggests what you consider to be a horrendous name. That name may grow on you with time.
- Think about whether you'll tell others what names you're considering. Do you want to keep it a secret, or would you rather ask for lots of opinions about your possible choices? If you tell, be prepared for people to respond with comments such as "I hate that name! I went to school with a kid by that name, and he was a jerk!"

Baby school

You know the old saying: Babies don't come with instruction booklets. Luckily, most hospitals and birth centers offer a variety of classes for expectant moms and dads. Classes aren't mandatory, of course, but they can be a great help because they instill you with confidence about your ability to manage your pregnancy, the delivery, and the beginning of your baby's life. Some hospitals offer classes for free; others may charge a nominal fee. Your obstetrician may have information about classes in your community.

Childbirth education. Learning about labor and delivery beforehand can help relax you by taking away some of the unknowns. Classes are usually taught by a nurse or midwife and are offered in the evenings for several successive weeks or on a weekend. The best time to take a childbirth class is in weeks 34–36 of pregnancy; that way you can complete it 4–6 weeks before your due date.

week 26

During a childbirth class you'll learn how to know you're in labor, what to take with you to the hospital, what happens once you check in to the hospital, relaxation and breathing strategies for coping with pain, information about delivery, details about pain medication, instructions for fathers/coaches, and explanations of unexpected events that may occur during labor and delivery.

Most classes also include a tour of the hospital's maternity area and delivery rooms. This is a great time to ask questions and familiarize yourself with your hospital's procedures. Many hospitals offer a class for first-time parents and a refresher course for those who already have a child but would like to update their knowledge. Some even offer classes for siblings and for first-time grandparents.

Your hospital might also offer classes about specific topics such as vaginal birth after cesarean (VBAC), planned cesarean, natural childbirth (giving birth without pain medications), and giving birth to multiples.

Baby-care education. Classes that teach about infant care can be instructive and fun for expectant parents who have little experience with newborns. An infant-care class will cover such topics as how to give your baby his first bath, how to take care of the umbilical cord stump and circumcision site, the many colors of infant poop and what they all mean, what to do when a baby cries, and so on. Classes in infant/child CPR and baby massage might also be available.

Breastfeeding education. It may sound ridiculous that you would need to learn how to breastfeed—isn't it a natural experience that comes easily to baby and mother? Unfortunately the answer to that question can sometimes be "no." Learning about breastfeeding beforehand can save you and your baby from the stress of trying to figure things out in the hospital and during the first few weeks postpartum. During a class on breastfeeding you'll learn about the benefits of breastfeeding, what happens during first feedings, how to get a baby to latch on to the breast, different ways to position the baby during breastfeeding, what medications are safe and unsafe for nursing mothers, how to use a breast pump and store milk, how to prevent plugged milk ducts, and what to eat (or avoid) while nursing. You may also receive information about how to get in touch with a lactation consultant if you need help after your baby is born.

Many hospitals offer breastfeeding classes. You can also turn to La Leche League (www.lalecheleague.org), an international organization that promotes breastfeeding, or your pediatrician's office for more information.

Your social life

You can't drink alcohol, you feel too tired to stay out late, and you find it hard to listen to what others are saying because you're so focused on your baby. Pregnancy can certainly put a crimp in your social life, and that's perfectly normal. But spending time with your friends and family is still important. You need their support now, and you'll need it even more in a few months, after your baby is born.

Work around your limitations. If you dislike going out to a restaurant and nursing a club soda while everyone else is hoisting mugs of beer, meet your friends for a movie or a walk instead. If you have trouble keeping your eyes open past 9 p.m., invite friends over in the afternoon. And if all you can think about is babies, set up dates with new mothers and friends who are expecting. Or push yourself to talk about topics that aren't related to your baby— sometimes it's good to step back from pregnancy and focus on other subjects for a while.

Diet & Exercise

A lesson on fats

Many people have grown up thinking all fat is bad. You may be thinking you should eliminate as many fats as possible from your diet in order to keep your weight gain in check. That's not really the best plan because fat is an essential nutrient that is vital to you and your baby. Fat supplies the body with energy and transports vitamins A, D, E, and K into the bloodstream.

Good fats. Unsaturated fats (mono- and polyunsaturated fats) have earned the title of "good" fats because they are believed to raise levels of helpful cholesterol (HDL) in the blood.

These fats are found in vegetable oils, avocados, nuts, olives, and other plant foods.

Bad fats. The so-called bad fats are cholesterol, saturated fat, and hydro- genated fats, also called trans fats. Saturated fat and cholesterol are found in animal foods such as fatty meat, poultry skin, bacon, butter, egg yolks, and full-fat dairy products. That's right—all the tasty stuff. These "bad" fats can damage your heart by increasing levels of harmful cholesterol (LDL) in the blood and decreasing levels of HDL. You can cut down on these fats fairly easily by choosing non-fat dairy foods and leaner types of meat, fish, and poultry; limiting eggs to about one a day; and cutting down or eliminating your butter intake.

The other fat to avoid is hydro- genated fat, which contains trans fatty acids, or trans fats; these are even worse for the heart than saturated fats or cholesterol. The current federal dietary guidelines advise people to keep their intake of trans fat very low—just a couple of grams daily. That's not easy: Hydrogenated fat is often an ingredient in commercially prepared foods such as cakes, cookies, crackers, and fast-food french fries and fried chicken.

If a food label doesn't show how many grams of trans fats the food contains, look for words such as "partially hydrogenated vegetable oil" or "vegetable shortening," which indicate that trans fat is present. The best way to reduce your intake of trans fats is to cut down on commercially prepared foods and eat more unprocessed foods.

Eat a rainbow

Dietitians recommend eating the colors of the rainbow, and they're not talking about all of the different hues of jelly beans. Intensely colored fruits and vegetables are full of nutrients. They provide vitamins as well as antioxidants and other phytochemicals that fight cancer, strengthen the immune system, and promote heart health. Make them a part of your diet during pregnancy and beyond. Check out the "Colorful, Nutrient-Rich Fruits and Vegetables" chart (below), which lists the many colors—and health benefits—of produce.

Fatigue during exercise

Walking up a single flight of stairs may leave you as winded as you would have felt climbing five flights prepregnancy. You might find yourself

Colorful, Nutrient-Rich Fruits and Vegetables

Color	Foods	Nutrients, Benefits
Dark orange	Carrots, pumpkins, sweet potatoes	• Vitamin A, beta-carotene, and other antioxidants
Yellow/light orange	Citrus fruits and juices (oranges, grapefruit, lemons), cantaloupe, corn, bananas	• Vitamin C and other antioxidants in citrus fruits • Vitamin A in cantaloupe • Lutein in corn (promotes eye health) • Zeaxanthin in citrus fruits (fights cancer) • Vitamin B6 in bananas • Bioflavonoids in citrus fruits (fight cancer, strengthen the immune system)
Red	Red peppers, strawberries, tomatoes	• Fiber • Vitamin K
Light green	Cabbage, lettuce, green peas, asparagus, Brussels sprouts	• Fiber • Vitamin K • Indoles in Brussels sprouts, cabbage, and asparagus (fight cancer)
Dark green	Spinach, collard greens, mustard greens, broccoli	• Vitamin K • Folic acid • Zeaxanthin and other antioxidants • Sulforaphane in broccoli (may reduce risk of breast cancer)
Purple/blue	Blueberries, blackberries, grapes	• Vitamin C in berries • Antioxidants in grapes

huffing and puffing halfway into an exercise routine that you used to be able to breeze through. That's OK. During the 3rd trimester, it's normal to become easily fatigued by activities that you could easily do a couple of months ago. You're carrying around more weight than before, which can tire you out. And if you're uncomfortable in bed or waking up constantly to go to the bathroom, you may not be getting enough high-quality sleep.

The best way to respond to fatigue is by slowing down. If you ignore it and push yourself to exhaustion, it's not good for you or your baby. Put your feet up and relax. Go to bed early, sleep late, ask your partner to take on more of the household chores. Listen to your body and give it what it needs.

Being thirsty, hungry, or hot can amplify feelings of fatigue. You may feel less worn-out if you stay hydrated, eat frequent mini-meals and snacks, and keep cool air flowing while you exercise. Choose snacks that offer a mix of protein and carbohydrates, such as cheese and crackers. Carbohydrates give immediate energy; the protein hangs on and fuels you after carb energy runs out.

When to stop exercising

Stop exercising and call your doctor if you experience any of the following:
- Bleeding or leakage of fluid from your vagina
- Difficulty breathing, even at rest
- Dizziness
- Headache

- Chest pains
- Muscle weakness
- Calf pain or swelling
- Decreased movement of the fetus

Common Questions

Q. Why am I kicking my partner while I sleep?

A. No, you're not experiencing some kind of subconscious animosity that plays out while you slumber. You may have restless legs syndrome (RLS), a condition that gives you a physiological urge to move, jerk, or kick your legs in response to sensations in your legs. Pregnancy doesn't cause RLS, but the hormonal changes that occur while you're expecting can worsen it. RLS is sometimes a symptom of iron deficiency anemia or diabetes. It can be exacerbated by stress.

Some people are aware that they have RLS because they feel a compelling need to move their legs, particularly late in the day and while they lie still in bed. They describe having a creeping or crawling feeling in their legs that can be relieved only by moving their legs. (Sometimes the feeling is a tingling, cramping, burning, or painful sensation.) Others notice no such sensation, and the only way they know about their nighttime kicking is from the reports their sleeping partners give them.

If you have RLS, you may feel unexpectedly tired during the day; all that kicking and jerking can prevent you from sleeping soundly.

There isn't much that can be done for RLS during pregnancy because the drugs

week 26

used to treat it—anticonvulsants, tranquilizers, opioids, and Parkinson's disease medications—are not recommended for pregnant women. Reducing stress, meditating, or walking before bedtime may help.

Ask your doctor about safe alternative medications such as vitamin E. The good news is that your kicking will probably stop after you have your baby.

Week 27

Your Baby

The inside story

Your baby is getting downright chubby as fat deposits continue accumulating beneath her skin, which looks pink because blood vessels are so close to the surface. She'll rely on those fat deposits after she's born to provide energy and insulate her against cold. By the end of this week, she'll probably weigh more than 2 pounds. The placenta is now almost fully developed.

Your baby is still kicking so much that you might worry if she's suddenly quiet. Don't. How much a baby kicks has more to do with her personality than with her health. If you want to reassure yourself that everything is fine, you can do an average "kick count." Lie on your left side—usually early evening after you've eaten is the best time—and check to see how long it takes to feel 10 movements. Do that every day for a week; then average the number of kicks to see what you should expect. Remember too that your baby's movements will naturally change as you enter your 9th month and her bedroom becomes more cramped.

Your Body

Pelvic bone pain

Toward the end of your pregnancy, you may feel pain in the area below your belly, just above your pubic hair. You may have "pubic symphysis separation." Although it won't affect your baby's health, it can be quite painful.

Your pelvis is a bone that encircles the lower abdomen and almost meets in the middle in the front. The gap between the two edges of the front of the pelvis is bridged by a flexible cartilage called the pubic symphysis (PS). The PS stretches like a rubber band so the pelvis can move and expand to make room for your baby. In rare cases the PS expands so much that it actually separates, which is what causes pain. A woman whose PS separates often has trouble walking, especially going up stairs.

Rest, heat, and wearing a maternity belt (a stretchy belt worn around the lower part of the belly for support) can sometimes offer relief. If the pain is very bad, your doctor may refer you to a physical therapist.

Be patient. This pain will go away within a few weeks of your baby's birth as the PS moves back into its prepregnancy position.

week 27

Hepatitis and pregnancy

Hepatitis is an inflammation of the liver that can cause fever, jaundice, abdominal pain, swelling, scarring of the liver, and, in some cases, permanent liver damage that can lead to life-threatening liver failure. It is most commonly caused by a virus, although drugs, alcohol, metabolic diseases, and autoimmune diseases can also cause it. It is dangerous because it may cause vague flulike symptoms or no symptoms at all, so you can be infected without realizing it. The virus can remain in your blood for months or years, causing liver damage.

Hepatitis can be confusing because various types exist. Each type is given a letter name to differentiate the virus that has caused it. Here's a quick look at the hepatitis alphabet:

TYPE OF HEPATITIS	DESCRIPTION
A (also known as infectious hepatitis)	Mild flulike symptoms such as nausea, a low-grade fever, headache, loss of appetite, and weakness. Passed via food or water contaminated by infected feces. Usually clears up on its own without treatment.
B (also known as HBV)	Symptoms similar to those of hepatitis A or, in some cases, no symptoms at all. Can lead to cirrhosis, liver cancer, and liver failure. Spreads through contact with infected blood and body fluids. Can also be passed from a mother to her newborn. Infection can be sudden and acute or chronic and long-lasting. More than a million Americans carry the HBV virus in their blood, many without knowing it.
	In pregnancy, hepatitis B causes the most concern. If a woman has the hepatitis B virus in her blood, there is a 75 percent chance that she will pass it on to her baby. Most babies who are infected by their mothers become lifelong carriers of the virus and are at high risk for liver diseases when they grow up. Doctors routinely test for hepatitis B early in pregnancy. If you test positive, immunoglobulin and vaccination of your newborn can prevent transmission of the virus to your baby.
C (also known as HCV)	The most dangerous kind of hepatitis. Four million Americans have been infected with it. Spreads through contact with infected body fluids. More likely than other kinds of hepatitis to cause life-threatening liver diseases. Difficult to treat. Is the most common reason for liver transplantation in the United States.
	Pregnant women are not routinely screened for hepatitis C, so if you think you might be infected, ask your doctor about being tested. The infection passes from mother to baby less than 10 percent of the time. Mothers who require treatment for HCV immediately postpartum are sometimes advised not to breastfeed.
D (also known as delta hepatitis)	Uncommon. Affects people who already have hepatitis B. Can cause serious liver damage.
E (also known as epidemic hepatitis)	Spreads through contaminated drinking water; more common in countries with poor waste disposal systems. Outbreaks have not occurred in the United States.

Beyond hepatitis

Several other liver diseases can strike during pregnancy:

TYPE OF LIVER DISEASE	DESCRIPTION	CAUSE	SYMPTOMS	TREATMENT
ICP (intrahepatic cholestasis of pregnancy) Affects fewer than 1 percent of women in the United States	Causes abnormalities in the flow of bile, a digestive chemical produced by the liver; those abnormalities allow bile acids to accumulate in the mother's blood and deposit in the skin. ICP may be associated with stillbirth.	Unknown; possibly hereditary or caused by estrogen.	Itchy skin all over the body, especially on the palms of the hands and soles of the feet, and jaundice, a yellowing of the eyes and skin.	Medications to decrease bile acids and anti-itch medications to decrease symptoms. Fetal monitoring may be recommended.
HELLP syndrome Affects fewer than 1 percent of pregnancies in the United States	A variant of severe preeclampsia, it's characterized by hemolysis (the breakdown of red blood cells), low platelets, and elevated liver function tests (showing inflammation of the liver). May or may not have high blood pressure and proteinuria, the classic signs of preeclampsia.	Unknown.	Nausea, vomiting, headache, pain in the upper right abdomen, and a general feeling of unwellness.	Delivery of the baby. The disease usually stops soon after delivery.
Acute fatty liver of pregnancy Affects 1 in 13,000 pregnant women in the United States	A very rare buildup of fat in liver cells. Risks are coma, organ failure, and death of mother and baby.	Unknown, although a small number of cases are linked to the baby having LCHAD (long-chain 3 hyroxyacyl CoA dehydrogense deficiency), a serious metabolic disorder that could be checked for at birth. It may not be part of your newborn screen.	Same as in HELLP syndrome. Possible jaundice, a yellowing of the eyes and skin.	Treatment is complicated. Includes immediate delivery of the baby followed by support for the mother.

week 27

Your Self

Avoiding accidents

Right now, while your baby is inside you, one of the best ways to take care of her is to take care of you. That means avoiding accidents, which happen far too often. Accidents are the fifth-leading cause of death in the United States. Reduce your chance of accidents with these suggestions:

Drive safely. Car crashes are the number one cause of death among Americans between the ages of 4 and 34. Obey the speed limit, don't use a cell phone while driving, pull off the road if you feel sleepy, and never get in the car with an impaired driver. (See "Auto safety and accidents," page 275.)

Always wear a seat belt. Seat belts save 11,000 lives a year. Don't worry that the seat belt will hurt your baby in a car crash—the main danger to your baby is an injury to you! To wear a seat belt safely and comfortably, place the lap belt below the baby, snugly across the hips and against the upper thighs. (Don't wear the lap belt across your belly.) Place the shoulder belt over your shoulder and in the middle of your chest, between your breasts. If it feels too tight at your neck, adjust the seat or the position of the belt feeder above the car door; lowering the belt feeder may help. Never wear the shoulder belt under your arm or behind your back because it won't protect you adequately in a crash.

Be aware of your surroundings. Avoid deserted parking garages, dark stairwells, and other isolated areas where someone could be waiting to ambush you.

Be a smart pedestrian. Look both ways and cross at the crosswalk. In short, follow all the rules you'll be teaching your child in a few years.

Install smoke detectors in your home. If you already have them, check the batteries. Fires kill more Americans each year than all natural disasters combined.

Reduce risks in your home. Secure loose handrails, remove throw rugs that may slide out from under you, and place a slip-preventing mat in your bathtub or shower. Store guns, weapons, and poisonous chemicals and cleaners safely. Post emergency phone numbers next to the telephone. If you swim, practice water safety.

Handle food safely. Improper food storage and preparation can cause illness. Remember to wash your cutting board with hot, soapy water.

Wash your hands frequently to stop the spread of germs. Use soap and very warm water. Lather up and rub your hands for as long as it takes to sing "Happy Birthday" twice.

The mid-pregnancy blues

You're more than halfway through your pregnancy, but you may feel as if you've been pregnant forever—and will remain pregnant forever. Feeling restless and anxious mid-pregnancy is normal. There's no way to zoom to your due date, but here are a few things you can do to soothe those mid-pregnancy blues:

Take a walk. Exercise invigorates your body by speeding up your circulation and improves your mood by triggering the release of feel-good brain chemicals. Grab a friend or neighbor, tell her you'd like to talk about anything but pregnancy, and set off. Tired of the same old walking route? Drive someplace different, park the car, and set off from there.

Create a distraction. See a movie, focus on your favorite hobby, spend the day with a good friend, or get caught up in a project in your community or church.

Read something besides pregnancy books. As important as it is to educate yourself, it's also good to put aside pregnancy and baby books sometimes. Grab the latest best seller, a trashy novel, or a fascinating nonfiction book. The same goes for television: Skip the televised show-everything vaginal and cesarean deliveries on the health channels.

Sign up for a class that's not related to pregnancy. Learn how to grow perennials, do your own taxes, put up wallpaper, shoot better photos, improve your computer skills, salsa dance, or trace your ancestry; learn something new, no matter what you choose. Classes are offered almost everywhere, from community centers and home-improvement superstores to crafts stores and camera shops.

Go away for the weekend. A change of scenery might be exactly what you need—and it's a nice time to rekindle some passion with your partner.

Don't forget your partner

Your identity changes during pregnancy, particularly if it's your first pregnancy. You start it as a woman and you end it as a mother. That's a transformation that's so big and encompassing that you might forget sometimes that your partner is making a huge transformation too. Your relationship with each other changes during pregnancy too as you make the shift from being a couple to being a family (or a bigger family, if you have other children).

Although it's not the case with every couple, women tend to think more about life changes before they happen; men are more likely to respond to them after they occur. You and your partner may be at different stages in your thoughts about parenthood.

It's important to communicate about what you're going through. Talk with your partner about the expectations and fears you both have of parenthood. Let him know what you're thinking and feeling and ask him to reveal his thoughts and feelings too.

One of his fears may be that when you become a mother, he'll have to share you with the baby. He may also worry that when you have a baby you'll have less interest in the sexual part of your relationship. It's best to talk openly and patiently about these issues before your baby is born

week 27

because life gets pretty hectic after delivery, and finding time to sit down for a heart-to-heart isn't as easy.

Diet & Exercise

Staying hydrated

Drinking plenty of fluids is more important now than at any other time in your pregnancy. Staying fully hydrated can help prevent uterine tightening, headaches, constipation, and dizziness. If you're well hydrated when you go into labor, you'll have more stamina than you would if your body lacked fluids. And remember that your baby needs water for her body and the fluid-filled amniotic sac where she lives. If you're hydrated, she will be too.

Eight glasses (64 ounces total) of water a day will keep you hydrated. Drink a few extra glasses if you exercise or if the weather is warm and you're perspiring heavily. If you're drinking enough water, your urine will be nearly clear; if you're not, it will be deep yellow.

Water is the best way to hydrate, but other fluids count in your daily tally, including milk, fruit juice, and decaffeinated coffee or tea. Most fruits and vegetables contain water. Tomatoes, for example, are 94 percent water by weight, and apples are 85 percent.

10 water alternatives

Bored with water? Wake up your taste buds with these substitutes:

- Seltzer flavored with a squeeze of lime or lemon juice or a splash of cranberry juice.
- Decaffeinated iced tea with a slice of fresh lemon and mint leaves.
- Orange juice blended with ice chips.
- A tropical fruit juice mocktail made with ½ cup of seltzer, ½ cup of juice (orange juice, papaya juice, pineapple juice, lime juice, or any combination of the four), and plenty of ice.
- Frozen flavored ice. Choose ones made with 100-percent fruit juice.
- Snow cones.
- Ice-cold water flavored with a drop of vanilla, cherry, or peppermint. Use only a drop, though, because these flavorings are strong and contain a small amount of alcohol.
- Iced café au lait made with decaffeinated coffee blended with skim milk and ice. Make it a mocha with a half spoonful of cocoa powder.
- Hot chocolate. Make your own non-fat, less sugary version with a cup of skim milk, a tablespoon of sugar, and a teaspoon of cocoa powder (100-percent-pure cocoa, not hot cocoa mix).
- Fruity iced tea. Try decaffeinated tea that's chilled with ice cubes made of orange juice and crushed strawberries or raspberries.

Common Questions

Q. What type of infant car seat is best?

A. When you're ready to take your bundle of joy home from the hospital, your baby will need to ride in a car seat. Some hospitals actually send a nurse down to your car with you to confirm that you have one. If you've checked out car seats in baby superstores, you know there is a bewildering variety to choose from. Which should you buy?

Choose rear-facing seats. According to the National Highway Traffic Safety Administration (NHTSA), the safest way for infants to ride in a car is in the backseat facing the rear of the vehicle. Never put the car seat in a front seat where an air bag is present; if the bag inflates, it could crush and kill your baby. Rear-facing car seats protect a baby's head, neck, and back in a crash. A baby should ride facing the rear until at least 1 year of age and 20 pounds, and longer if possible. If you want to keep an eye on your rear-facing baby, you can attach a mirror to the backseat, positioning it in the view of your rearview mirror. Some experts discourage the use of these mirrors, however, because they distract the driver from watching the road and can become deadly projectiles in a car accident.

There are two kinds of car seats for babies. Small, lightweight, infant-only seats are one option. Larger convertible seats safely hold a baby facing the rear and can be turned around and converted into a safety seat for a toddler or preschooler weighing up to 35 pounds. Both kinds of seats are equally safe, so the kind you choose depends on personal preference.

Pay attention to installation. Closely follow the directions that come with the seat. If it is not installed correctly, or if the baby is not properly harnessed into it, the seat may not protect the baby in an accident. You may want to install your car seat and then drive to an inspection check-point to verify that you've put it in correctly. Local police stations, hospitals, and car dealerships often provide this service free of charge.

Do the paperwork. When you buy a car seat, fill out the registration card that comes with it and send it to the manufacturer. That way the manufacturer will be able to contact you if the seat is recalled.

Q. Can I use a secondhand car seat to save money?

A. A car seat should not be used after it is involved in a moderate to severe crash. Even if it looks fine, its internal structure may have been weakened by the impact of the crash. Never buy a used car seat at a secondhand shop or tag sale because you have no way of knowing whether it was involved in a crash.

If a friend offers to lend you a car seat, and she's sure it's never been in a crash, ask her these questions. If all of the answers are yes, go ahead and borrow it.

- Is the seat less than 6 years old? (Ordinary wear can reduce a seat's protective abilities.)
- Does the seat have all its parts? (If not, you may be able to order missing parts from the manufacturer.)
- Does the seat have labels stating its

week 27

date of manufacture and model number? (You'll need these to find out if the seat has been recalled or if it is too old.)

- Does the seat have its instruction booklet? (If not, you may be able to request a copy from the manufacturer or download a copy from its website.)
- If the seat was recalled, has it been properly repaired? (The manufacturer should have recall details. Or call the NHTSA's Auto Safety Hotline: 888-327-4236. Sometimes a problem on a recalled seat can be fixed.)

Week 28

Your Baby

The inside story

Your baby can open and close his eyes at will now, and he'll suck his thumb if he's so inclined. He's probably close to 2½ pounds. If your baby is a boy, his testes will soon descend into his scrotum.

Your baby's brain is developing rapidly right now. An ultrasound of your baby at 28 weeks shows a head that is large in proportion to his body; at birth a human baby's brain accounts for a whopping 12 percent of his body weight. Your baby already has the 100 billion or so brain cells he'll have at birth. However, he still has to build connections between them to form the neurological network that will give him control over everything from his footsteps to his speech.

During the first year of life, a baby's brain grows faster than the brain of any other mammal. This burns a lot of calories; your baby will require a diet that's 50 percent fat to fuel all that growth. Luckily, breast milk and formula are both designed to offer that balance. It's a good thing that this brain-building process takes place after birth; otherwise your baby's head would be too large to fit through your pelvis.

The placental blood flow is increasing dramatically to support your baby's rapid growth during the 3rd trimester, and the placenta itself is growing. For example, the placenta weighed only about 6 ounces during your 20th week of pregnancy, but by now it's probably close to 15 ounces.

Your Body

Amniotic fluid levels

Sometimes amniotic fluid rises too high if there's a birth defect in your baby, such as a gastrointestinal blockage (pyloric stenosis). This is rare, affecting only 1 in 500 to 1 in 1,000 babies. Other times the baby is normal but is surrounded by more than the expected amount of amniotic fluid. Most women go on to deliver healthy babies even if their amniotic fluid is high, but your provider will discuss all the possibilities with you if the fluid is too high. Many times a chubby baby will have a little more fluid than a smaller baby.

If your amniotic fluid is too low, it could indicate a problem with the placenta or a tear in your amniotic membrane. If your baby doesn't have enough amniotic fluid, he runs the risk of sitting on his umbilical cord or not having enough room to kick around; this may result in premature delivery, poor lung development, and feet that are turned inward. This too is a rare condition. It happens to less than 5 percent of all women. You'll know you're at risk for it if, for example, your belly is smaller than it should be or you are leaking fluid. Your doctor will monitor your condition closely through the rest of your pregnancy and may ask you to drink extra water.

3rd-trimester screening

During the 3rd trimester, you'll likely have these tests:

Glucose testing. Sometime between weeks 24 and 28, your doctor will test to see if your body is using sugar correctly. You'll drink a very sugary liquid and then, an hour later, you'll have a blood test. You do not need to fast before this 1-hour glucose test, but don't have a doughnut on your way to the doctor's office either. If there is excess sugar in your blood, your doctor will order additional bloodwork to determine whether you have gestational diabetes. (See "Gestational diabetes," page 231.)

Hematocrit. This blood test determines whether you have anemia, a shortage of iron in the blood.

Syphilis screen. A woman can have syphilis without knowing it, and she can unknowingly pass the infection on to her baby. If she tests positive for the bacteria, she can be treated with

antibiotics during pregnancy, and her baby will receive antibiotic treatment shortly after birth. Without treatment, some babies who are infected in the uterus die within a few days of delivery. Those who survive are at very high risk for blindness, brain damage, hearing loss, and problems with bones, skin, and teeth.

Rh factor. Your blood was checked for Rh factor at your first prenatal visit. (Rh factor is a protein that is found on red blood cells. Most women have this protein, but about 15 percent of Caucasian women and 7 percent of African-American women don't. They are considered to be "Rh-negative.") Many doctors will repeat the Rh test sometime in weeks 26–28 to confirm your Rh status, particularly if you tested Rh-negative earlier in your pregnancy and if the baby's father is Rh-positive. In such cases, there is a chance your baby will have Rh-positive blood and your body will build up antibodies to it during pregnancy. If your body does develop these antibodies, they could jeopardize future pregnancies. (See "Rh incompatibility," page 128.)

If you are Rh-negative, you will get a shot of Rhogam (Rh-immune globulin) at 26–28 weeks as a precaution; it fights those antibodies if a small amount of Rh-positive fetal blood has mixed with your blood.

If you are Rh-negative and your baby is Rh-positive, you will receive an injection of Rhogam (RhIg) within 72 hours of delivery to help prevent an immune response against

Gestational diabetes

Around this point of the pregnancy, doctors test women for gestational diabetes, which affects approximately 3–5 percent of pregnant women. Here's what you need to know:

What is it? Diabetes is a disease in which blood glucose levels are too high. Glucose levels soar because the body does not produce enough insulin, the hormone that converts sugar, starches, and other foods into the fuel that is needed for daily life. Or the body may produce enough insulin but fails to use it properly. Diabetes that occurs during pregnancy is called gestational diabetes.

How does it affect a pregnancy? If a woman with gestational diabetes does not receive treatment, her fetus will receive too much blood sugar and may grow very big. Large babies are difficult to deliver and often require a cesarean delivery. Babies born to mothers with uncontrolled diabetes may have breathing difficulties, low blood sugar, and jaundice during their first few weeks of life. Gestational diabetes can also raise a woman's risk of high blood pressure during pregnancy.

Who gets it? You are at increased risk if you:
- Have a sibling or parent with diabetes.
- Are African-American, Native American, Asian-American, Hispanic American, or a Pacific Islander.
- Are over age 25.
- Are overweight or obese.
- Have had gestational diabetes before.
- Have given birth to a baby weighing more than 9 pounds.
- Have been diagnosed with prediabetes, a condition in which blood glucose levels are higher than they should be but not high enough for a diagnosis of diabetes. It's also called "impaired glucose tolerance" or "impaired fasting glucose." (Unless they make lifestyle changes, most people with prediabetes develop diabetes within 10 years.)

How is it diagnosed? Simple blood tests can measure the glucose in your blood.

How is it treated? Sometimes making diet and exercise changes is enough. How you eat affects your body's ability to use insulin, and exercise can lower blood glucose levels. If lifestyle changes are not enough, you need to give yourself injections of insulin or you may be offered an oral hypoglycemic medicine. You'll also learn how to test your blood glucose levels using a small device known as a blood glucose meter.

Will it go away? In most cases it will go away after delivery. However, if you have gestational diabetes you have a 50 percent chance of developing type 2 diabetes later in life. Your doctor will test your blood glucose level 2–6 months after delivery to make sure it has returned to normal.

What can I do to reduce my risk of developing type 2 diabetes after my baby is born? Weight, exercise, and diet all contribute to diabetes risk. Ask your doctor to refer you to a diabetes educator or to a registered dietitian who can help you make effective lifestyle changes.

Rh-positive blood. If your baby turns out to be Rh-negative, then you will not need this injection.

Increased heartburn

Indigestion can get much worse during the 3rd trimester. Some women have it throughout pregnancy; others escape it until the 3rd trimester. (The luckiest ones never get it.) Over-the-counter antacids such as Mylanta, Maalox, and Tums provide relief for minor indigestion, but stubborn 3rd-trimester indigestion that keeps you up at night calls for stronger medicine. Two types of drugs can help reduce acid production and damage to the stomach and esophagus: H2 blockers (Pepcid, Tagamet, Zantac) and proton pump inhibitors (Prilosec, Protonix). These medications are believed to be safe for your baby. Some of these are available without a prescription, but it's best to consult your doctor before taking them.

Multiple sclerosis

Why talk about multiple sclerosis (MS) in a pregnancy book? MS is more prevalent in women of childbearing age than in any other group. Pregnancy doesn't cause MS, but because MS targets women between the ages of 20 and 50, some women happen to be pregnant when their MS is diagnosed.

What it is. Multiple sclerosis is an autoimmune disease that affects the brain and spinal cord. People with MS experience a range of symptoms from mild (numbness in the limbs, muscle weakness) to severe (paralysis, tremors, and vision loss). Although it is not a fatal disease, it is chronic, so people who have it will have it for the rest of their lives. Symptoms may come and go for months or more.

Unless symptoms are severe, MS can be difficult to diagnose, particularly during pregnancy. Some of the symptoms of MS—numbness, problems with bladder and bowel function, fatigue, mood swings, inability to concentrate, and forgetfulness—are similar to some of the ordinary side effects of pregnancy.

Treatment. Scientists have discovered several medications that help modify the natural course of MS. These medications are most effective if taken early in the disease. If you experience any MS-type symptoms, tell your doctor.

How MS affects a pregnancy. Here's some good news for women who start pregnancy with MS or develop it during their pregnancy: Studies show that MS does not harm a pregnancy. In fact, pregnancy appears to have a protective effect on some women with MS. During pregnancy—particularly in the 2nd and 3rd trimesters—women with MS tend to experience fewer flare-ups than when they are not pregnant.

A woman with MS generally needs no special care during labor or delivery. After a woman with MS gives birth, flare-ups may be more common, rising in the first 3 to 6 months postpartum. However, long-term studies have found that women with MS who have babies suffer no more MS-related disability than those who don't give birth.

Bed rest

If you have certain complications, your doctor may advise you to curtail your activities or to spend part or all of the remainder of your pregnancy in bed. This is called "being on bed rest." A doctor puts a pregnant woman on bed rest if he or she feels that everyday activity puts the health of the mother, baby, or both in jeopardy. It can be very hard to put your life on hold for a few weeks or months, but if you keep in mind the important goal—delivering a healthy baby—it is bearable.

Likely candidates. Bed rest makes sense with certain complications, including placenta previa (the placenta is low and may be covering the cervix), preeclampsia (high blood pressure), and placental abruption (separation of the placenta from the uterus). It is sometimes prescribed for preterm labor and intrauterine growth restriction (IUGR), although there is no scientific data to support it as a useful treatment.

Risks. Right now the thought of spending a few days lounging around in bed or on the couch may sound wonderful. However, it does carry some risks, so it should be recommended only when necessary. Without any activity your muscles can stiffen and lose strength. Gaining excess weight is a problem for many women on bed rest. Boredom pushes them to eat more than they need, and their inactivity reduces the number of calories they burn. Women on bed rest may become depressed. The

digestive system slows down and stool moves more slowly through the intestines and rectum, making constipation more likely to occur. The most serious complication of limited movement is an increased risk of blood clots.

Ask the right questions. If your doctor advises bed rest, ask exactly what that means. Should you stay in bed all the time, have someone bring you your meals, and get up only to use the bathroom? Should you rest in bed several times a day and perform your ordinary activities between resting periods? Or does your doctor want you to spend your days on the couch and your nights in the bedroom, while still allowing you to go to the kitchen a few times a day for meals and snacks?

Your Self

Coping with bed rest

Although staying in bed for a couple of months can be challenging, make the most of it by doing things you've never had time for until now. Here are some suggestions:

Log on. If you don't have a computer and an e-mail connection, now is a good time to get them. E-mail will help you keep in touch with friends and feel less isolated. If you can access the Internet, you can join virtual support groups with other bed-resting women.

Work. If you have the kind of job that can be done in bed, see if you

week 28

can telecommute. Some jobs can be done easily with a phone, a fax machine, and a computer. If your job doesn't lend itself to telecommuting, perhaps you can help out a friend who's running her own business and needs assistance with the paperwork.

Raise money. Your favorite charity may need someone to do phone work.

Launch a project. Now may be the perfect time to put 10 years' worth of photos in albums, read through all your high school journals, create a scrapbook, or type up all of your favorite recipes.

Set a reading goal. Not too many people can say they've read all of the works an author has written. Set a goal of reading all of Shakespeare, Sue Grafton, Arthur Conan Doyle, Robert Ludlum, Jane Austen, J. K. Rowling, or whoever suits your taste.

Set a movie goal. If you have someone to go back and forth to the video rental store, plan on watching sets of movies—everything that Johnny Depp has been in, for example, or all of the Elvis movies.

Call in all your favors. You'll need help with cooking, cleaning, shopping, and childcare, if you already have a child. Ask friends and family to help, and when people say, "Can I do anything for you?" have specific answers in mind—make dinner, go to the library, wash a load of laundry.

Ask for visitors. Having someone stop by to say hello can brighten a day on the couch or in bed. When you invite people over, ask them to bring just themselves and not gift boxes of candy or tins of homemade cookies.

Learn to knit or crochet. In no time you'll have a blanket for baby or a sweater for yourself.

Do whatever exercise you're permitted. It may be fine for you to lift light arm weights or do some simple yoga stretches. Ask your doctor what exercise, if any, is safe; then do what you can to maintain strength and flexibility.

Avoiding STDs

Just because you're pregnant doesn't mean you can't get a sexually transmitted disease (STD). In fact, pregnancy is one of the worst times to pick up an STD because some can cause birth defects or severe neonatal illness. To protect yourself and your baby, follow the rules of safe sex: Have sex with only one partner who has no other partners, doesn't have HIV, and doesn't use injectable drugs. If you have any doubts, use a male or female condom. If you have any question or concern that your partner may have an STD, never let that person's blood, urine, semen, vaginal fluid, or feces get into your anus, vagina, or mouth.

Planned cesarean delivery

One in four deliveries in the United States is a cesarean delivery (also called a "C-section"), which is the birth of a baby through a surgical incision in the mother's lower abdominal wall and uterus rather than through the vagina. Doctors usually turn to cesarean delivery after labor has begun either because of an unexpected complication or because labor is failing to progress.

Sometimes, however, cesarean deliveries are planned in advance because of certain complications, including the following:

Placenta previa. If the placenta is positioned abnormally low within the uterus, there is a chance that the placenta will block the cervix. This could prevent the baby from advancing through the birth canal and could cause severe bleeding or hemorrhaging in the mother.

Size. If the baby is very large, a cesarean can sometimes be the safest way to deliver.

Position. Babies who are breech (presenting buttocks first or feet first) or traverse (side or shoulder first) sometimes require cesarean delivery.

Medical problems in the mother. Long-standing diabetes or active genital herpes can make vaginal delivery dangerous to mother or baby.

Previous cesarean. Some women with previous cesareans can deliver vaginally, but for others, another cesarean is the safer choice.

Birth defects. Depending on the situation, a baby with a major birth defect may have a better outcome if delivered by cesarean.

Multiples. Twins and triplets may be delivered vaginally or by cesarean, depending on the situation. The more babies you are carrying, the more likely it is that your doctor will recommend a planned cesarean.

Elective cesarean delivery

What if you simply prefer the idea of a cesarean delivery over a vaginal birth? Can you choose an elective cesarean delivery? It's not a great idea, and your doctor may not agree to it anyway.

A cesarean poses more potential risks to a woman and her baby than a vaginal delivery does. These risks are worth taking when mother or baby has a health problem or complication, but they are not worth taking in an otherwise normal pregnancy in a healthy woman. Most doctors consider it unethical to choose the higher-risk cesarean procedure without medical cause, and so does the American College of Obstetricians and Gynecologists (ACOG). "If the physician believes that performing a cesarean would be detrimental to the overall health and welfare of the woman and her fetus, he or she is ethically obliged to refrain from performing the surgery," says an ACOG opinion statement.

Performing a cesarean delivery

The anesthesiologist will explain the different pain medications available. Most use an epidural, a spinal block, or a combined spinal-epidural block; these will leave you awake but numb from below your breasts to your toes. (See "Pain relief during labor," page 244.) You can discuss the possibility of having a small amount of morphine in your spinal or epidural as well; this may help control pain after the procedure for up to 24 hours.

week 28

Once you have anesthesia, the nurse will put a catheter in your bladder to drain urine before surgery begins; this lowers the risk of injuring your bladder during the procedure and makes it easier to deliver the baby. She'll then shave the lower part of your abdomen and clean your belly with antiseptic solution.

The doctor will drape you with sterile sheets and put up a low screen across your chest to prevent you from seeing the surgery; however, in some institutions, you're allowed to have a mirror or you can request that your view not be blocked.

If your partner wants to accompany you to the operating room, he will have to put on hospital scrubs, booties, and a mask. He will sit beside your head, so he can talk with you, hold your hand, and give you support during the procedure.

For most cesareans, the doctor will make a horizontal incision in your abdomen along your bikini line; in some emergency situations the cut will be made from your navel down to your pubic bone. The doctor will then make another horizontal or vertical incision in your uterus, depending on the position of the baby and the placenta. Afterward she will break the amniotic sac, if it is not already broken, and allow some fluid to escape. She'll then gently put her hand in to lift the baby out through the incision, headfirst. The tugging and pushing you may feel occur as the head emerges through the incision and the surgical assistant is pushing at the top of your uterus to expel the baby.

The doctor will clamp and cut the cord, then hand the baby to a pediatrician or skilled nurse who will examine the baby immediately and then wrap her up and hand her to your partner.

After delivering your baby, your doctor will bring the placenta out through the same incision; then she'll massage your uterus. The actual delivery of your baby will happen only 10–15 minutes after the start of the procedure. The rest of the surgery—stitching up the two incisions and getting you into recovery—takes approximately 30 minutes more. Throughout the procedure you won't feel much more than tugging or pulling sensations.

After a cesarean, you'll be taken to a recovery room where your blood pressure, bleeding, pulse rate, and respiration will all be monitored. The catheter may remain in for about 12–24 hours after surgery, and you'll continue to get fluids through an IV until the next day. You may stay in bed the first day, though you'll be encouraged to change positions, roll over, and sit up in bed. You should be able to breastfeed your baby by laying a pillow across your abdomen to help support him in your arms as he nurses, and you should be walking within 24 hours. Your doctor will give you pain medication for discomfort, and you will be released from the hospital in about 3 or 4 days.

Diet & Exercise

Say yes to yogurt

Yogurt is a nearly perfect pregnancy food. It is rich in calcium and protein, low in fat (if you choose low-fat varieties), and filling. Some yogurts contain live active cultures, which are beneficial bacteria that are believed to enhance digestion, improve nutrient absorption, boost the immune system, and inhibit the growth of harmful bacteria in the digestive system. (Check the label for cultures such as *L. bulgaricus, S. thermophilus, L. acidophilus, Bifidus, L. casei,* and *L. reuteri.)*

Yogurt can be eaten plain or dressed up with fresh fruit or crunchy nuts. Blend it with berries to make a smoothie or spoon it onto cereal instead of milk. Mix it with peeled, chopped cucumber, fresh dill, and minced garlic to make an elegant sauce for fish or chicken. Or combine a cup of plain yogurt with ½ cup of salsa for a tangy, spicy vegetable dip.

Say no to low-carb diets

Eating plans that encourage you to eat lots of meat and to avoid most carbohydrates are no good for you or your baby. Carbohydrates are an essential part of your diet, providing energy quickly and efficiently. If you give up carbohydrates you'll be cutting out many high-fiber, nutrient-packed foods.

High-carbohydrate foods worth choosing include fruits, vegetables, beans, and whole grain breads, pasta, and cereals. Pass up cake, white bread, soda, and other high-carbohydrate foods that offer nothing but empty calories.

Common Questions

Q. Should I bank my baby's umbilical cord blood?

A. Umbilical cord blood contains a large number of stem cells that can be used to treat several pediatric cancers, blood diseases, and genetic disorders. Typically the umbilical cord blood is discarded after birth. In recent years, however, parents have had the option of saving some of their baby's umbilical cord blood in case the baby—or a family member—needs stem cells sometime in the future.

Parents who choose to save their baby's cord blood arrange to have it collected immediately after birth and stored by a commercial blood bank. This can be expensive: Collection costs as much as $1,750, and parents are charged annual storage fees of $50 to $100.

Storing cord blood makes sense for parents who have a family history of certain kinds of genetic diseases, immune disorders, or cancers. However, for people with none of these diseases in their family, the chance of needing a transplant from cord-blood stem cells is only 1 in 20,000.

Parents also have the option of donating their baby's cord blood to a public bank so it can help others who need stem cell transplants. This option is available only in certain parts of the United States; ask your doctor if there is a public bank in your area. (For more information on public cord banking, contact the National Marrow Donor Program at 800-627-7692 or www.marrow.org.)

The American Academy of Pediatrics (AAP) considers cord-blood stem cell transplantation to be an encouraging area of research but still in the investigative stage. Storing blood privately as biological insurance for your child's use in the future is not worth doing, the AAP says. However, the AAP does endorse the collection of cord blood from babies with siblings who have conditions such as leukemia or other blood diseases. The AAP also encourages public banking of cord blood.

The decision to save cord blood is both personal and financial. If you think it's the right choice for your family, discuss it with your doctor or a genetic counselor. Do not feel guilty if you decide against it.

Childbirth classes for mom and partner

Most childbirth classes welcome fathers as well as mothers. The classes are helpful to fathers because they provide information on what part a partner can play in the labor and delivery process. They also provide the father an opportunity to be more involved in the pregnancy. Your partner can serve as a second set of ears in class, which is helpful because there can be a lot of information to absorb.

What if you would like your partner to attend childbirth classes with you, but he can't or won't? If you really want him to come with you, talk with him about it. Tell him that you would like his support and that you will both benefit from the classes. Ask him why he won't go. Is he concerned that it won't fit into his schedule? Is he nervous about participating in the birth? Does he think he'll feel out of place when women's biological functions are discussed openly? After determining what's holding him back, look for ways to get around his roadblocks. Check the class times at various hospitals to find one that fits his schedule. If he is worried that he'll feel out of place, remind him that there will be other men in the class who may feel uncomfortable too. Offer him an out by telling him that you don't mind if he takes restroom breaks when the discussions get too graphic. If he continues to be reluctant, ask him to go with you to the first class and then decide whether to continue attending.

If you can't convince him to go with you, consider taking along a good friend or relative to share the experience.

Week 29

Your Baby

The inside story

Your baby's hearing is so well developed by now that she will startle at loud noises. Soon she'll start turning her head to listen to sounds outside your body.

By now your baby weighs well over 2½ pounds and most likely measures about 15 inches long. She's beginning to store enough fat beneath her lovely pink skin that she may already have those baby dimples on her elbows and knees. If your baby is a girl, she'll probably weigh less at birth than if you are carrying a boy; either way, your baby will probably weigh between 7 and 7½ pounds at birth. If this is your second or third pregnancy, you can expect this baby to weigh more than your last.

As she runs out of room, your baby may bow her head down toward her knees, curling as she did when she was very tiny. She's long enough now that you'll notice her kicks more. Forget those little fluttery motions. This feels more like someone is elbowing you for space on the subway! Play "guess that body part" with your partner as you try to distinguish a knee from a heel.

Your Body

Fatigue returns

You're carrying around a noticeable amount of extra weight now, and you're waking more often at night because of your baby's cartwheels and your full-to-bursting bladder. That means you may be exhausted during the day—perhaps nearly as tired as you were during your 1st trimester—and you may feel that you're experiencing pregnancy wilt instead of pregnancy glow.

Combat 3rd-trimester fatigue by making yourself as comfortable as possible at night and resting more during the day. This will benefit your health and your baby's, especially if you work outside the home. Researchers have found that expectant working moms who report on-the-job stress and fatigue run a higher risk of having their amniotic sac or membranes break early.

To rest better during the 3rd trimester, lie on your side, bend your legs, and put a pillow between them. Put another pillow under your belly. You can also invest in full-length body pillows to support your body and ease stress on your back and breathing. During the day, nap at least

week 29

Babies in the breech position

At one of your prenatal visits, your provider might tell you that your baby is in a breech position, which means that he's sitting upright, with his legs folded in the lower part of your uterus, instead of in the head-down position most babies assume before delivery. Don't let this worry you. Many babies are doing somersaults up until the 36th week of pregnancy. Your baby will probably turn around on his own before your due date.

Identifying a breech baby. If your baby is still breech a few weeks from now—a diagnosis usually made by feeling your baby through your abdomen and uterus—you may have an ultrasound to confirm the baby's position. Most babies flip between weeks 34 and 37. But a small percent—about three out of every 100 full-term babies—never get around to it. Your chances of having a breech baby are higher if you previously gave birth to twins or have too much or too little amniotic fluid, a uterine abnormality like multiple fibroids, a premature delivery, or placenta previa (placenta covering the cervix).

Possible complications. A breech presentation can raise the risk of injury to your baby, especially if you go into labor early. In most vaginal births, the baby is born headfirst, and because his head is the biggest part of him, it stretches the birth canal enough that the rest of his body can slip out easily. A breech baby is born feet- or buttocks-first, and because his skinny body slides out so quickly—especially if he's premature and hasn't accumulated much fat—the birth canal hasn't stretched to accommodate his head. The head may then have trouble delivering.

Another possible complication is umbilical cord prolapse when your water breaks. In this situation the cord might slide to the bottom of the uterus and become squeezed as the baby's butt and legs move downward. The pressure on the cord cuts off your baby's supply of blood and oxygen. Many hospitals require babies in the breech position to be delivered by cesarean.

Your best bet at this point is to wait to see if your baby flips in his own sweet time. If he still hasn't turned by your 37th week, discuss your options with your provider. You may need special exercises or manual manipulation (external version) to turn your baby before labor begins. (See "Singleton breech babies and version," page 300.)

20 minutes every afternoon. If you can't find the time (or don't have the inclination) to actually sleep during daylight hours, take 5-minute breaks every hour to put your feet up and flip through a magazine. You can always catch up on work in the middle of the night when your baby is doing his gymnastics.

Balancing acts

In addition to being spacey, you can expect to be clumsy. Your uterus has grown to the point where you can't see the tips of your toes if you're standing up straight, so it's hard to notice curbs and rumpled throw rugs.

Pregnancy also changes your center of gravity. Center of gravity is the average location of the weight of an object. Before pregnancy, your weight was pretty solidly above your feet; now a fair amount of it is in front of you. A change in your center of gravity shakes up your sense of balance because you now have to balance your body's weight in a different way than you did before. As your belly grows you may find yourself tripping or dropping things like never before.

Hormones are making your hands, feet, and legs feel heavy and water-logged. As if that weren't enough, your ligaments are continuing to stretch and soften in preparation for childbirth, and you might suffer from a numbness and tingling sensation in your fingers. It's a symptom of carpal tunnel syndrome, which occurs when that extra fluid causes swelling in your wrist and hand, pinching the nerve beneath the ligament and leading to pain that can radiate from your fingers to your shoulders. This usually is a temporary condition during pregnancy and goes away after childbirth (see "That tingling in your hands," page 252).

The reality is that you really can't do as much now as you could before pregnancy, so you might as well accept that and slow down a bit. When you do exercise, maintain good posture and place your hands and feet carefully in the correct positions to keep your balance. Spend a few minutes with your feet up every day to reduce the ankle and foot swelling that makes you feel as if you're wearing gravity boots. Take extra care when climbing stairs or walking on unfamiliar sidewalks.

Now is also the time to keep both feet planted solidly on the ground. Stand up slowly or you're likely to feel dizzy. Leave the ladder ascents and step-stool climbs to someone else. If there's something in a high cabinet that you use regularly, ask someone to move it down to an easier-to-reach location. Keep floors clear of toys, shoes, boots, and area rugs that can slip out from under you. Get a good grip on small objects before carrying them; otherwise you'll fumble them to the floor. And given your slippery fingers, let someone else do the dishes.

This all may make it seem as if you're living life in slow motion. But it will soon pass, and you might as well enjoy the chance to cruise in low gear while the house is still relatively peaceful and your time is still more your own.

Best positions for labor

Researchers have now confirmed what most moms seem to know instinctively: If you move around during labor, or at least sit in an upright position, you can help your baby progress downward. The added pressure of your baby's head on your cervix can help you dilate faster too. Studies have shown that most women, when given the freedom to labor in any position they choose, prefer to stay on the move when contractions prevent them from resting. They walk, sit, squat, or lean on whatever is available. They rock with

Premature rupture of membranes (PROM)

When you go into labor, your membranes—also known as your "bag of waters"—will weaken and break, allowing amniotic fluid to leak out of your body as your baby is born. That fluid has been keeping your baby well protected against infection and injury while in utero. If your water breaks before labor actively begins, it's called PROM, or premature rupture of membranes.

PROM is fairly common, occurring in one out of every 10 pregnancies. About 90 percent of women whose membranes rupture near their due dates will go into labor within 24 hours, and 50 percent of preterm women will go into labor within that time. No matter how far along you are, though, your risk of infection—and your baby's—increases as more time elapses between your water breaking and your baby being born.

What to do. If you suspect that your membranes have ruptured, call your health care provider immediately. She will most likely want to examine you to determine if the fluid leaking from your vaginal area is from the amniotic sac, a urine leak, or some other type of vaginal discharge. If your membranes have ruptured, the next event will be determined by your baby's maturity and whether your provider suspects an infection.

After 36 weeks: If you're past your 36th week of pregnancy, your provider will probably wait at least 6–12 hours to see if you go into labor. Some providers will wait longer if your baby is moving and you have no signs of infection. Your doctor may allow you to wait at home, or she may ask you to come into the hospital. If you're not in active labor, she may then induce labor with Pitocin (a synthetic oxytocin that stimulates contractions) to decrease the chance of an infection occurring in you or your baby.

Between 32–36 weeks: Your provider may test your amniotic fluid to see if your baby's lungs are mature enough for him to breathe on his own. If they are, your provider may induce labor. If not, she may try to prolong your pregnancy through bed rest. She will induce labor if you show any signs of infection, such as fever or uterine tenderness; she may also give you steroids to improve your baby's lung function. In most cases, babies born after the 32nd week of pregnancy have few long-term complications.

Before 32 weeks: Your provider will almost certainly try to prolong your pregnancy unless there is evidence of active labor, infection, or abruption. She will probably admit you to a hospital with special perinatal services if her own hospital doesn't provide those. You may be given antibiotics to ward off infection and prolong the time from membrane rupture to delivery and steroids to promote your baby's lung development.

Risk factors for PROM:

- Amniocentesis
- Cervical surgery during pregnancy
- Cigarette smoking
- Certain congenital anomalies
- Infections
- Maternal trauma
- Multiple gestations
- Prior PROM
- Prior preterm delivery
- Vaginal bleeding during the 2nd trimester
- Cervical incompetence

the contractions or even get down on hands and knees.

Although there's no need for you to practice labor positions before your due date, it's well worth trying different ones ahead of time to see what's most comfortable for both you and your partner. (This might also help your partner suggest positions when you're in the throes of labor and can't think of anything much beyond the moment.) It's also worth asking ahead of time what your hospital or birth center provides as birthing props. Do they have showers, tubs, birthing balls, squat bars, birthing beds, or rocking chairs? If they don't have something that you find particularly comfortable, like a birthing ball (basically a great big rubber ball like the sort you might see people use to exercise with in a gym), you can buy one to take with you to the hospital when you deliver.

Ultimately, the labor positions you choose while having your baby will depend on what kind of labor you experience. Here are some you can consider and try out. Improvise to make them your own:

Kneel and rock. Labor may be easier with props. (See illustration, right.) Using a rocking chair, a regular chair, or a birthing ball, kneel with your arms resting on the chair or ball for support. You can lean on your elbows or cross your arms and put your head down, as if you're a kindergarten student at rest time. When a contraction comes, rock forward as you breathe in and rock backward as you breathe out. Keep your back flat as you rock. This position takes very little muscle, won't tire you or your partner, and will help make gravity your friend.

Walk and lean. If you're upright and

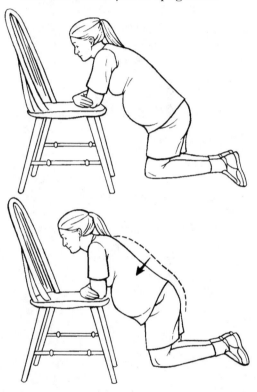

walking, the baby is headed in the right direction, and you'll have something to do to take your mind off labor. Lean on your partner, labor coach, or a nearby wall during contractions. Then take a deep breath and keep moving.

Lie on your side. You can't stay in constant motion because you'll get tired. When you do stop to rest, recline on your side. This can help ease a hard, fast labor during strong contractions. You can also lie on your side between contractions to rest until another one comes.

Sit on a ball or low stool. Sitting on something low that allows you to spread your legs helps open up your pelvis and put gravity to work (see illustration, below). You can also sit astride your birthing bed. If you have trouble keeping your balance, ask your partner to sit on a chair in front of you (or stand, if you prefer) so that you can reach out and hold on to his hands or reach his knees with your arms outstretched. If your hospital doesn't provide a birthing ball, bring your own with you; you can buy them at most sports equipment stores.

Squat. This move takes energy and

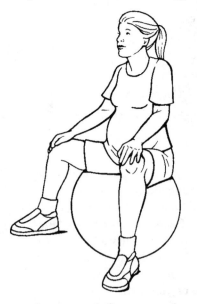

muscle; so save it for more active labor or even until it's time to push and deliver your baby. Ask your prac-

titioner for a squat bar, which most birth centers and hospitals have. This attaches to the birthing bed like a chin-up bar, and you can hang from it while you squat. You can also hang on your partner's neck if he braces his legs the right way. Loosen your abdominal muscles while you're squatting and place your feet a couple of feet apart as you slowly get into position. If you don't have a squat bar and want to get lower to the ground, have your partner sit on a stool and hold your hands while you squat in front of him.

Pain relief during labor

Many women dislike the idea of being drugged during labor—after all, you've waited 9 months for your delivery date, and you don't want to be in a total fog during these life-changing moments. However, you may also be afraid of the pain you may feel. The good news is that anesthesia has come a long way since the medical practices of the 1950s, when women were typically drugged into unconsciousness during labor and babies showed the effects of medication for many hours after birth. Now drugs can be administered locally and in smaller doses with little impact on the baby. While natural childbirth is often best for moms and their babies, anesthesia is a good choice if your pain—or your fear of it—impedes your labor from progressing because you're hyperventilating, exhausted, or suffering from other stress reactions.

If you're giving birth in a hospital,

the most common painkillers that are used are an epidural or opioid, such as Demerol.

Opioids. Opioids don't completely remove the pain, but they do dull it considerably. Unfortunately you may also feel very groggy as a result, and so could your baby. Short-acting opioids are usually given intravenously (IV) or intramuscularly (IM).

Epidural. Another option might be an epidural. Well over half of all pregnant women in the United States have epidurals now. That's more than double the number from 10 years ago, and the procedure is becoming increasingly popular as the techniques for administering epidurals improve.

If you choose to have an epidural, the anesthesiologist will ask you to sit up or lie on your side. She will first clean off a spot on your back with an antiseptic solution, then inject a local anesthetic under the skin in your lower back. Then she'll insert a thin tube (catheter) through a larger needle between the bones of your spine and near the spinal cord. The needle is removed, leaving the tube in the epidural space to deliver a local anesthetic continuously or every couple of hours or so.

In the past, epidurals were so powerful that they usually rendered women numb in the legs and pelvic region, making it impossible to move around and difficult to push when it came time to deliver the baby. Anesthesiologists now use a diluted anesthetic, usually combined with a low dose of an opioid drug, to relieve pain while leaving you less numb. In some hospitals, you might even be allowed to walk. Most epidurals won't prevent you from pushing when your baby is ready to make his appearance.

Combined spinal epidural (CSE). This option is gaining popularity for labor. It is administered much like an epidural. After a clean space on your lower back is prepared, a needle delivers an opioid and local anesthesia into the spinal fluid for immediate relief; a catheter is then put in the epidural space to deliver opioids and local anesthetics continuously.

General anesthesia. Prior to a cesarean delivery, general anesthesia may be used. With general anesthesia, the pregnant woman is temporarily put to sleep and has a tube in her windpipe to allow the delivery of oxygen. Most women want to be awake to hear their baby's first cry, so general anesthesia is usually reserved for emergencies.

Risks. There are risks with any procedure and with the use of opioids. When opioids are given intravenously, mom will feel sleepy, and most babies will too. The fetal heart rate pattern usually shows this by having fewer accelerations, but this resolves as the baby awakens. If the opioid is given close to delivery, some babies will be sluggish in their breathing and will need a boost.

The risks of epidural and CSE include spinal headache (severe headache after regional anesthesia that worsens upon standing up) for less than 1 percent of women. Many women will complain of low-back ache after delivery, but very few of those complaints are related to the epidural. Other women worry that a needle near their spinal cords will cause nerve damage. This is an extremely rare complication of regional anesthesia.

Common delivery room fears

Here is the truth behind many women's delivery room anxieties:

- "I'll be in labor for days." Not a chance. The average first-time labor is only 18 hours, and few providers will allow labor to last for more than 20 hours after your water breaks.
- "I'll totally lose control." Your ability to handle pain is greater than you know, and you'll be learning breathing and relaxation techniques before you deliver. In addition, it's seldom too late to ask for pain medication during labor if you really can't stand it.
- "My husband will faint." Very few men actually faint, and your partner will have a good idea of what to expect during labor if he goes to childbirth classes with you.
- "I'll have a cesarean delivery." You might, but the odds of having a vaginal birth are higher, especially if this is your first baby. Only 18 percent of first-time moms have cesarean deliveries.
- "I'll have an episiotomy, and it'll really hurt." Doctors perform episiotomies (surgical cuts made between the vagina and the rectum during labor) only about 20 percent of the time, and that number is dropping. Even if you have one, you won't feel it because of the pressure on your perineum from your baby's head and the light anesthetic your provider will administer beforehand.

Your Self

Conquering fears of childbirth

Birth is more than a natural biological process; it's a fundamentally loving, sacred act of creation. It's also a powerful rite of passage for many women, leading to deep transformations as they bring a new soul to life and discover hidden strength in themselves. Even if you've had a child before, it's natural for you to feel apprehensive, ambivalent, and even scared about such a momentous event as your due date approaches.

However, as many as 10 percent of all pregnant women feel such an intense fear about childbirth that their negative emotions interfere with labor and delivery. If you fall into this group, you may experience full-blown anxiety attacks heralded by symptoms such as heart palpitations, dizziness, shortness of breath, or a racing pulse. You may have nightmares too or problems focusing on anything but this looming terror of the unknown.

A little stress is good for you, sending endorphins into your bloodstream and putting you on alert when you meet new challenges. However,

Domestic violence during pregnancy

Though it's extremely unfortunate, domestic violence and abuse by a partner are not uncommon during pregnancy. In fact, according to the Family Violence Prevention Fund (FVPF) (www.endabuse.org), abuse is more common for pregnant women than gestational diabetes or preeclampsia.

Here are the facts, based on data from FVPF:

- Homicide is the leading cause of traumatic death for pregnant women and new mothers in the United States, accounting for about 31 percent of maternal injury deaths.
- Each year about 324,000 pregnant women in the United States are abused by their partners.
- A significant proportion of all female homicide victims are killed by their intimate partners.
- Women whose pregnancies were unplanned have 2–4 times greater risk of being abused than do those whose pregnancies were planned.
- Young mothers are particularly vulnerable: 26 percent of new mothers between the ages of 13 and 17 are abused during pregnancy or the first three months postpartum.
- A pregnant woman who is abused is more likely to suffer from low weight gain, anemia, infections, vaginal bleeding, miscarriage, preterm labor, and other pregnancy complications.

If you are being abused physically, sexually, or emotionally, there are ways to get help. If you are in immediate danger, call the police or go to the hospital. To find a domestic violence program near you, talk with your doctor or contact the National Domestic Violence Hotline (800-799-SAFE or www.ndvh.org). To get help and information about sexual assault, contact the National Sexual Assault Hotline (800-656-HOPE or www.rainn.org).

when you're too frightened, your muscles tighten up, stress hormones flood your bloodstream, your heart rate zooms, and your blood flow is redirected outward toward your limbs in a fight-or-flight response. If your fears about labor have put you in a constant state of panic, share those fears with your provider. She may clarify misconceptions or have suggestions to address your specific concerns.

Coping strategies. The best way to cope with childbirth is to learn not to fear it. Yes, some of labor will be uncomfortable, and some of it will hurt. But there are many avenues for pain management. You will get through it, just as many generations of women have gotten through it before you. And at the end of the day you will hold your baby in your arms. What you need now are strategies for diminishing your fear.

Figure out why you're so afraid. For instance, if your medical history includes a past miscarriage or stillbirth, a difficult delivery with a previous child, or excessive exposure to

week 29

traumatic labor stories, you need more information about labor and delivery and reassurance that your pregnancy is going well. Write down your concerns about medication, cesarean deliveries, and your baby's well-being. Share these fearful scenarios with your provider, who can help you work out strategies for coping.

Consider talking to a therapist. Research has shown that women with an intense fear of labor who talk to therapists may have shorter labors and fewer unnecessary cesarean deliveries than those who don't seek therapy. Your provider may be able to provide a referral to a good therapist.

Finally, shut out the negative stories. Steer clear of scary television shows on childbirth, and if your friends start regaling you with their own labor travails, ask them to change the subject. Learn relaxation skills and find a trusted midwife or doula to help you put them into practice during these final weeks of pregnancy. She will also stay by your side and ease your fears during labor and delivery.

A safe nursery

A little shopping therapy can take your mind off the aches and anxiety of these last weeks of pregnancy. As you start feathering your little one's nest, remember that nursery safety has to be your main concern. Injuries caused by baby equipment have dropped 20 percent since the early 1990s, thanks to safer products, but more than 71,000 children are still injured each year by products that are unsafe or used incorrectly. Before buying, read these tips on choosing safe baby furniture:

Cribs, bassinets, and cradles. Your first major purchase will probably be something for your baby to sleep in. More than 8,600 injuries—mostly from strangulation and falls—are attributed to cribs, cradles, and bassinets each year. If your baby's head is caught between crib slats that are spaced too widely apart, for instance, or if clothing catches on a corner post, he could strangle. Measure any bed you're considering for your newborn: There should be no more than $2\frac{3}{8}$ inches between slats. Also check for a snug-fitting mattress, corner posts extending no more than $\frac{1}{16}$ inch above end panels, a solid headboard and footboard with no cutouts, properly installed hardware, and a wide base if it's a bassinet or cradle.

Playpens. These are extremely useful for keeping your baby out of harm's way while you get dinner on the table or play with a toddler nearby. However, be aware that about 1,980 injuries are associated with playpens each year. If you buy a mesh model, for instance, and the drop side is left down, it can form a pocket that may suffocate your baby.

Alternatively, if you drop the side and don't lock it properly, it can collapse and strangle your baby. It's also possible for a baby's head to get caught if the mesh weave on the sides is too wide or if you have a wooden playpen with widely spaced slats. The safest playpen is a mesh model with top rails that lock automatically. The mesh netting should have openings of less than ¼ inch. Wooden playpens should have slats no more than 2⅜ inches apart.

Changing tables. Without a doubt, a changing table is a great item. It provides wonderful storage space, and it saves strain on your back because you don't have to bend over every time you diaper your baby. However, about 1,650 children a year are injured on changing tables, usually because their parents don't strap them onto the surface and they roll over and fall off. Choose a changing table with a safety strap and always use the strap. Also, look for a model that has drawers and shelves that will be easily accessible to you but out of your baby's reach.

Diet & Exercise

Chest and shoulder stretches

The weight of your growing belly can pull your shoulders forward, tightening the muscles in your chest. These stretches can help loosen up your tight chest muscles and relax your shoulders. Remember, stretch only to the point where you feel a mild tension; then relax as you hold the stretch. Never bounce. Breathe slowly and naturally while stretching and do not hold your breath.

Chest stretch #1. Stand with your head upright and with your back straight. Clasp your hands behind your back and, without leaning your shoulders forward, gently stretch your arms up and back to feel a stretch in the front of your shoulders and arms. Hold for 10 seconds; then relax.

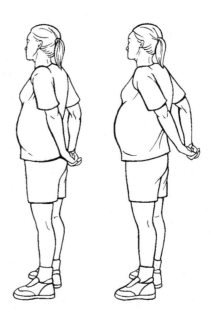

Chest stretch #2. Stand in front of a doorway. Place hands at shoulder height on either side of the doorway. Move your upper body forward until you feel a comfortable stretch. (Keep your chest and head up and knees slightly bent.) Hold for 15 seconds; then relax.

Shoulder stretch #1. Sit or stand with your arms hanging loosely at sides. Shrug shoulders up. Hold for 5 seconds; then relax your shoulders downward.

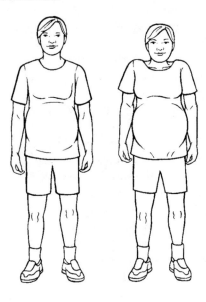

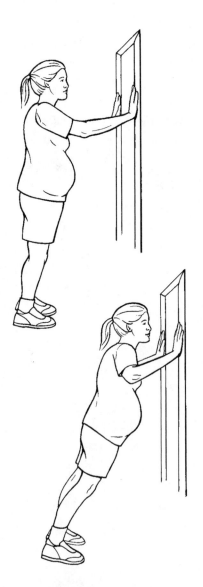

Shoulder stretch #2. Stand or sit. Place your right hand on your left shoulder. With your left hand, pull your right elbow across your chest toward your left shoulder. Hold for 10–15 seconds; then relax. Repeat on the other side.

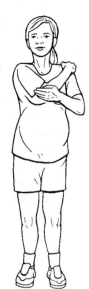

Common Questions

Q. I've heard that you can be hypnotized to make labor less painful. Is that really possible?

A. Silly television stunts and stage acts in which hypnotists wave pendants and command people to moo like cows or eat ice cream out of their shoes have given hypnosis a bad rap. In fact, hypnosis—also called hypnotherapy—is a respectable tool for overcoming fears and pain. The American Medical Association has approved of hypnosis as a medical intervention since 1958, and hypnotherapy is now used to conquer everything from smoking to migraine headaches. Hypnosis has been used routinely in many countries for more than 50 years to help women manage childbirth pain. It's now catching on in the United States as well. Many hospitals and birth centers now offer classes in "hypnobirthing," the term used to describe hypnosis during pregnancy and childbirth. Hypnobirthing helps women alter their conditioned or learned reflexes to pain.

How does it work? Basically, hypnobirthing teaches pregnant women how to achieve a state of focused relaxation so they can take advantage of the human body's natural ability to anesthetize itself against pain. This meditative trance isn't that different from what you experience if you do yoga or if you practice the breathing techniques taught in some childbirth classes. About a quarter of women who try hypnosis say they suffer no pain at all during childbirth.

Some researchers believe it's effective because, in a hypnotic state, the part of the brain that controls concentration is able to direct other areas of the brain to reduce or eliminate awareness of pain. In other words, if your brain isn't paying attention to what hurts, then you won't feel it. Researchers liken this to the ability some people have to study or read when there's a lot of noise and commotion around them.

If you want to add hypnosis to that bag of tricks you're planning to bring to the birth, sign up for a hypnobirthing class at your local hospital or find a certified private practitioner. Ideally, you should start learning hypnosis techniques several weeks before your due date to give you time to master them. You can find a hypnotist through the American Society of Clinical Hypnosis (630-980-4740; www.asch.net) or the American Psychotherapy & Medical Hypnosis Association (www.apmha.com).

Week 30

Your Baby

The inside story

Your baby weighs close to 3 pounds. He's growing so fast now that if he kept up this rate, he'd weigh more than 200 pounds by his first birthday! In order to accomplish his final growth phase during the 3rd trimester, he will continue to absorb nutrients from your body: calcium for his skeleton, protein for his muscle growth, and iron for his red blood cell production. You might feel more tired or suffer from anemia as a result.

Like most babies, yours probably has blue eyes right now. Once he's born, his eyes may turn brown after being exposed to the natural sunlight that will finalize pigments in the iris. The hair on his head may start to grow in now as he finishes losing that covering of fine, downy lanugo hair on his body.

Even though your baby is already about as long as he'll be at birth, he will continue to gain weight rapidly as he adds a layer of fat to his lanky limbs. His brain is almost as advanced as a newborn's at full term. However, your baby's brain will keep growing quickly as his brain cells continue to make connections that will allow him to develop speech, memory, and maybe even the ability to remember the Pythagorean theorem.

Your Body

That tingling in your hands

Just when you thought you couldn't get any clumsier, you may experience a numbness or tingling sensation in your hands, especially in your thumb and first three fingers. It might become painful to type or close your hand around your water bottle, or you may feel pain that radiates from your wrist to your neck and shoulder.

These are hallmark symptoms of carpal tunnel syndrome, another side effect of your increased swelling. Typically affecting people whose jobs demand repetitive motions such as typing on a computer keyboard, carpal tunnel syndrome is named for the carpal tunnel in the wrist, a hollow region that houses nerves and ligaments leading to your hand. When the tissue swells in this tunnel, it can press on the nerves and cause numbness, pins-and-needles tingling, or burning sensations.

Carpal tunnel syndrome can be especially aggravating at night, when fluid has pooled in your extremities.

Sleep with your hands propped up on a pillow to encourage fluid to drain to other regions of your body. If you work on a keyboard or do other repetitive motions on the job, examine your environment to see what you can do to rest your hands more. Take more breaks or alter your position to avoid putting pressure on the nerves in your wrist. For instance, lower your computer keyboard so that you type with your wrists angled downward. You can also wear a plastic splint (available in pharmacies) to stabilize your wrists and keep them straight. Shake your hands vigorously from time to time to dispel the tingling.

About 25 percent of women get carpal tunnel syndrome while pregnant. Although the condition can be painful, the good news is that, in all but 2 percent of cases, it goes away on its own after you've delivered your baby. (It might take a few weeks longer if you're nursing because hormone and fluid levels will fluctuate then too.) However, if you find that it's seriously impairing your job performance, sleep, or overall comfort, ask your practitioner about treatments and physical therapy.

Other causes of numbness

Some pregnant women experience a feeling of pins and needles in their hands that's not related to carpal tunnel syndrome. Some even feel it in their feet. This sensation is usually your body's way of telling you that your hands and feet are not getting enough blood or that a nerve is being compressed.

Why it happens. Babies sometimes find a favorite position in the uterus

Preeclampsia

About 7–10 percent of first-time moms develop preeclampsia in the late 3rd trimester of pregnancy. The cause of preeclampsia, which is also known as toxemia, is unknown. The diagnosis is made when your blood pressure goes up (usually to more than 140/90) and you spill protein in your urine or have swelling in your face, hands, and feet. Many women with preeclampsia feel fine, but others have symptoms of severe preeclampsia such as headaches, seeing spots, blurred vision, pain in the upper abdomen, or seizures (known as eclampsia). Women who are at higher risk include those with chronic high blood pressure, kidney disease, diabetes, obesity, and multiple gestations.

Treatment. The only treatment for preeclampsia is delivery. If you have severe disease, your doctor may recommend delivery even if your baby is early. If you have mild disease, you'll probably be evaluated with blood and urine tests; your doctor may recommend induction when your baby is full-term.

Detection. Although researchers have tried for years to find prevention strategies such as baby aspirin, low-sodium diets, and megavitamins, none have proven useful so far. Detection is the best strategy doctors can offer. Therefore, your weekly visits at the end of pregnancy are especially designed to try to catch this disease early.

week 30

that is quite comfortable for them but not so great for you because the uterus presses on your blood vessels, narrowing them and keeping blood from flowing freely. Other babies can sit directly on your nerves, sending zinging pain into your buttocks or down the back of your leg.

Getting relief. Numbness is sometimes relieved by shifting positions while sitting or lying down or by drinking plenty of fluids, which helps reduce swelling. Shaking the feet and hands (with fingers and toes pointed downward) can pump up the circulation to your extremities. And any kind of aerobic exercise—swimming, walking, stationary cycling—increases the blood circulation throughout the body.

If your hands or feet feel cold when numbness strikes, heat sometimes helps. When the body is cold, blood circulation to the arms and legs slows down in order to keep organs such as the heart and lungs warm. Soak your hands or feet in warm (not hot) water or warm them up with a hot-water bottle or heating pad.

If you experience any numbness, mention it to your doctor. In very rare cases it can be a symptom of diabetes, thyroid disease, vitamin B12 deficiency, heart disease, or multiple sclerosis.

Bellyaches

It's too soon for that bellyache to be labor. Or is it? Here are some possible causes—and solutions—for abdominal discomfort in late pregnancy.

Uterine growth. Your uterus is still growing to accommodate that bigger-by-the-minute baby of yours, and that means you're going to feel uncomfortable. The discomfort can range from a feeling of being too full to stabbing pains when you change positions—like getting out of bed too suddenly in the morning. That pain is caused by stretched ligaments around the uterus; you can ease it by slowly assuming different positions and breathing deeply as you move to get enough oxygen to the muscles. Or do a pelvic leg lift: Steady yourself by placing one hand on a table or stair railing while you bend your knee and lift one foot a couple of inches off the ground in front of you. Count to 10 and put your foot down again. Do this 10 times on each side.

Abdominal muscle separation. As your uterus expands, the long bands of muscles down the middle of your belly separate to accommodate its new size. The muscles pull apart (you can feel a hollow space when you push your fingers between them), and this can be uncomfortable. Usually the muscles resume position after your baby is born.

Constipation. Because pregnancy hormones slow down your digestion and your enlarged uterus increases pressure on the large intestine, waste products move more slowly through your body. That can cause abdominal cramps if you become constipated. Drink plenty of fluids and eat food with roughage (such as bran flakes and crunchy veggies), both of which will soften your stools.

Baby's antics. If your baby is now in the birth position, with his head toward the bottom of your uterus, you may suddenly be aware of pains in new places as he tap-dances against your ribs or plays the bongo on your bladder. Shift positions when this happens or pat your baby and sing to distract him.

False labor. At times you might feel as if you've been lassoed around the middle and someone is tightening the rope under your belly and around your back. These are Braxton Hicks contractions (see "Braxton Hicks contractions," page 214). If you have them often, you might think you're in labor when in fact you're not. The difference between false labor and the real thing can be difficult to diagnose: False contractions are mostly in the front of your belly, they don't get stronger over time, they feel more like pressure than pain, and they usually lessen in intensity if you put your feet up and drink lots of water. If the tightening persists, call your doctor. Checking your cervix is a quick way for your doctor to distinguish true from false labor.

Increased vaginal discharge

It's normal to have your vaginal discharge increase during pregnancy, especially in the last few months. Usually this discharge is milky and odorless. Called leukorrhea, the discharge may become heavy enough in the 3rd trimester for you to change your underwear more often or to wear pantyliners. Avoid vaginal deodorants, perfumed soaps, and douching because all of these things can upset the balance of bacteria in your vagina and cause an infection. Resist the urge to use pantyliners because they keep wetness against your skin.

If you notice that your vaginal discharge looks different or smells fishy, contact your health care provider and have her swab the area for a diagnosis. It's not normal for your vaginal discharge to be clear, for instance; that might signal a leak in your amniotic fluid. Pregnancy is not the time to fool around with self-diagnosis, no matter how easy it might seem from past experience.

Here's a list of the most common vaginal infections experienced by pregnant women; you can head off most of them by keeping your perineum clean and dry.

Yeast (candida or monilia) is easy to identify by the thick, cheesy vaginal discharge and the red color, soreness, or burning pain in your vaginal area. Your provider will probably suggest over-the-counter suppositories or cream containing imidazole medication. A yeast infection poses no risk to your baby, other than a greater chance of contracting thrush at birth, which is easily treated by ointment.

Trichomoniasis (trichomonal vaginitis) is an STD caused by parasites, and it may cause a persistent burning or itching sensation similar to a yeast infection. The key difference is that trichomoniasis causes a frothy white, yellow, or green discharge that smells like day-old fish.

week 30

There is no risk to your baby from this infection, but it can make you feel miserable. Your provider might suggest metronidazole pills.

Bacterial vaginosis is the result of too many "bad" bacteria knocking off the "good" bacteria in your vagina. Vaginosis affects about 20 percent of pregnant women, and it can cause an increased creamy-looking discharge and mild irritation. Your provider will probably prescribe oral antibiotics to treat it because if left untreated bacterial vaginosis can increase the risk of premature delivery.

The role of a doula

Women have been helping each other through labor throughout history. Before modern hospitals, when a woman gave birth at home, a female family member, friend, or neighbor might have assisted her. If you'd like to have another woman by your side to offer emotional support, advice, and encouragement during labor, you might hire a doula. *Doula* is a Greek word that means "woman's servant."

Services. A doula is not a midwife. Rather, she is a paid labor coach. Doulas are trained to provide physical, emotional, and informational support to women and their partners during labor and birth, according to Doulas of North America (DONA). DONA is an organization that trains and certifies doulas.

A doula guides a woman through breathing techniques and suggests positions that help labor progress. She may offer massages, breathing exercises, and advice, both before you go to the clinic or hospital and after you're admitted. A doula is not medically trained; she does not perform medical exams, make diagnoses, or actually deliver the baby. She does not take the place of a doctor, nurse, or midwife. Some doulas also offer postpartum care such as breastfeeding support, newborn care, and household help for a new mother.

Who may benefit. Doulas are especially great for women without partners or women whose partners will be uncomfortable in the delivery room. A doula also can be helpful if you've decided to have your baby naturally, with no medical interventions or pain medications.

Choosing a doula. There are good doulas and bad doulas. A good one supports the mother and her partner, helping them make medical decisions based on the doctor's recommendation and the couple's desires. A bad one makes the partner feel unneeded, argues with the doctor about issues such as pain medication, gets in the way of the nurses, and stresses the mother rather than helps her.

Before you hire a doula, ask her about her birth philosophy to see if it agrees with yours. If you feel strongly that you want to have epidural pain medication, avoid hiring a doula who is against medication during labor and who will argue with you about your choice. It's also important that you click with your doula on a personal level—you may end up spending a lot of time with this woman, so you'd better like her.

Some doulas work independently; others are employed by hospitals or doula agencies. Either way your health insurance is unlikely to cover the cost of a doula, although it's worth asking. To find a doula, ask your doctor or friends for a referral. Or contact DONA (www.dona.org), which maintains a list of certified doulas in the United States.

Fees. You'll need to pay a doula somewhere in the range of $300 to $1,500 in most places. That amount usually covers several prenatal visits, her stay with you throughout labor and delivery, and a follow-up meeting. Always discuss your decision to hire a doula with your midwife or obstetrician; some providers find the presence of any sort of labor coach intrusive. Other providers might be able to offer you some good referrals, and you may benefit from the extra support.

Your Self

Protecting your job

Wondering how much time off you can take without putting your career in jeopardy? Under the Family and Medical Leave Act (FMLA) of 1993, the government mandates that you're entitled to take up to 12 weeks of unpaid, job-protected leave every 12 months for specific family and medical reasons. If you're planning to cover your maternity leave through

FMLA, here are some things to keep in mind:

- The FMLA requires you to give written notice of your intention to take a leave at least 30 days in advance. Do this anyway, out of common courtesy, even if this Department of Labor act doesn't apply to your employer.
- Your employer has the right to request occasional status reports while you're on leave under the FMLA. Talk to your supervisor and the people covering your job about how often these will be expected. E-mail is usually the easiest way to stay in touch with people at work, but your supervisor might ask for more formal written communications as well. Avoid doing anything by phone; if you do file or receive communications from your office by phone, make notes in a log.
- The FMLA allows you to take your leave in different segments. For instance, you might want a month off to recover from child-birth. Then you might return to work for a couple of weeks to catch up on pressing items and take the rest of your leave after that. Be aware that federal law dictates that you must use all of your leave within a year of your baby's birth. Work out your staggered leave with your employer ahead of time. Your employer is also allowed to move you into a job where being absent won't make as much of an impact.

- The FMLA stipulates that if you choose to take more than 12 weeks of leave, your employer is under no obligation to give you your job back or to continue your health insurance benefits. Some employers may offer you more leave than this out of their individual company policies or sheer goodwill. However, get this agreement in writing to protect your job.

If your company doesn't fall under the Family and Medical Leave Act of 1993 (see "Maternity leave laws," page 144), which grants all parents (that includes dads) 12 weeks of leave after giving birth, you most likely still qualify for an unpaid or partially paid "maternity disability" or medical leave, usually lasting 6 weeks after a vaginal birth and 8 weeks after a cesarean. If your employer isn't bound by any leave laws, check out the Pregnancy Discrimination Act of 1978. This act states that if your company has more than 15 employees and has held a person's job for some other type of medical disability—such as a heart attack—it must reinstate you after medical disability due to pregnancy.

Maternity leave options

The phrase "maternity leave" is bandied about so freely that working women naturally assume they're entitled to one. The truth is that most companies don't pay for your maternity leave. Many women aren't even eligible for leave under family leave laws, either because they haven't been working long enough or because their company has fewer than the requisite 50 employees. Even if your company does grant family leave, you may not be in a position to take it if it's unpaid, or you may want to finance a longer maternity leave. Either way, it's worth exploring all of your options.

Explore your options for disability insurance too. Several states have state-run temporary disability plans that cover the weeks you're medically unable to work. These plans usually compensate for about 60 percent of your pay during the first 6–8 weeks postpartum that you're medically unable to work.

Beyond these federal- and state-mandated leave laws, you can use accrued vacation, sick days, or personal days to help finance your time off. You might also ask if you can borrow paid leave against future time off. Adjust your tax withholding at work now to reflect your extra dependent if the baby will be born in the current tax year. That way you'll benefit from the deduction now.

Diet & Exercise

Emotional overeating

Hunger is only one of the many reasons people eat. Boredom, depression, stress, loneliness, spiritual emptiness, fear, and even happiness can send you to the refrigerator too. If you eat for emotional reasons, however, you may eat too much, particularly during the 3rd trimester when emotions intensify. Your pregnancy will be healthier if you gain the recommended amount of weight and no more.

Emotional hunger draws you into a cycle in which emotions trigger overeating, overeating triggers emotions, and so on. You eat when you're stressed and you gain too much weight. Then you feel stressed because you're gaining too much weight. Then you eat even more, and the cycle continues.

How can you break the cycle? Dieting won't do it. What works is understanding why you overeat. Once you know which emotions trigger overeating, you can work on soothing those emotions in other ways.

Start by keeping a food log. Be completely honest and write down everything you eat for a week, along with when you ate it, what was going on at the time, and how you felt before and after you ate. After a week, go back to your log and look for patterns. Maybe you overeat whenever your partner works late or when you have a difficult day at work.

Once you identify patterns, think of what you can do in place of overeating. If you eat when you feel lonely, for example, make a list of things to do instead of eating, and when loneliness strikes reach for your list instead of a piece of cake. Call a friend, go for a walk, play solitaire, do a crossword puzzle—whatever works.

If you've been an emotional eater for a long time, you won't be able to stop overnight. But you can think of pregnancy as a time to begin taking your emotional eating seriously and looking for ways to rely less on food for comfort.

Exercise and heart rate

Even when you're at rest, your heart is working hard to pump blood through your body. During pregnancy your extra weight and your baby's oxygen needs make your heart work even harder. Exercise demands even more of your heart because your muscles need plenty of oxygen when they are at work.

As you progress through your 3rd trimester, you'll be asking your heart to work continuously harder. That's all right—your heart can take it, as long as you don't have heart disease. There's no need to curtail your exercise if your heart rate increases; it's normal that if you work hard, your pulse will go up.

"Vigorous" exercise means different things for different people. Vigorous exercise for a sedentary woman may be only a warm-up for a marathoner. What's important is that you avoid pushing yourself too hard; "too hard" means to your own point of discomfort. It's OK if you notice your breathing speeding up as you exercise, but you shouldn't be pushing so hard that you can't talk. Listen to your body. Any kind of movement is good, even if it's slower and less intense than your prepregnancy and early-pregnancy activity.

week 30

Common Questions

Q. I'm nervous about childbirth, but I'm even more scared about my baby dying after he's born. I've heard that babies can actually die in their sleep for no reason at all! How often does this happen? Is there any way to prevent it?

A. The condition you describe is called SIDS (sudden infant death syndrome), and it's the number one cause of death in infants 1–2 months old. It's also one of the most tragic and frustrating conditions because doctors don't know what causes these babies to die; they only know that the babies stop breathing for some reason, usually when they're asleep. To minimize the risk of SIDS, the American Academy of Pediatrics suggests the following:

- Always put your baby to sleep on his back. Researchers believe that babies who sleep facedown run the risk of breathing in their own exhaled air, which contains toxic carbon dioxide. What's more, experts believe that SIDS babies may have an area in the brain that's underdeveloped. That area of the brain might be the one responsible for arousal and breathing; this would explain why a SIDS baby fails to wake himself up and gulp fresh air if he starts to suffocate.
- Don't sleep with your baby in your bed because your baby might be suffocated by blankets or trapped between your headboard and your mattress; you might also roll onto your baby if you've been drinking alcohol or if you've taken any medication that makes you sleep more heavily than usual.
- Make her crib as safe as possible. The crib should have a firm mattress and no blankets, pillows, or stuffed animals. Don't overdress your baby for bed or keep her room too warm either because that might make arousal more difficult.
- Eliminate your baby's exposure to tobacco smoke. One of the toxic tobacco by-products might be responsible for that underdeveloped brain area and your baby's inability to wake himself up if he has trouble breathing, experts say. They base this theory on the fact that moms who smoke during pregnancy have twice the risk of a baby dying of SIDS.

Q. I love the idea of a family bed. My husband is adamantly opposed to this; he says our baby should learn to sleep in his own room immediately or he won't be independent and we won't have any privacy. Who's right?

A. This is a tough and very personal decision. The American Academy of Pediatrics argues against sleeping with your baby in your bed because it might increase the risk of SIDS (see previous question). Most research shows that co-sleeping poses a negligible risk by itself. What really puts babies at greater risk in a family bed isn't the fact that they sleep with their parents, but other factors, such as parental smoking or alcohol use, getting trapped beneath a comforter or against a headboard, or being put down on their stomachs so that they can't pick up their heads and turn them. If you do sleep in a bed with your baby, keep in mind that your bed doesn't meet the same safety standards as a crib. Take care that your baby sleeps on her back, use light blankets instead of soft quilts and comforters, and don't let your baby sleep with her head on a pillow.

Some researchers have demonstrated that babies who co-sleep with their parents cry less and have an easier time stabilizing their nervous systems after birth than babies who sleep alone. In any case, the first few months of your baby's life is not the time to teach him independence, but rather a time to teach him that his needs will be met when he requires comforting for any reason. You can't spoil a newborn. On the contrary, some studies show that children who sleep with their parents are more confident and independent than children who do not. The truth is that most parents sleep with their children at least sometimes, whether they have an "official" family bed or not, simply because of the frequency with which they have to get up to tend their infants. (In other words, exhaustion sometimes forces the issue of where your baby will sleep.)

The best solution is to keep a safe baby bed next to your own bed for the first few months. That way you can keep baby close without worrying about rolling over on him or burying him in adult-size bedding. When you are awakened in the middle of the night, you won't have as far to go to feed or comfort your baby.

If it's sex your husband is worried about, or watching TV in your room while the baby sleeps, there's no need to be concerned. Newborns sleep through almost anything. In fact, some sleep better with a certain noise level, and it's absolute quiet that wakes them instead.

Your partner: Preparing him for delivery

You're going to be the one panting and pushing, but your partner is probably afraid too—of letting you down, of seeing you in pain, of something happening to the baby during birth, or of having to make tough medical decisions on his own. Prepare your partner to participate in the delivery room by discussing his fears and offering ideas for making delivery as easy and memorable as possible.

Tell him exactly how to help. Before you go into labor, give your partner specific instructions on the kind of assistance you'd like during labor. If you're planning to give birth naturally, give him information on how to support your early labor and help you breathe. Ask him to advocate for you if the medical staff suggests interventions—such as an IV or fetal monitor—that you'd rather not have unless there's an emergency. Of course there are always situations where a cesarean delivery will be necessary, but your partner will be best able to talk to the medical staff and make medical decisions on your behalf if he knows your wishes ahead of time.

Warn him. All of those TV movies with pregnant women screaming "I hate you!" at their partners are based partly on fact. Women do feel intense pain during childbirth at times, and that can lead to primal outbursts of anger or fear. Let your partner know, here and now, that you don't know what you might say and do during labor but that some of it you might not be able to control.

Suggest distractions. Labor can take a long time, and much of it might be boring for both of you. That may be especially true if you've had an epidural and your partner doesn't need to support you physically the way he might during a more active, medication-free birth. Let him know what you'd like to do during breaks. Want him to read you a trashy novel? Play cards with you? Bring along your favorite CDs? A portable DVD player? Ideally most of the less active time will be spent in the luxury of your own home.

Drop hints about your post-baby celebration. Whether you want him to bring you roses or fudge, let him know or you'll set yourself up for disappointment. Tell him what would make you feel extra special when it's time to celebrate.

Have him pack a bag for the hospital. You're not the only one who's going to spend hours in the hospital. Your partner may want to pack a few things for himself:

- Bottled water
- Call list of relatives and friends
- Books or magazines
- Snacks
- Toothbrush, deodorant, and comb
- Razor
- Cash
- Comfy footwear
- Change of clothes
- Portable music player
- Pictures of labor positions
- A notebook and pen (questions for providers, notes from partner)

Week 31

Your Baby

The inside story

You may notice that your baby moves more when you talk to him. You'll probably start feeling different kicks now as his body continues to grow, but the kicks you do feel will be harder. They might even hurt, especially if he's practicing karate chops on your groin.

Your baby may weigh 3½ pounds this week, and he should be 16 inches in length. His belly is Buddha-like, round and hard because his liver is busily producing red blood cells. Some babies have a full head of hair by the 31st week of pregnancy, while others are bald as eggs. It's common for babies to hiccup at this stage and for the hiccups to be strong enough to wake you in the middle of the night.

If you want to have some fun, shine a light on your stomach to see if your baby changes his movements. (If he doesn't, he might be napping; try it again in a few hours.) You can also press against your abdomen to see if he answers you with a kick. Or rest a book on your belly and marvel when he objects to the encroachment on his home turf by kicking the book right off your stomach.

Your Body

Will baby fit?

Your due date is fast approaching, bringing less-than-tactful comments about your size and impending birth experience. "Boy, with hips like that, your baby's going to fall right out of you," some women may hear, while others wince as "friends" tell them that they'll have to have a cesarean delivery because they're too slim for a baby to pass through the pelvic area.

Ignore these comments. It's impossible to tell how easily a woman will deliver by looking at her. Even if you have a large build, you may still have a narrow pelvis (which means your pelvic bones are close together) or an android pelvis (a pelvis shaped like a heart around the opening). Either of these features can make it harder for your baby to slide through. If you are a small woman, you may still have a generous-size pelvis.

Chances are that you, like more than 80 percent of women, have a perfectly adequate pelvis: well-rounded and now starting to loosen for childbirth, no matter how slim or broad you were before pregnancy. Determining "fit" depends on more than your pelvis too. "Fit" depends on the baby's size and the position of her head.

Easing pelvic pressure

You've probably been feeling some pressure and discomfort in your pelvic area all along. However, once your baby descends in preparation for birth, you may feel both pressure in your pelvis and sharp, stabbing pains in your pelvic and groin area. This is caused by a shifting in your pelvic bones, as your body opens a bit to deliver your baby, and by ligaments stretching to allow these bones to shift. You may feel these sharp pains in the middle of your pelvic bone, in your lower back, or even down your thighs. The discomfort might be constant, or you might notice it most when you cough, sneeze, or laugh.

The best way to relieve pelvic pressure and these shooting pains—which you'll most often feel if you lift your leg to pull on a boot, for instance, or as you get up out of a chair—is to shift positions when it happens and to keep exercising until your due date. It bears repeating that any exercise is good, even if it's a walk or a slow swim.

If you get to the point where pelvic discomfort prevents you from doing any exercise, talk with your doctor about using a more high-tech maternity support belt or visiting a physical therapist. A physical therapist can probably offer you some relief by helping you balance the weight of your belly better.

Genital changes

Your partner may be startled to discover that things don't just feel different on you at this point; things look different too.

Your genitals are much larger than they were before pregnancy. This is due to hormones and increased blood flow, both of which cause veins to enlarge and your swollen labia to darken in color. As a result of your new, generous proportions, you may find that penetration during intercourse is more pleasurable thanks to your swollen tissues and increased vaginal secretions. Or you may find it's less pleasurable for you because engorgement makes a tighter fit for your partner. All of these things are perfectly normal. Your genitals will return to their original proportions and color after childbirth.

Relaxing for a better birth

Research has demonstrated that relaxed moms who feel less frightened during labor and delivery have shorter labors and are more likely to deliver healthy babies. This may not be only a psychological effect but a physiological one as well. When a mom is frightened during labor, she may respond by clenching her teeth, grabbing the side rails of the bed, and curling her toes as if she's steeling herself against the pain or even fighting it. This can happen with the pain of a contraction or the fear of another one coming. She may also be afraid of the unknown.

Unfortunately, this response may

physically inhibit your baby's birth. When you tense up in response to your contractions, your body produces adrenaline, the hormone that surges through you when you face situations that cause you fear or pain. When your body produces adrenaline, that chemical response inhibits the production of oxytocin, the hormone that causes your uterine muscles to contract. In effect, your fear of pain during labor can prevent your body from doing the work it needs to do to move your baby through the birth canal and into the waiting arms of the people who already love him.

Thinking ahead to labor

Many books and providers divide labor into three stages (see "Labor and delivery," page 343). To you, labor will be a continuous experience, and you will probably think of it only as "early" and "active" labor according to how intense the contractions are. However, because your practitioner and labor nurses may divide the labor into stages when talking to you or to each other, it's useful to know the definitions:

Stage 1. This is the longest part of labor, usually defined as that part of labor where the cervix thins and opens (effaces and dilates). This stage is further divided into "early" and "active" first-stage labor. During early first-stage labor, your cervix will dilate from 0 to 4 centimeters; during active first-stage labor, you will dilate to about 8 centimeters. Then there is a transition phase as your cervix

finishes dilating to 10 centimeters in preparation for birthing your baby. During transition, the rhythmic, cyclic pattern of your active labor may be disrupted. Now the contractions might be much more erratic and powerful, with less time between contractions for you to rest.

Stage 2. Contractions are shorter, more intense, and more frequent during second-stage labor as your uterus pushes your baby down the birth canal and out of your body through the opened cervix.

Stage 3. You will deliver the placenta and membranes in the third stage of labor.

The placenta

About 5 minutes after you give birth, when your partner and the nurses and anyone else who happens to be in the room are admiring your baby, your uterus will still be at work, squeezing out the placenta. After a few mild contractions, you'll deliver the placenta (also called the afterbirth, for obvious reasons).

The placenta is the organ that connects you and your baby. It develops from the outermost layer of cells on the fertilized egg. It takes oxygen and nutrients from the mother's bloodstream and supplies them to the fetus. It also removes the baby's waste products, depositing them in the mother's blood for elimination by the kidneys. The baby is connected to the placenta by the umbilical cord.

Watch for signs of placenta previa

(page 268) and placental abruption (page 269), two problems that can occur with this critical organ. Talk to your provider about any concerns you may have.

Practicing for labor

Believe it or not, you're only about 8 weeks from your due date, and this is the perfect time to start practicing relaxation and breathing techniques that you'll use during childbirth. Even if you have already decided to have an epidural or opioids to relieve pain—or if you change your mind about natural childbirth and ask for pain medication midway through your delivery—these techniques can help you manage any discomfort you do feel and actively participate in your baby's birth. Use these techniques, in addition to those you learn in childbirth class, to teach yourself to work with your body and make labor easier on yourself and your baby.

These techniques may be especially useful in early labor. If your baby is moving and you haven't broken your water, stay at home for early labor.

Relaxation techniques for early labor. One of the best ways to relax during labor is to learn to isolate different muscle groups in your body. Your uterus must contract to push the baby down and retract the cervix over the baby's head. If other muscles are tight during contractions, you're wasting energy and oxygen. By learning to relax the rest of your muscle groups, you can focus on allowing most of your oxygen to travel to your uterus.

To learn how to relax your body during contractions, work with your partner or labor coach. Prop yourself up against the pillows in your bed or lie on your side. Starting with your toes and moving up toward your head, focus on relaxing each individual set of muscles in your body.

Have your coach issue different commands, one at a time, asking you to contract different muscle groups. For instance, if your coach says, "Contract your left arm," raise that arm and make a fist. Your coach should check to see that the rest of your body is relaxed by lifting different parts of your body. They should feel heavy and loose in his hands. Then have your coach say, "Relax your left arm." You should focus on letting that arm fall slowly until it's heavy enough for him to feel the weight of it in his hands.

The goal here is to learn how to relax your entire body while one muscle contracts. Ideally, during early labor your coach will be able to help you relax your entire body when your uterus is contracting. How long you will be able to keep doing this throughout labor depends on how skilled you are at relaxing your muscles and the type of labor you are having.

Breathing techniques for labor. No matter what your birth experience, breathing techniques can help make it faster and easier. Practicing them for several weeks before your delivery can delay or eliminate the need for pain medication during childbirth.

You will no doubt learn Lamaze or other breathing techniques if you take a childbirth class. Although there are variations, the point of most of these exercises is to teach you to focus your energy and work with your body as your baby makes her way into the world.

Paced breathing. Once labor contractions get so regular or intense that you have to stop a conversation or halt your activities, it's time to start your paced breathing. Practice paced breathing techniques every day, starting at least 2 months before your due date:

- Take a deep breath to fill your lungs completely and exhale it.
- Channel your energy by focusing on one spot on the wall, ceiling, or floor (depending on your position).
- When your coach says, "Contraction begins," take 5–10 deep breaths for a minute. As you inhale, place your hands on the lower part of your abdomen and stroke gently upward toward your ribs. As you exhale, let your hands glide back down. Massaging the uterus during a contraction can help ease the discomfort, much like massaging a cramp in your leg. Your coach should count out a minute in 15-second intervals so that you can track the time and peak of each contraction: "15, 30, 45, 60."
- Breathe normally when your coach says, "Contraction ends."
- Practice your paced breathing exercises in all of the basic labor

positions—sitting in a chair, reclining on pillows, lying on your side, standing, and kneeling against a large ball or bed.

Modified paced breathing. In active stage 1 labor—when your cervix has dilated about 5 centimeters—the slow, deep breaths of paced breathing may no longer be enough to get you through a contraction. Then it's time to modify your paced breathing to keep up with the pace and intensity of labor. Practice modified paced breathing, starting at least 6 weeks before your delivery date. Doing it daily will help you master conditioned responses to your labor coach's commands:

- Take a deep, relaxing breath.
- When the coach says, "Contraction begins," start with your slow breathing. Accelerate your inhale-exhale pattern as the contraction builds and peaks, using faster, lighter breathing. It will help if your coach counts out each contraction for a minute, "15, 30, 45, 60 seconds," so that you'll know when to start slowing your breathing again. Generally your contraction will peak around 30 seconds, and you can slow your breathing after that.
- There is no one right time to start modified breathing, or one right pace. Generally you'll be breathing at twice your normal rate. The important thing is that your breathing should be regular, and you should take in the same amount of air that you exhale. If

you feel light-headed, that means you're breathing in more oxygen than you're exhaling; if you find that your breaths are shallow, you're probably letting out more air than you're inhaling.

- You may still find that massaging your uterus, as described on the previous page, helps you keep time and get through the contraction. However, some women find the extra sensation too overwhelm-

Placenta previa

The placenta has been hard at work throughout your pregnancy, transporting nutrients and oxygen from your blood to your baby via the umbilical cord. Normally this organ is attached high on the wall of your uterus; problems may occur if instead the placenta grows over the cervix, a condition called placenta previa.

What's normal. During childbirth, the baby arrives before the placenta, traveling through your cervix and vagina. Within half an hour of your baby's birth, you will deliver the placenta when it separates from the wall of your uterus. This sequence of events is necessary because your baby relies on the placenta to provide life-sustaining oxygen until he can breathe on his own.

What's abnormal. If the placenta grows low in the uterus, it may partly or completely block the opening in the cervix that leads to your vagina. This happens in about 1 in 200 pregnancies. You're more at risk if you're older, if you've had several babies, if you've had a prior birth by cesarean, or if you smoke cigarettes.

Concerns. Placenta previa can heighten the risk of life-threatening hemorrhage, either before or during labor. This severe, uncontrollable bleeding can happen because, as your cervix thins out and opens in preparation for delivery, the placenta's attachments to the uterus can more easily become damaged due to its lowered position. If this happens you might start bleeding without any pain. Your provider will do an ultrasound to determine the cause of the bleeding. An ultrasound at 18–20 weeks may show a low-lying placenta or a placenta previa. The ultrasound will be repeated in the 3rd trimester, when most low-lying placentas will no longer be low because the uterus has grown larger. If the placenta still completely covers the cervix at the time of the 3rd trimester ultrasound, most of the time it stays there. Placenta previa is usually diagnosed during the last 2 months of pregnancy.

Treatment. Treatment is determined by the length of your pregnancy, whether the placenta has started to detach from the wall of the uterus, and your baby's health. The treatment goals are to prevent bleeding and lessen the risk of premature delivery. If placenta previa is diagnosed but there is no bleeding, your provider will probably tell you to go on bed rest or limit your activities to lessen the danger of bleeding until your baby is big enough to safely deliver by cesarean. If you start to bleed, you will be admitted to the hospital; how long you remain in the hospital depends on several factors. Cesarean deliveries are almost always necessary because the placenta would be torn from its roots during a vaginal delivery, causing life-threatening bleeding for mom and lack of oxygen for the baby.

Placental abruption

As noted in the description of placenta previa (previous page), your placenta usually implants high on the uterine wall, and it doesn't detach until after you deliver your baby. This allows your baby to continue receiving oxygen from the placenta until she can breathe on her own. If, however, your placenta separates from your uterus before your baby is born, this condition is called placental abruption. It puts you and your baby at risk.

Risk factors. These factors put you at risk for placental abruption, which affects 1 out of every 200 births: cocaine abuse, high blood pressure, preeclampsia, abdominal trauma, and a history of placental abruption during a prior pregnancy.

Symptoms. It's imperative to alert your practitioner to any symptoms such as bleeding from your vagina, severe pain in your abdomen or back, tenderness in your uterus, or strong contractions every minute. In most cases of abruption, a portion of the placenta separates. In rare cases, placental abruption is complete and the baby usually dies. You may suffer from hemorrhaging or organ failure—or you may die—if the condition isn't treated.

If you have bleeding after 24 weeks' gestation, you will be evaluated in the hospital to determine if the placenta is separating. Your doctor will monitor your blood pressure and pulse and the baby's heart rate, and he will perform an ultrasound and a pelvic exam. How and when you deliver will depend on your health and your baby's health; you may deliver vaginally or by cesarean, and you may deliver immediately, within hours, or even days later.

ing and have to stop at this point. Ask your partner to massage your thighs or back instead.

Breathing through transition and pushing. The point of controlled breathing during transition and second-stage (also called "expulsion") labor is to keep yourself from bearing down and pushing—no matter how much you might want to—until the doctor or midwife tells you that your cervix is fully dilated and ready. You'll feel a lot of pressure in your rectum, almost as if you need to move your bowels, and you'll need to use some special breathing to distract yourself from wanting to answer this call to push your baby into the world. This is important because if you push too

soon you may have more swelling and tearing of your cervix. Try the following techniques:

- When your coach says, "Contraction begins," take a deep breath; then pant several times.
- When your coach says, "Urge," instead of exhaling in one breath, imagine a candle in front of your face. Make an "O" with your mouth and try to blow it out.
- Repeat this pattern of breathing several times for each urge to push. Many educators describe this pattern as "six pants, one blow" so that you're saying something like "hee, hee, hee, hee, hee, hee, who!" Blowing air outward makes it impossible to strain downward to

push your baby out.

- When it's time to push, you're going to use your entire body to bear down with your uterine contractions, so take deep breaths and lean into the contraction.
- Bear down with all your might, slowly exhaling and grunting or groaning as you tighten your abdominal muscles and exert more pressure on your diaphragm. Visualize your baby moving downward and assume a position that will work with gravity instead of against it.
- Don't push or bear down between contractions. Use that opportunity to rest and wait for the next urge.
- Practice these pushing breaths in the different labor positions to choose the ones that feel most comfortable for you. But don't push—it's way too early!

Your Self

Will I bond with my baby?

If you've had one of those pregnancies riddled with problems, in which you seemed to move from constant nausea to backaches to carpal tunnel syndrome and swollen ankles, you may have begun to wonder if disliking pregnancy means you'll dislike your baby too. After all, it seems strange that you'd fall in love with someone you've never met who is making you sick to your stomach, keeping you up all night, kicking you when you're down, making you take

time off from that exciting project at work, and giving you a belly that rivals Santa's.

However, for most women, the pregnancy itself will be forgotten the minute they finish giving birth. That doesn't mean that love will come easily. Predicting when and how much moms will love their babies is an inexact science because once again your body is at the mercy of hormones. Endorphins—the same hormones that make you feel so good after a sweaty run or workout—are released during childbirth, infusing you with good feelings. You also produce oxytocin and prolactin, and levels of those bonding hormones will be even higher if you nurse your baby. So falling in love with your baby may come naturally as chemistry kicks in.

However, there are also parents who struggle not to feel resentful of their newborns. Some of these parents may have been ambivalent about the pregnancy to begin with or have an inadequate family support system. Some are also disturbed to see that their babies aren't picture-perfect after birth, but red-faced, bald, squinty-eyed creatures covered with goo. Others are so overwhelmed or depressed by new responsibilities that they feel numb or angry (see "Postpartum emotions" and "Postpartum depression," page 376). These post-baby emotions can affect you whether you're a teenage mom or an over-40 mother who's had infertility treatments because she wanted to have a child.

Don't worry. So long as you go through the motions of feeding and rocking your baby, talking to her, and meeting her various needs, those feelings of love will materialize because you're repeatedly acting in a loving way. Research shows that even babies whose parents initially feel resentful of them turn out fine as long as they're well cared for during this adjustment period. Eventually your baby will smile at you or babble in response to your conversation, and that love light will shine. If after time you think the bonding simply isn't happening, talk to your obstetrician or pediatrician.

Doing it all is overrated

If this is your first child, you may wonder what all the fuss is about caring for a teeny baby. After all, you're a modern, independent woman who's been working out of the house or spending her weekends rock climbing. Really, how difficult can caring for a baby be?

Very. Depending on whether you've had a vaginal birth or a cesarean delivery, you will be back home only two to four days after delivery. Your body will be sore, you won't be sleeping, your hormones will be running riot, your breasts will be so engorged that they feel like a pair of cement blocks strapped to your chest, and your mood swings will be active throughout the day. Factor in feedings every 2 or 3 hours, diapering a dozen times a day, a mountain of laundry, and no chance to take a

shower or get to the grocery store by yourself, and you're looking at hard days ahead.

In the United States, people often measure accomplishments by what they are able to check off a "to do" list; after your baby is born, you'll be lucky to microwave dinner. Even if this is a second or third child and you think you know the drill, every baby is different. This one could be a crier, or your toddler may suddenly regress and become the stick-to-your-leg kid now that he has a little competitor for your attention.

This is not the time to wing it solo. The best thing you can do for your new baby is arrange the support you'll need so that you can take care of him. Accept that you're human and don't be afraid to ask for help.

Start by making a list of all the things you'll need to do when you come home with your new baby. Who's going to manage the housework? The cooking, grocery shopping, yard work, bill paying, dry cleaners? Who can watch the baby so that you can grab a shower, take a nap, or get back to your walking routines to ease your body back into your favorite jeans? Who's going to give you breastfeeding tips to help your baby latch on? Who will keep you company on those days when you're feeling so isolated you want to scream?

Make a list with your partner of what you think you'll need, not just for the first week after baby comes home but for the first year. Then make a companion list of your support network. Include family, friends, babysitters, and professional organizations like La Leche League or temporary nanny and housekeeping services. You may want to be at home alone with your baby for the first week or so, especially if your partner can stay home from work too. That will give you both a chance to get to know your baby without interference. After that, you'll want to tap into your support network, so start communicating with everyone on your list about the hopes or expectations you have regarding their involvement. Be very clear about what you want—and very grateful— and come up with a plan for your post-delivery life that will allow you and your baby to sail through your first months more smoothly.

Diet & Exercise

Desk posture

If you sit at a desk all day, maintaining good posture will help prevent back and shoulder tightness and pain. When sitting, keep your back in a normal, slightly arched position. Use a chair that supports your lower back; if your chair doesn't, use a thin pillow or a folded towel for support. Keep your head upright, your chin level, and your shoulders erect and relaxed. (You may notice that when you feel stressed, you unconsciously pull your shoulders up toward your ears.) Rest your arms comfortably at your sides.

Place your feet flat on the floor. If you can't reach the floor comfortably, use a footrest. (The best footrest is one that is slightly angled down toward your heels.)

If you use a computer, bend your elbows at a 90-degree angle and keep your wrists straight over the keyboard. The keyboard height should be just below your elbow height, and the monitor should be 18–22 inches from your forehead. The top of the screen should be at eye level.

Pull your chair in as close to your desk as you can manage. (If the chair's armrests get in the way, see if you can remove them—many office chairs have removable armrests.) If your belly gets in the way, lower your chair slightly. If you're still farther away from your desk or keyboard than you'd like, do the best you can, but take breaks every 20 minutes or so to get up, walk around for a minute, and even do a couple of shoulder and chest stretches. (See "Chest and shoulder stretches," page 249.)

Proper portion sizes

Even if you eat the most nutritious food in the world, you'll still gain excess weight if you eat too much of it. That's why eating proper portion sizes matters. Of course eating sensible portions can be hard in a world of 32-ounce sodas, ½-pound burgers, and "single-size" bags of chips that contain enough for three people. At home you can read labels to find out portion sizes, but when you're away from home, you have to guess. Here are a few handy guidelines to follow:

- 1 cup of dry cereal = the size of a baseball
- 3 ounces of meat, fish, or poultry = a deck of cards
- 1 serving of thin fish = a checkbook
- 1½ ounces of cheese = four dice
- ¾ cup of frozen yogurt or ice cream = a tennis ball
- ½ cup of fruit, rice, pasta, or cooked vegetables = half a tennis ball
- 1 cup of pasta = a closed fist
- 1 2-ounce bagel = a hockey puck
- 1 teaspoon of butter = the tip of your thumb
- 2 tablespoons of peanut butter = a roll of film

Common Questions

Q. This is my second child, and I'm worried that I won't make it to the hospital on time. During my first labor, my doctor told me to wait until the contractions were 5 minutes apart, and by the time I got to the hospital, I was already fully dilated. This made my delivery feel rushed. Should I come in sooner this time?

A. Every labor and delivery is different. First-time moms can usually expect to labor for several hours at home and still have many more hours ahead of them at the hospital, which is why that 5-minutes-apart rule is the standard. In general, everything is faster with a second pregnancy, so don't wait too long. Still there's a great deal of variation in how quickly a woman moves from early labor to active labor (when contractions are no more than 4 minutes apart), and that's what makes things so unpredictable.

In addition to timing your contractions, consider how far away you are from your birth center or hospital and how dilated your cervix was at your last prenatal visit. Also consider how quickly your contractions intensified last time. How long did it take you to go from contractions that were 5 minutes apart to the transition phase of labor or to contractions that were only 1–2 minutes apart?

You'll also need to consider getting to the hospital sooner if your membranes have ruptured or if you're extremely anxious or in more pain than you think is normal for early labor. You are the best judge of when to go to the hospital, so go when you think it's time. If you think you'd feel more comfortable, or at least less anxious, if you spend part of that early labor in or near the hospital, then go. The worst that can happen is that they'll send you away for a while. In that case, you can walk around the hospital neighborhood until it's the right time.

Week 32

Your Baby

The inside story

Your baby has definite sleep-and-wake cycles, but she probably sleeps about 70 percent of the time. Ultrasounds reveal that sometime between 32 weeks and 36 weeks babies develop the ability to dream. They have definite periods of REM (rapid eye movement) sleep and non-REM sleep. Your baby also has periods of quiet alertness in which she listens to the exciting sounds beyond her dark room.

At almost 4 pounds, your baby is definitely big enough by now to survive outside the womb. Her lungs are maturing, and her heart rate is starting to slow down a bit. However, research shows that the fetal heart rate speeds up if the mother is stressed, so stay as relaxed as you can to help your baby stay peaceful.

Your baby is still kicking, and all of that kicking is good practice for what she'll instinctively do if she's put on your belly after birth: She'll scramble her way up your belly to your breasts, where she will latch on and nurse.

Your Body

The truth about due dates

You may have calculated your due date using the exact date of your last period, or your practitioner may have made a prediction based on an ultrasound and measurements of your uterus. Either way it's unlikely that you'll have your baby on exactly that day. Believing that due dates are real is just one more comforting fantasy we humans hold dear.

In reality most women deliver healthy babies anywhere between 37 and 42 weeks after getting pregnant—a pretty broad window—with no more than 5 percent of women actually having their babies on their due dates.

The calculations. You and your provider formulated this magical date by taking the first day of your last menstrual period and adding 280 days, or 40 weeks. However, this method assumes that your periods are a tidy, predictable 28 days long, when in fact they might be 23 days or 32 days or so varied that you don't even bother keeping track. Typically, if you have longer menstrual cycles, you're more likely to deliver your baby after your due date, but you can never know for certain ahead of time. In fact, even a 1st-trimester sonogram—the most trustworthy way to calculate a woman's due date—has to be taken with the proverbial grain of salt because nobody really knows what triggers labor.

Educated guesses. So how do you know when your baby will arrive? You really don't until the Big Day. Until then you can make an educated guess. For instance, if this is your first pregnancy, you're likely to deliver early if your mother did. Caucasian mothers tend to have the longest pregnancies, and so do women under 30. Girl babies are more likely to be born early than boys. The most popular birthday in the United States is Tuesday, if that's any help, while weekends have noticeably lower birthrates—probably because cesareans and induced births are typically scheduled during the workweek for the sake of the doctors performing them.

If your pregnancy extends to 41 weeks, your practitioner will probably perform weekly nonstress tests, but many won't intervene until 42 weeks as long as you and your baby seem to be doing fine. So relax and enjoy a few more romantic dinners when you don't have to tote along an infant seat, a bulging diaper bag, and—oh, yes—a baby!

Auto safety and accidents

It isn't always easy to drive when you're reaching for the steering wheel around the 25-pound obstacle your belly has become. Most women continue driving until the end of their pregnancies. However, studies have shown that expectant mothers are more apt to be involved in car accidents than women who aren't pregnant. Researchers believe this probably has something to do with driving under the influence of pregnancy hormones, which can make you feel dizzy, fatigued, nauseous, or unfocused. Although driving is safe for most women even in the last weeks of pregnancy, this is a good time to take extra safety precautions:

- Wear a seat belt with a shoulder harness. Fasten the seat belt snugly beneath your belly and adjust the shoulder belt so that it doesn't rub against your neck. If you're in a car accident during your 3rd trimester, the added weight of your baby will give you greater forward momentum, so you'll fare better in a fender bender if you're buckled in.

- Follow the "stop, stretch, and stroll" rule, which is appropriate throughout pregnancy. That means taking frequent breaks to wake yourself up with a brisk walk, refocus your concentration, and use a restroom.

- Drive before or after rush hour, rather than through the thick of things. Fewer cars on the road around you mean fewer possibilities for mishaps behind the wheel.

- If you are in a car accident, your baby will probably be fine; infants are well protected within the

Emergency cesarean deliveries

In their most hopeful moments, women visualize giving birth gracefully, breathing through the pain, perhaps even smiling as they make that last push to give their babies the miracle of life. Many work hard to ensure that they can deliver naturally by choosing providers with low cesarean delivery rates, taking childbirth classes, exercising during pregnancy, maintaining a moderate weight gain, and perhaps even hiring a doula to accompany them to the delivery room. Yet the U.S. cesarean rate is higher than it has ever been—26.7 percent—even though few women imagine that they will need one.

Handling the emotions. No matter how many preventive steps you've taken or how healthy and low-risk your pregnancy has been, things do happen that might cause you to have an emergency cesarean. You will feel disappointed. You might even feel like a failure. However, it's important to maintain perspective. It's true that a cesarean delivery carries the inherent risks of any major surgery, such as internal bleeding, blood clots, infection, or damage to your organs. Some babies also have brief respiratory problems following a cesarean. However, thanks to improved anesthesia and surgical techniques and better antibiotics, cesareans carry fewer risks than ever, and having a healthy baby is far more important, in the long run, than delivering vaginally.

Causes. One of the most common reasons for an emergency cesarean is a surprise breech baby (one that's positioned feet or buttocks over your cervix) or a baby that's lying sideways in labor. Another is arriving in labor with heavy bleeding and concern that the placenta has separated or a previa has begun to bleed. The most common cause of an emergency cesarean is that the baby doesn't tolerate labor; if the fetal heart rate pattern shows cause for alarm, a cesarean may be the quickest and safest way to deliver the baby.

Procedure. It can be a chaotic scene with everything happening at once. You'll have your lower abdomen prepped for surgery. It will be washed and perhaps shaved, and you'll be given antibiotics and other fluids through an IV. You will either have your labor epidural dosed up to cesarean level or have a quick spinal or even general anesthesia. If you have an epidural or spinal anesthesia, you will be numb from your chest down; you will be awake, but you won't feel the doctor make the incision. You probably won't see it either because there is typically a surgical drape to shield your abdomen from your view—and because your baby is out before you know it!

muscular uterus and amniotic fluid. The main risk posed by any sort of car accident is separation of the placenta (see "Placental abruption," page 269), which might cause you to experience vaginal bleeding, severe pain, or contractions. Even if you do not experience these symptoms, call your doctor. She'll examine you, monitor your baby's heartbeat, and may even do an ultrasound to confirm that all is well. If you had a direct trauma to your belly and

week 32

are Rh-negative, you may also need a shot of Rhogam.

- Move the seat back, put a small pillow between your belly and the seat belt, and adjust the headrest so that you're as comfortable as possible while driving.
- Stay close to home. If you're going to travel more than 30 miles from home, take a cell phone and a companion with you.

Can the umbilical cord knot?

The umbilical cord is a critical lifeline that looks like a white, twisted telephone cord. Its two arteries and single vein transport nutrients and oxygen from your body through the placenta to your baby. The umbilical cord grows as your baby does, so by the time you deliver the cord will probably measure about 2 feet long. That's just the right length to allow you to hold your baby in your arms and begin nursing her even before you deliver the placenta.

Before birth. Many parents worry unnecessarily about knots in the umbilical cord. The truth is that most babies can do all sorts of somersaults and wave their umbilical cords around like jump ropes without doing any harm to themselves or the cords. A true cord knot can occur when a baby passes through a loop of umbilical cord. This usually happens early in pregnancy, though, when your baby is still small enough to move about freely. Most of the time the knot stays loose and does nothing to impede the baby's development.

Cord prolapse. Another potential—but extremely rare—problem is a cord that slips out of the uterus into the vagina either before or during labor. This can lead to the baby's oxygen supply being cut off if the cord is compressed. You may feel the cord protruding yourself if the cord descends into your vagina. This most often happens when a baby is breech or premature, especially if your water breaks, because the baby's head is not in position to prevent the cord from being carried into your cervix by the rush of amniotic fluid.

If you should feel the cord protruding, support it with a clean towel while you lie on your side and phone your emergency room and provider immediately. You will probably be sent to the hospital where you will be prepared for a cesarean delivery.

Cord abnormalities. Abnormalities in cord length can be associated with risk factors to your child's health. For instance, a short cord may prevent the baby from going deeper into the pelvis during labor. A cord that's overly long poses a higher risk of knots and tangles around the baby's neck either before or during delivery. If at birth only one artery and one vein are visible in the cord (instead of the usual two arteries and one vein), there's a chance that your baby may suffer health problems related to his cardiovascular or gastrointestinal system; that's why your doctor will examine the cord carefully after delivery. Remember that these abnormalities are extremely rare.

Stillbirths

A baby who dies in utero after 20 weeks of pregnancy, or one who dies during delivery, is stillborn. Any family death is devastating, but a stillborn baby can be especially tragic because it often happens suddenly and can occur in a previously uncomplicated pregnancy. However, it is extremely rare. Only 1 percent of pregnancies end in stillbirths, and more than half of those occur before the 28th week of pregnancy.

There are many complex reasons why a baby might be stillborn, from genetic abnormalities to problems with the placenta. Sometimes there appears to be no explanation at all, even after the baby is delivered and examined. The most common medical conditions associated with stillborn babies are infection (10 percent) and placental abruption (14 percent). Older mothers, mothers who smoke or drink alcohol, and mothers who are obese are more likely to have stillbirths.

If your baby dies before you go into labor, you will probably know it without a doubt. Your uterus will feel still and heavy without the usual movements of your baby. If you notice any significant decrease in your baby's activity—fewer than 10 movements in 2 hours is certainly cause for concern at this stage in your pregnancy—contact your provider immediately to see if you need a medical intervention to save your baby's life. Your provider will immediately check for your baby's heartbeat.

If your baby dies, you will probably start labor naturally within a couple of weeks. You may want to carry your baby for as long as possible. Many women, however, are too upset to continue the pregnancy. If that is how you feel, your provider may suggest inducing your labor right away or in a day or so when you've had a chance to prepare yourself. A vaginal delivery is still preferable to a cesarean, which poses more health risks.

During the labor and delivery, you may ask for pain medicines, such as opioids or an epidural when you need it. Don't be afraid to ask for information from your nurses, your provider, and whoever examines your baby and the placenta following birth. Although very difficult to think about at the time, autopsy and examination of the placenta may yield important data. Some research suggests that the more information a woman has about her stillbirth, along with a chance to name her baby and hold her to say good-bye, the better able she is to grieve afterward.

There is no single way to accept this dreadful loss. You and your partner will want support from friends and family. It may help to join a bereavement group or see a therapist. A memorial or funeral service will help you and your families to grieve, though you may find that many people, even those caring for you most directly, feel awkward. They may encourage you to "move on," but of course you won't be able to for a long time. To you this child was a real presence, a life within you, and you'll have a long way to go before the pain lessens. Keep a journal and a few mementos of this life you carried—a footprint, a lock of hair, a photograph—and don't be afraid to look at them from time to time. This baby was a part of you and a part of your family, however briefly, and deserves to be remembered.

week 32

Monitoring baby. Most cord problems cause no harm to your baby. The best way to know if there's a problem with your baby's umbilical cord is by charting your baby's activity. If you don't notice at least 8–10 movements in 1 hour, then count for a second hour; you may have been counting while the baby was asleep. If you still don't detect any movement or the baby's movements have decreased, call your doctor. She will likely ask you to go to the office or hospital for either an ultrasound or nonstress test. They may tell you that all is well, but it's important to know for sure while there is still time for a cesarean delivery should it be necessary.

Your Self

Preparing for baby's arrival

Your first few weeks after delivery will be easier if you prepare as much as possible now. If you stock up on all of the baby supplies you'll need, you'll save yourself the aggravation of running out of diaper cream in the middle of the night. Stocking up can also save you money if you buy in bulk at discount stores or sales.

Diapers. Newborns go through 10–12 diapers in a 24-hour period, so do some quick math and see how many you'll need to have on hand. If you choose disposable diapers, shop around to find the best prices. Don't assume brand-name diapers are the best; many mothers find less

expensive store-brand diapers to be every bit as good. Take this helpful hint: Major manufacturers of diapers send money-off coupons to customers who register at their websites, so log on today. The companies also send coupons to parents of multiples.

If you prefer cloth diapers, buy them several weeks before your due date, because they should be washed several times before use. Advocates of cloth diapers say babies who wear them develop fewer cases of diaper rash than babies who wear disposables, because cloth allows more air circulation. This helps prevent rash-causing bacteria from multiplying. They say cloth diapers feel more comfortable, cost less, and are better for the environment.

Cloth diapers are easier to use now than they were in your mother's day. They now come pin-free, with options such as Velcro closures, disposable liners, and colorful covers. If you choose to use cloth diapers, you can wash dirty diapers yourself or use a diaper service. If you plan to wash them yourself, buy enough to last between washings. If you plan to launder cloth diapers every four days, buy at least 48 diapers for your newborn. Diaper services rent diapers to clients and usually come once a week to pick up soiled diapers and deliver clean ones. To find a diaper service near you, contact the National Association of Diaper Services (610-971-4850; www.diapernet.com).

Wipes. Disposable wipes are an easy way to clean your baby's bottom. For a newborn's tender skin, choose unscented wipes. Cloth wipes are also available and are sometimes sold by companies that sell cloth diapers. Or you can use paper towels and warm water.

Diaper cream. Every baby gets diaper rash, so it's a good idea to have diaper cream on hand. There are two basic kinds: petroleum ointment, which is good for minor diaper rash, and white zinc oxide, which is thicker and better for more stubborn cases of diaper rash. It's also stickier and messier than petroleum ointment.

Bath supplies. You'll need a baby bathtub, gentle baby soap, no-tear shampoo, and soft washcloths.

The ABCs of daycare

At this point you might be having trouble believing your due date will ever arrive, so it may not have occurred to you to start looking for someone to care for your baby when you return to work. However, as any experienced working parent can tell you, searching for the right daycare solution is a tough task. It's difficult both logistically and emotionally. You're going to have to find a loving caregiver whose schedule and values match your own.

Luckily, there are more options than ever, and the past two decades of research has shown us that high-quality daycare is actually beneficial for most children. While some research, including a study conducted recently by the National Institute of Child Health and Human

Development, suggests that children who spend more than 30 hours a week in child care are more likely to be aggressive and disobedient by the time they reach kindergarten, that same research also pointed to daycare gains, like better language, problem-solving skills, and memory development. The view held by most researchers is that the most critical influence on a child's behavior is his home environment, whether he's in full-time daycare or at home with his mother.

So how do you find the right daycare for you? Here are some options to consider:

Au pairs and nannies. We'd all love to have Mary Poppins floating in on her umbrella to tidy up the nursery and have the baby asleep by sunset. If you have an extra bedroom and don't mind sharing your living space, an au pair can be ideal. An au pair is typically a foreign woman, working through an agency, who gets a small

Questions to Ask a Daycare Provider

- How long have you been doing daycare?
- Can I visit my baby anytime?
- How often do you let babies cry themselves to sleep?
- May I give you breast milk in bottles for my baby?
- How do you usually spend your day with a baby?
- What credentials and references do you provide?
- Do you have infant CPR training?

salary and room and board in exchange for daycare. If you don't have the space to house an au pair, or want more privacy and don't mind shelling out the extra money, a day nanny might be the solution, especially if you also have an older child who needs to be driven to various preschool classes and activities.

Pros

- Hours can be more flexible than daycare centers
- One-on-one care for your baby
- Some housekeeping services and cooking
- Baby can stay home, so there's no need to carry supplies to daycare— or bring viruses home

Cons

- Difficult to meet in advance if au pair is from a foreign country
- Someone else is running your house
- Her professional training might be limited
- May have to pay taxes for a nanny
- May have to tack on an agency fee

Daycare centers. If the daycare center has a high-quality staff, your child will probably develop an early zest for learning and great socialization skills. However, daycare centers can be financially out of reach for many parents of infants unless they're subsidized or associated with your workplace. That's because state laws require such small infant-to-caregiver ratios (as well they should) that rates charged for newborns can be double the rate charged for toddlers.

Pros

- Trained staff
- On-site perks for older infants and toddlers like art supplies, computers, toys
- May be subsidized or convenient if affiliated with workplace
- Structured routines make it easier to keep baby happy at home

Cons

- Have to commute to daycare before commuting to work
- Babies have to go with the center's nap and feeding schedule
- May have waiting list

Family daycare. Family daycare doesn't necessarily mean your own family but a family-like setting, where a licensed daycare provider takes children into her home. For young infants, family daycare can offer the perfect mix of a calm family environment with the stimulation of other children. The downside for parents is sometimes a feeling of guilt that it's not you staying home—or discomfort with the way someone else is "mothering" your child.

Pros

- Usually less expensive than daycare centers or an at-home nanny
- Close, loving bonds among caregiver, other children, and your baby
- Relaxed environment

Cons

- If your caregiver's own kids get sick, you might be out of daycare
- Quality of care is highly variable from one caregiver to the next
- You might feel competitive with her

Finding the Best Daycare

Your best bet for finding the highest-quality daycare is by word of mouth: Ask your friends, your family, your provider, and your workplace colleagues for suggestions. You can also contact the organizations below.

Daycare centers:
National Association for the Education of Young Children
800-424-2460
www.naeyc.org

Child Care Aware
800-424-2246
www.childcareaware.org

Au pairs:
The U.S. Information Agency cultural-exchange page
http://exchanges.state.gov

Day nannies and family daycare providers:
Yellow Pages, word of mouth, bulletin boards in pediatricians' offices or churches, and the employment section of your local newspaper

The right fit for feet

Are you struggling like Cinderella's stepsister to get your shoes on? Are they pinching your toes so much that you kick them off under your desk at work? Toward the end of your pregnancy, you may find that your shoes simply don't fit. Like the rest of you, your feet are growing. This isn't necessarily due to your weight gain. It's more likely the result of that 40 percent increase in blood and body fluids moving through you and causing tissues to swell. In addition, your uterus is now large enough to press on the veins through your pelvic area, slowing down blood flow in your lower body. Your feet might expand to fill an extra shoe size by the end of your pregnancy.

Your foot size will diminish again after you give birth, though it may never be as petite as your prepregnancy measure. Stay comfortable in the meantime by investing in a couple of pairs of shoes in a larger size. It's best to buy canvas, cotton, or leather shoes to keep your feet cooler; stay away from flats because they can strain your back. Of course, with your new proportions you should skip the stilettos, too, and settle for that happy medium—a heel between ½ inch and 2 inches is probably the most comfortable. It's also wise to buy shoes with either elastic sides or buckles that can expand with you throughout the day. You'll soon find out that bending over to tie shoes will take massive effort, so slip-ons are a great idea. Carry a pair of elasticized slippers with nonskid soles to work and have another pair by your door to put on the minute you're home.

Diet & Exercise

9 ways to get more calcium

If you're a milk drinker, getting the calcium you and your baby need is relatively easy. If you don't like milk, you can still get plenty of calcium if you're creative. Here are some ways to sneak calcium into your diet:

- Add low-fat or fat-free shredded cheese to your salads or cooked vegetables.
- Use plain non-fat yogurt as a base for salad dressings.
- Mix powdered non-fat dry milk into smoothies.
- Eat high-calcium vegetables such as broccoli, okra, kale, mustard greens, and collard greens.
- Drink hot cocoa made with skim milk instead of water.
- Add milk instead of water to canned soups.
- If you like coffee, order a decaf latte with skim milk.
- Drink calcium-fortified orange juice.
- Experiment with calcium-fortified soy products, such as soymilk and tofu.

Simple leg stretches

Your legs are working hard carrying you and your baby around all day. If your leg muscles feel stiff or achy, loosen them up with these stretches. Remember, stretch only to the point of mild tension, never bounce, and breathe slowly and naturally while you are stretching:

Ankle stretch. Stand and hold on to something for balance or sit comfortably in a chair. Lift your right foot a few inches from the ground. Rotate foot and ankle 8–10 times clockwise, then 8–10 times counterclockwise. Repeat on other side.

Front-thigh stretch. Stand a little way from a wall and place your left hand on wall for support. Standing straight, bend your left leg at the knee and grasp the top of your left foot with your right hand. Pull your heel toward your buttocks. Hold 10–20 seconds. Repeat on other side.

Outer-thigh stretch. Sit on the floor with your right leg straight out in front. Bend your left leg, cross your left foot over, and place it outside your right knee. Pull your left knee across your body toward the right shoulder. Hold 10–20 seconds. Repeat on other side.

Inner-thigh stretch. Stand with your feet pointed straight ahead, a little more than shoulder width apart, and your hands on your hips. (If necessary, hold on to a chair to avoid tipping over.) Bend your right knee slightly and move your left hip downward toward the right knee. Hold for 10–15 seconds. Repeat on other side.

Common Questions

Q. I feel so huge that I don't think I can get any bigger at this point. How can I tell if my baby is still growing at the right rate?

A. Even now, during each prenatal visit your practitioner will measure your fundus (top of the uterus) to check your baby's growth rate. This may seem like an incredibly low-tech way of measuring your uterus because it's being done from the outside of your body, but it's quite accurate.

The uterus is amazingly stretchy, starting from the size of a tennis ball in your

1st trimester and ballooning to just beneath your rib cage by your due date. By the time your baby is born, your uterus will have a volume 1,000 times greater than before your pregnancy, and it will weigh about 2 pounds all by itself. No matter where you are in your pregnancy, the length of your pregnancy should correspond nicely with the distance in centimeters between the top of your uterus and your pubic bone. If they correspond, your baby is growing at a normal rate.

Q. During my last prenatal visit, my midwife measured my uterus and said that I'm a little small. Now I'm worried that something is wrong. What causes this?

A. If your midwife didn't order another diagnostic test, such as an ultrasound, and if she didn't seem concerned about the baby's heart rate or activity level, there's nothing to worry about. Some women may measure smaller than expected for many reasons: The baby may be small because you are small, the baby may be transverse, or the baby's head may be positioned deep in the vagina.

If your baby doesn't gain adequate weight in the 3rd trimester, however, you may have a condition known as intrauterine growth restriction (IUGR). This describes any baby that consistently measures smaller than he should given the length of the pregnancy. It's most common in situations where the expectant mother suffers from a chronic health condition such as high blood pressure or when there are twins or more. It can also be a sign of abnormalities in the baby or the placenta.

Typically, a practitioner who suspects IUGR will first carefully review the gestational age, which in most cases was based on a sure last menstrual period, early pelvic exam, and/or an ultrasound prior to 20 weeks. Due dates do not get shifted at this late date based on the baby's size unless there was a mistake made early on.

If the due date is accurate and the baby simply isn't growing, the next step is an ultrasound to measure the baby's head, long bones, and abdominal circumference. This will show an estimated fetal weight and where your baby is on the growth curve. The ultrasound also allows the doctor to see if your baby is small but healthy and moving around or if your baby is small and sluggish. If he is healthy, the doctor may tell you to be patient and let your baby grow in his own time. If he is too small or not perky enough, the doctor may order more fetal testing. He may even decide to deliver the baby, especially if you are at 37 weeks or later.

Week 33

Your Baby

The inside story
During these final weeks of pregnancy, your baby enters his "finishing period." This is exactly what it sounds like: Your baby's organs, skeleton, and body are well formed, but he needs a little more time to finish getting ready to take on the world. By now he weighs a good 4½ pounds and measures more than 17 inches long, pushing the height of your uterus nearly to your rib cage. His toenails have completely grown in, as has any hair on his head.

Your amniotic fluid level is at its highest about now. The placenta is still providing oxygen to your baby through the umbilical cord, but your baby is practicing his breathing regularly, swallowing amniotic fluid as he opens and closes his mouth and exercising his diaphragm muscle. He continues to store iron in his liver, and the connections between his brain cells keep spreading like tiny tree branches. Neurons and synapses are developing between those brain cells, forming connections so that he'll have the skills to thrive as an infant.

Your Body

Belly geography
Line up a half-dozen similar-size pregnant women who are all at the same point in their pregnancy and who have all gained the same amount of weight, and you're likely to see a half-dozen different ways of carrying the pregnancy. One woman will carry low, another will carry high. One will be carrying only in front, and another will look pregnant from the sides, front, and back. One woman's entire front will stick way out, and another's will look more like a wide, flattened ball. All are normal.

The contours of a growing belly vary based in part on your baby's size and position, your height and build, and where your extra weight happens to settle. Carrying a certain way doesn't indicate the gender of your baby, even though people will swear that they know whether you're having a boy or girl based on how high or low you're carrying.

When breastfeeding may not be an option
Not everyone should breastfeed. You should bottle-feed if you are extremely underweight; if you abuse

Delivering a special-needs baby

If your baby has been diagnosed with a birth defect, discuss delivery options with your doctor and any of the specialists you've consulted with regarding your baby's condition. Although many special-needs babies can be delivered vaginally, some are better off being born by cesarean delivery. Where and how you deliver depends on your baby's situation. For example, if your baby has a congenital heart defect, he can probably be delivered vaginally. If the baby has spina bifida, he might fare better if delivered by a cesarean because a vaginal birth could cause additional damage to his spine. If your baby has a cardiac defect, delivering in a specialty hospital may make sense because there will be experienced medical staff on hand to provide specialized treatment.

Your doctor may recommend a scheduled cesarean delivery in week 37 or 38, before you go into labor. If so, your doctor may perform an amniocentesis; by analyzing a teaspoon or two of your amniotic fluid, he can check for a substance that is present only when your baby's lungs are mature. At this point in pregnancy, the risks from an amniocentesis include causing labor or breaking your water; miscarriage is not one of the risks.

drugs or alcohol; if you take medications that could pass into your breast milk and harm your baby—for example, certain drugs for cancer or hypertension; or if you have a serious medical condition such as HIV/AIDS, or a deficiency of prolactin, the hormone responsible for milk production. If you have had major breast surgery or breast implants, talk with your health care provider about whether you can breastfeed.

Your Self

Developing a parenting plan

What kind of parent will you be? Overprotective? Authoritarian? Indulgent? Controlling? Affectionate? Permissive? Strict? Playful? Distant? Do you feel strongly about how much television your child will watch, how much junk food he'll eat, or what musical instrument he will play? Do you want to be very involved in your child's life, or would you rather he be independent? Do you believe in punishing bad behavior or rewarding good behavior? All these questions and more run through most expectant parents' minds as they think about how they will raise their children.

Pregnancy is a good time to talk with your partner about what expectations and ideals you each have about parenting styles. Both of you bring very different experiences to the parenting table based on how you were raised, whether your feelings about your childhood are positive or negative, and thoughts you may have about what you wish your parents had done differently. You also may have formed opinions about parenting by watching how your friends and family members are raising their children. Talk about these opinions and experiences and draw from them a rough outline of what kind of parenting you would like to provide for your child.

Parenting philosophies influence your actions even when your child is a baby. If, for example, you believe in being very attentive to your child's needs, and your partner believes that children should grow up being self-sufficient, these different parenting styles may clash as you disagree over whether to let your baby cry himself to sleep. You may feel strongly that you should go to your baby and comfort him; your partner may feel that it's time your child started to find ways to comfort himself and put himself back to sleep in the middle of the night. Neither strategy is completely right or wrong, but they are different. Life may be easier if you discuss such things now, rather than in the middle of the night.

You can't predict now how you will both react to various parenting situations in the future, but you can initiate a discussion about your overall philosophy and priorities. This will be the beginning of a conversation that continues until your baby grows up. If you are both open-minded, flexible, and willing to communicate, you'll find ways to meld different approaches into one cohesive parenting style that feels right to both of you.

Sanity-saving secret weapons

Beyond the nursery basics (the crib, bedding, a changing table, a stroller, diapers, and one-pieces), stock up on these must-haves to make life easier after baby:

- **Fun reads.** Keep a few paperback novels or celebrity magazines near the places where you plan to feed your baby so that you'll have something to do when the novelty of counting your newborn's eyelashes wears off.
- **Water (if you are breastfeeding).** Always have bottles of water on hand—especially in your car or stroller—in case you're caught somewhere and don't have another source of liquid. Drinking plenty of water while breastfeeding helps your body produce ample supplies of milk.
- **Dimmer switch or three-way lamp.** If you want to read but keep things peaceful for baby, put a book light on the table next to the rocking chair where you plan to sit during night feedings.
- **White noise.** Many babies—and moms too—sleep better with a fan or a CD of ocean sounds to help mask intrusive noises, especially during nap time.
- **Stain remover.** You'll have more laundry than you ever thought possible once your new addition arrives. Having some spray-on stain remover can keep those baby duds bright and beautiful.
- **Whiteboard or chalkboard.** Hang a whiteboard in the kitchen to help communicate daily events to your partner and other members of your family, including what's in the

freezer to cook for dinner, when grandmother is making her next appearance, or reminders to put out the trash and buy diapers.

Dressing your baby

Need a guaranteed pick-me-up? Head out shopping for baby clothes. Should you get the pretty pink dress with ruffles? Or is that mini aviator jacket calling your name? It's smart to wait until this latter part of pregnancy to stock up on clothing because you'll likely receive all sorts of baby clothes as gifts. Leave tags on any clothing you buy so that if you receive duplicates as gifts, you can return the items you bought for a refund or credit. You'll be amazed how quickly your baby outgrows newborn-size clothing, so consider saving money by borrowing clothes from friends or by shopping in discount or outlet stores.

Babies go through a lot of clothing. Diaper leaks and spit-up can soil or dampen a couple of outfits a day, and leaving a baby in wet or dirty clothing can cause skin rashes. Buy or borrow enough clothes so that you won't have to do laundry every day. Here are some estimates of what you'll need:

- 5–7 one-pieces: These one-piece outfits are comfortable, easy to wash, and simple to put on and take off. Most parents find that one-pieces and one-piece sleepers suffice for stay-at-home days.
- 5–7 undershirts: short-sleeve or long-sleeve, depending on the season. Choose undershirts that snap at the crotch; they won't ride up on your baby.
- 1 pair of cotton mittens: While moving their arms, babies may scratch themselves with their fingernails. Mittens help prevent scratches. An alternative to mittens is long-sleeve undershirts with built-in hand-hugging flaps.
- 2 one-piece pajamas: Choose warm footed styles if the baby's sleeping area will be cold; if the room will be temperate, drawstring-bottom sleeping bags can make middle-of-the-night diaper changes easier. On very warm nights, your baby can sleep in an undershirt that snaps at the crotch.
- 5 pairs of socks: On cold days, socks worn under one-pieces or one-piece pajamas can help keep baby's feet warm.
- 2–3 nice outfits for dress-up days.
- A sun hat with a chin strap.
- Outerwear, if the weather is cold: a sweater, jacket, or fleece (zip-up is easier to put on than over-the-head); a warm coat or baby bag that fits into the car seat; and a hat.

Storing baby clothes

Your baby showers were more wonderful than you could imagine, and now your nursery is full of adorable outfits that'll clothe your baby until he's two years old! As you likely discovered, when people give baby clothing as a gift, they often buy larger sizes that your baby won't grow into for months. And when friends offer hand-me-downs, they usually give you a big box or bag of all sizes.

week 33

Babies outgrow clothing quickly, and the window of time that they fit into outfits is often small. Most mothers with older children remember taking a brand-new outfit out of the drawer, tags still hanging off it, and discovering that their baby had already outgrown it.

Do yourself a favor and sort clothing by size. Use cardboard or plastic boxes and label them with various sizes: 3–6 months, 6–9 months, 9–12 months, 12–18 months, 24 months. Keep newborn-size clothing close at hand in a dresser or closet, and when it starts getting tight, grab the 3–6 months box. Keep a box or bag in the closet for outgrown clothes that you'll either save for your next baby or pass along to a friend.

Baby clothes can shrink, so when you're sorting hand-me-downs by size, go by looks rather than labels. The outfit that fit your friend's baby at 6 months may fit yours at 4 months. Also keep in mind that since baby clothes are sized by age, if your baby is especially large or small, clothing for his age may not fit.

Diet & Exercise

Feeding your baby's brain

By the end of this trimester, your baby's brain may be three or four times larger than it was at the start. To support its astonishing leaps in size and function, his brain demands extra nutrients. One of the most important is DHA, an omega-3 fatty acid commonly found in fish. This vital substance helps your baby's brain cells grow larger and develop a crucial insulating sheath of myelin, which helps speed up communication pathways in the brain. Fatty acids are uniquely concentrated in your baby's brain during the 3rd trimester, so this is a great time to boost your baby's DHA levels with extra helpings of fish, canola oil, or flaxseed.

Food safety

Admit it: You don't think twice about sampling a few spoonfuls of cookie dough before it makes its way into the oven. While eating foods with raw eggs in them is not a good idea any time, it's an especially bad idea now that you're pregnant. Every year, 76 million Americans get sick from contaminated food, and pregnant women are among the most vulnerable. The illnesses range from mild—producing flulike symptoms such as upset stomach, diarrhea, cramps, and headache—to fatal. Approximately 5,000 people in the United States die each year from food-borne illness.

Food-borne illness occurs when you eat food that is contaminated with bacteria, viruses, parasites, and toxins. Bacterial contamination is most common. You can't avoid harmful bacteria completely, but if you follow these steps, you can help prevent them from making you and your family sick:

- Wash your hands before preparing foods and after changing diapers, using the bathroom, touching pets, coughing or sneezing, taking out the garbage, and handling raw meats, fish, or eggs.

- Cook meats thoroughly. Use an oven thermometer to determine the internal temperature of cooked foods. Roasts and steaks should register at least 145 degrees F; whole poultry, 180 degrees F; and pork, ground beef, and casseroles, 160 degrees F.
- Reheat leftovers thoroughly.
- Wash fruits and vegetables well.
- Avoid raw eggs and egg products and foods that contain raw eggs. When cooking eggs, cook them thoroughly until the yolk is hard.
- If you take leftover food home from a restaurant, be sure to refrigerate it promptly.
- Check expiration dates and toss old food in the trash.
- Clean your refrigerator regularly to remove any trace of bacteria that may spread onto food.
- Wash countertops, cutting boards, and utensils with hot, soapy water.
- Use one set of cutting boards and utensils for produce and another for meat.
- Throw away moldy foods.
- Set your refrigerator at 40 degrees F or below to prevent bacteria from multiplying. Set your freezer at 0 degrees F or below.
- Refrigerate hot foods as soon as possible, at least within two hours after cooking.
- Defrost food in the refrigerator or microwave oven. Never defrost at room temperature.
- If a food has been sitting out for more than 2 hours, throw it away.

Common Questions

Q. Do I have to have an episiotomy?

A. The majority of women don't have an episiotomy, which is a small cut made into the perineum (the area between the vagina and the rectum) to widen the vaginal opening. Episiotomies are performed to make delivery easier or to prevent tearing of the vaginal tissue.

Although episiotomies were performed routinely for nearly a century, they occur less frequently now. Between 1983 and 2000, the episiotomy rate fell from about 70 percent of all vaginal births to about 20 percent, according to the American College of Obstetricians and Gynecologists.

Episiotomy rates can vary widely, however. A 2003 study found that women who deliver their babies attended by physicians in private practice are seven times more likely to undergo an episiotomy than women whose babies are delivered by OB/GYN residents or hospital faculty physicians. The researchers suggested that the higher rates among private physicians may reflect the period in which they trained.

Years ago episiotomies were believed to prevent tearing of the vagina and damage to the pelvic floor. However, recent studies have shown that vaginal tears cause less pain and bleeding than episiotomies and that pelvic floor damage is more likely to occur with an episiotomy than with a tear. Feel free to inquire about your doctor's and your hospital's episiotomy rates. If you don't want to have an episiotomy—and who does?—discuss your feelings with your doctor.

Preventive measures. Studies show that perineal massage can reduce the need for an episiotomy. Massage can help make the perineum more flexible and stretchy, so when the baby comes out, the perineum is more likely to stretch than tear. To do perineal massage, sit in a warm bath and gently massage the area around the opening of the vagina for about 10 minutes a day, beginning around week 34. This won't guarantee you an episiotomy-free or tear-free delivery, but it may help.

When an episiotomy is required. Episiotomies may be necessary in some situations: if your baby's heart rate drops and delivery is expedited by cutting the perineum, if she is being delivered by forceps or vacuum suction, or if her shoulders are too wide to fit through the birth canal.

The procedure. If you have an episiotomy, your doctor will give you a shot of local anesthetic to numb the area before cutting, unless the area is already numb from your epidural. The cuts range from superficial to deep: An episiotomy is said to be first-degree if only the skin is cut; second-degree if the skin and underlying tissue are cut; third-degree if skin, underlying tissue, and the muscle around the anus are cut; and fourth-degree if the cut goes through the rectal mucosa as well as the other three layers. Usually only a second-degree cut is made, but the baby's head extends the cut to tear the muscle or rectum. After your baby is born, your doctor will stitch the episiotomy and other tears with dissolvable sutures.

Q. Should I videotape my baby's delivery?

A. Video cameras tend to get in the way in the delivery room. In order to get a decent view, the cameraperson has to move intrusively from here to there and back again, which can be annoying for doctors, nurses, and midwives. If your partner is running the camera, he may focus so much on getting a good shot that he won't be able to give you the support you need. Plus he may end up watching his child's birth through the viewfinder of his video camera rather than seeing it with his own eyes. Pack a still camera and have your partner take occasional snapshots if you really want to preserve your delivery for posterity.

Q. Can I breastfeed if I have flat or inverted nipples?

A. If you have flat nipples (nipples that don't protrude) or inverted nipples (nipples that seem to point in rather than out), you probably can breastfeed, according to some lactation experts. Wearing breast shells inside your bra during pregnancy can help draw out flat or inverted nipples. When placed over the nipple, these two-piece plastic shells put pressure on the nipple and cause it to protrude. Once your baby is born, using a breast pump or other suction device just before feeding may draw out your nipples too. To find out more, talk with a lactation consultant, obstetrician, or your baby's pediatrician.

Week 34

Your Baby

The inside story

Most of the weight your baby gains now is stored as fat, which will help insulate her against the chilly world when she's born. She now weighs close to 5 pounds, and she has nearly run out of room to move. That doesn't mean that she'll stop moving, but you may notice a change in the way she bumps and thumps against you. By now she's closing her eyes when she's asleep and keeping them open when she's awake. She has also learned to blink.

At this point your baby's brain is so well developed that she has the ability to see, hear, learn, and remember. She is her own person— and very soon now, you'll have the pleasure of meeting her face-to-face.

Your Body

(More) nausea and vomiting

A morning sickness-like nausea and vomiting sometimes make an appearance during the 3rd trimester. Nausea can result when the uterus compresses the stomach or when the normal contractions of the stomach slow down. Eating a few crackers or limiting yourself to tiny portions at each meal usually helps. If it doesn't, you may have a stomach bug, which will make you feel crummy but won't hurt the baby.

Several rare liver problems cause nausea, vomiting, and a kind of general, overall ill feeling (see "Hepatitis and pregnancy," page 222). If your nausea is constant and nothing you do offers relief, talk with your doctor. Liver problems are rare, but they're serious, so it is wise to

---

Signs of trouble

Certain signs should not be ignored. Call your doctor if you notice the following:

Sudden swelling of your feet, face, or hands. If swelling is gradual and progresses as the day wears on, it's likely the ordinary swelling of pregnancy. However, if swelling occurs suddenly, it could be a sign of preeclampsia (see page 253). Call the doctor right away.

Decreased movement of the fetus. If your baby seems to be moving less than usual, do a kick count (see "Reduced fetal movement," next page). If after 2 hours you don't feel normal movement, call the doctor because the baby may need to be evaluated.

Reduced fetal movement

As your baby grows, you may start to feel that she's less active. The truth is that if she's healthy, she's moving as much as she did when she was smaller, but her movements feel different because she's all folded up and wedged in your uterus. Your baby has about as much space to move as you would if you were trying to swim in a bathtub.

If you're concerned because you notice a big difference in your baby's activity rate, you can count kicks. After eating a meal or snack, sit or lie down comfortably in a quiet place with no distractions, check the time, and count how many times your baby moves, kicks, twists, or pushes an elbow into your lungs. (Don't count hiccups.) You can count how many times she moves in an hour, or how long it takes for her to move 10 times. If you don't feel much movement, try again later on—your baby may be sleeping. It should take her no longer than an hour to kick 10 times, although you may find that you feel 10 movements long before an hour passes.

Write down your baby's kick rate and then count again the next day at about the same time. Overall you should come up with approximately the same number of movements from day to day. If your baby's activity level drops dramatically, call your doctor. It simply may be that your baby may not be feeling well or she is a less active baby, but in either case you should check with your doctor.

investigate whether your nausea is related to a liver condition.

When your baby "drops"

As you approach your due date, you may feel a change in the way you're carrying your baby as she drops lower in your pelvis, a process called "lightening" or "engagement." However, don't worry if your baby doesn't descend yet. Not all babies travel downward before labor begins, especially if this isn't your first pregnancy.

Your Self

Feeling beautiful

OK, so you may not fit into the little black dress in the back of your closet, but you can still look and feel beautiful. Start with your clothes. Have you gotten into the habit of wearing the same two or three maternity outfits all the time? Treat yourself to a new blouse even though you'll only wear it for a few more weeks. Or dress up your old clothes with a bright-color scarf or some pretty jewelry.

Next, look at your fingernails (and your toenails, if you can still see them). Pregnancy hormones make nails grow faster than usual. If you've been so busy preparing for your baby's arrival that you've neglected your nails, treat yourself to a manicure and pedicure at a beauty salon. Or do your own manicure, but spring for the pedicure; a good pedicurist will give you a soothing foot massage.

Now for your skin. If you're lucky, you have the beautiful, rosy glow of pregnancy that some women have. If you're not so lucky—and most women aren't—you look ruddy and puffy. Minimize puffiness by avoiding salt and drinking plenty of water. Makeup will help with the ruddiness, and a free makeover is as close as your nearest department store cosmetics counter. Many dermatologists suggest nontoxic chemical peels to improve your mood and your skin.

How's your hair? Though you may be tempted to spring for a drastic haircut, resist the urge and get a trim instead. Your face may be bigger now than it will be a few weeks after your baby's birth, so wait until your non-pregnant face returns before making any big change.

Gear for leaving the house

Whether you're going to jog through the neighborhood with your new baby in tow or cruise the aisles of your grocery store, having the right gear makes outings easier and more comfortable for you and your little one.

Before you buy anything, talk with your friends and family. Borrowing gear can save a lot of money. If you buy, advice from friends is invaluable. They can clue you in to their best buys—and their biggest mistakes. Here are some things to consider:

Diaper bag. The kind of diaper bag you choose depends mainly on how much stuff you like to carry around with you. Some moms like the ready-for-anything style that has room for clean bottles, toys, a change of clothes, and a blanket for baby to crawl around on. Others prefer smaller styles that are just big enough for a couple of diapers and a pack of wipes. Diaper bags differ widely in stylishness too. You can buy a leather bag made by a top designer for several hundred dollars or an inexpensive plastic pack for only a few dollars. Aside from size, consider how you want to carry a diaper bag—over your shoulder, on your back like a backpack, with handles, or a mix of all three. Color may matter too: If your partner is going to be toting the diaper bag around, you may want to buy a neutral color rather than a flowery, feminine design. Some mothers also find that having two diaper bags comes in handy.

Stroller. There are so many different kinds of strollers that your head may start to hurt just thinking about them: car seat/stroller combos, umbrella strollers, bassinette strollers, joggers, upright strollers, double strollers, and strollers in which the baby sits up front and an older sibling can hitch a ride on the back. The kind you buy depends completely on personal preference; different styles are suitable for different functions. It's important to test-drive a stroller before buying. During the test-drive, notice if the handle is at a comfortable height for you, if the wheels maneuver easily, if it is light enough for you to lift in and out of a car trunk, if it folds easily (if you want it to fold), whether the seat reclines for napping, and how much storage room it has. Strollers come in a huge range of prices, but price doesn't necessarily equal quality, so choose with a blind eye to high-status brand names.

Jogger stroller. Which jogger stroller you buy depends on what activity you'll be doing. Will you be walking in the neighborhood on cement sidewalks or running on unpaved paths? Do you want a jogger that will fold easily and tuck away in your trunk? Would you like a jogger that converts into a bike trailer? Your options also include wheel size (the larger the wheels, the smoother the ride off-road), suspension (the better the suspension, the smoother the ride off-road), front wheel style (a wheel that is fixed in place is better for runners; a wheel that swivels is better for less athletic pursuits such as maneuvering through malls and grocery stores), and price (from under $100 to more than $500). Other options include a reclining seat, cup holders, and rain hoods. Joggers are available for one, two, or three babies.

Backpack. Choose a backpack that suits your lifestyle: Hiking up mountains calls for a more rugged backpack than strolling through malls. Not all backpacks fit all people, so be sure to test the backpack in the store, preferably with a baby in it, to determine whether it fits on your back comfortably. Other things to consider include cushioning for your baby, padding on shoulder straps (to keep your shoulders from getting

sore), ease of putting it on and taking it off (particularly if you'll be using it alone without another person to lift a loaded pack onto your back), and storage space.

Convertible frontpack/backpack. These packs convert from frontpack to backpack. Some parents complain that switching from one to the other is too complicated; try them out in the store before buying.

Convertible stroller/backpack. These can be a godsend for travelers, city dwellers, and anyone else who needs to alternate between stroller and backpack. Look for a model that allows you to do the converting easily without removing baby or needing a second person to help out. Try them out in the store before buying to be sure that the model you choose isn't too heavy and awkward to be a good backpack and that its wheels work well enough to be a good stroller.

Sling. Slings allow you to carry a baby or toddler on your front, hip, or back in upright or reclining positions. They allow for discreet nursing but can be used by dads as well as moms. Slings come with or without padding.

Front carrier. A front carrier is a great way to keep your infant close while leaving your hands free. A good front carrier is comfortable, cushions your baby well, doesn't cut or pull your shoulders, is adjustable for use by you and your partner, and is reversible, allowing a small baby to face toward you with the back of her head supported and an older baby to face out and see the world.

Preparing your call list

Your grandmother, girlfriends, and neighbors will be waiting on pins and needles for news of your baby's birth, but the last thing you and your partner will feel like doing after delivery is calling all 100 friends and relatives to let them know the good news. Take time now to set up a phone tree. First, make a list of everyone who would like to be contacted. Then figure out a "tree" of connections. For example, you call your parents and your partner's parents. They call all of your respective siblings. One of your siblings calls your best friend, your next-door neighbor, and your favorite coworker. Your best friend calls all of your other friends, your neighbor spreads the news in the neighborhood, your coworker calls your work friends, and so on.

A phone tree is successful only if everyone has a list of names and phone numbers ahead of time. Double-check phone numbers a few weeks before your due date to save friends and relatives the trouble of having to track down phone numbers.

You may prefer to notify people by e-mail. If you do, get everyone's e-mail addresses ahead of time, set up a group list, and test it. Also set up a phone tree for people who don't use e-mail or have access to it only at work but won't want to wait until Monday to hear that you had your baby Saturday morning.

Some hospitals will post babies' pictures on their websites for your friends and family to view. Others have a service on the postpartum ward by which you can do it yourself. Check with your hospital now to see if it offers this service and whether special arrangements have to be made beforehand.

Diet & Exercise

Excessive weight gain

It's best not to gain excessive weight during pregnancy. But what if you have already gained more than you or your doctor would have liked? Although excessive weight gain can increase your risk for gestational diabetes, back problems, and a cesarean delivery, the majority of women who gain more weight than they should have no serious problems during pregnancy, and they deliver healthy babies. If the weight is still coming on fast, take a careful look at the reason for your weight gain. Have you given yourself permission to eat whatever you like? Have you abandoned your exercise program? Once you figure out why you're gaining, try to make some changes.

It's never too late to start eating smart. Begin to learn and practice good nutrition habits now, and you'll keep your weight gain down for the rest of your pregnancy. You'll also know how to eat after your baby is born when you're trying to lose your pregnancy pounds.

Energy boost between meals

During the last weeks of pregnancy, when your baby is growing bigger and bigger, eating five or six mini-meals every day makes more sense than two or three big meals because big meals can cause heartburn. For energy-boosting snacks, choose foods that provide protein as well as carbohydrates. Reach for snacks such as leftover chicken on a slice of whole wheat bread, yogurt and fruit, cheese and crackers, cereal with milk, trail mix made with nuts and raisins, a glass of milk and a piece of fruit, apple slices spread with peanut butter, or beans and rice.

Fast, fabulous beans

Beans are nutritional powerhouses filled with protein and lots of fiber. If you're finding constipation a problem, as many pregnant women do, the large amount of fiber in beans can help relieve your constipation. But finding ways to include beans in your diet can be a challenge: There's a limit to how much chili you can eat! For variety, try one of these super-fast, super-delicious recipes.

Black bean salsa. Mix 1 can black beans (drained) with 1 can of corn. Add a 12-ounce jar of your favorite salsa and mix together. Serve over grilled chicken, tossed with pasta, or with cut-up pita bread for dipping.

White bean dip. Put 1 can cannellini beans (drained), 1 teaspoon minced garlic, 1 teaspoon dried rosemary, and 1 tablespoon extra-virgin olive oil in a food processor. Process until smooth, adding water if needed to make a smooth puree. Serve as a dip for thin slices of French bread, vegetables, or cut-up pita bread.

Common Questions

Q. Should I have an ultrasound in my 3rd trimester?

A. Ultrasounds during the 3rd trimester are not routinely done. However, some situations call for them: if your baby seems too big or too small, if the doctor is unsure whether your baby is breech, if your doctor is concerned that your placenta is too close to the cervix, or if your baby has a fetal malformation that requires evaluation before delivery.

If an ultrasound is performed to determine whether your baby is in the right position, it will likely be done during the 36th week. That way, if the ultrasound shows that your baby is breech, there is time to do a version (a procedure in which the baby is turned from feetfirst to headfirst). If your pregnancy is complicated at all by health conditions like diabetes or hypertension, your practitioner may want you to have ultrasounds every 3–4 weeks to carefully monitor your baby's progress.

Q. What is back labor, and why does everyone say it's so horrible?

A. Ordinarily, if you are lying on your back during delivery, your baby will be facing down toward the floor. (This is called the occiput anterior position.) Some babies face up toward the ceiling (occiput posterior position). Laboring with a face-up baby causes more back pain and is known as back labor.

Back labor usually lasts longer and may require more pushing than an ordinary labor if the baby remains in the occiput posterior position. Pain is concentrated in your low back because the back of the baby's head is pressing against your tailbone or spine. Some women who have experienced back labor say it is excruciatingly painful. Others find that the pain of back labor isn't worse than ordinary labor, merely different.

Most babies in a posterior position will rotate the necessary 180 degrees on their own as labor progresses, especially if mom's pelvis is not completely relaxed with epidural anesthesia. Sometimes a doctor or midwife will attempt to rotate the baby with her hand. If the baby stays in a posterior position, he can be delivered that way if he fits through the birth canal. However, if a posterior baby is angled in such a way that he needs a little extra space, and there is not enough room in the birth canal, the doctor may recommend a cesarean delivery.

To reduce pain during back labor, try changing positions—kneeling on all fours, rolling onto your side, or squatting. Your labor coach or doula can apply ice or heat to your low back, massage your low back, or press on it with a tennis ball or other round object. This is called counterpressure, and it sometimes reduces the pain of back labor. Pain medications or an epidural will also help.

Week 35

Your Baby

The inside story

Now more than 5 pounds, your baby might be more than 18 inches long and seriously competing for space with every other organ scrunched into your torso. Your abdomen may be stretched so large that you're starting to worry your baby is too big, but nature usually does a good job of matching up babies and moms. In any case it's hard to accurately assess a baby's weight at this point because as your baby grows, your amniotic fluid level rises and the placenta grows too.

You may notice that your baby's behavior is becoming increasingly structured, with definite sleep-and-wake cycles. His periods of increased movement may last as long as 20 minutes.

The air sacs of your baby's lungs are becoming lined with surfactant, a chemical substance that keeps lungs expanded after each breath. This will help your baby breathe on his own outside the uterus.

Even without an ultrasound, your provider should be able to tell by now how your baby is "presenting"—whether he is positioned upside down, which means his head is ready

to come out first, or if he is breech, which means he'll come out bottom-first. That's partly because your baby's skull, once so soft and pliable, is hardening as calcium is deposited there. His brain still isn't completely closed over with bone, though. His head has fontanels, which are "soft spots" where the skull bones don't completely join together. The largest one is diamond-shape and slightly toward the front of his head. This is the anterior fontanel, and it's the "soft spot" everyone talks about. There is one other noticeable but smaller fontanel toward the back of your baby's head.

Your Body

Labor length

If this is your first baby, you may have heard that you'll be in labor longer than with your next baby. It's actually true. First labors tend to last longer than other labors. On average, a first labor takes 12–24 hours, and subsequent labors last somewhere in the neighborhood of half as long as your first labor. That's not true for everyone, though, so don't be surprised if your second labor is as long as or longer than your first!

week 35

Singleton breech babies and version

Babies are ordinarily born headfirst, which is known as vertex presentation. They may float around freely in the uterus during the early and middle months of pregnancy, but most move into the head-down position by about the 37th week. If by week 37 your baby is in a feetfirst or buttocks-first position, it is called a breech presentation (see "Babies in the breech position," page 240). Breech presentation occurs in about 3 percent of full-term births.

Risks of a breech birth. Doctors prefer not to deliver breech babies vaginally because they are more likely than vertex babies to suffer from complications during delivery. The baby's feet and umbilical cord can get tangled. Very rarely, the slim body comes out but the head gets stuck. These complications are rare, but your doctor must act quickly to avoid problems for the baby.

When version may be used. If at week 37 your doctor suspects that your baby is breech, she may send you for an ultrasound to find out for sure. If the ultrasound confirms the diagnosis, your doctor may recommend a version (also called an external cephalic version), which is the manual turning of the baby into the head-down position. Your doctor may offer to do the version that day or within a couple of days, but she won't wait long because within a week or two the baby's bottom may be so low in the pelvis that a version will not work.

A version may start with an intravenous shot of a uterus-relaxing drug for you and a nonstress test or biophysical profile for your baby (see "Biophysical Profile," page 419). If your baby is moving normally, the version will begin. Using ultrasound to guide her and to monitor the health of your baby, the doctor places her hands on your abdomen and applies pressure, pushing the baby's bottom up and guiding the head to encourage a somersault. She is literally trying to turn the baby upside down. After the version, your doctor will do another nonstress test or biophysical profile to ensure that your baby tolerated the move.

Having a version can be uncomfortable. Because it carries a very small risk of placental abruption, premature rupture of the membranes, tangling of the cord, or starting labor, it should be done in a hospital where an emergency cesarean can be performed.

If the version is successful, your baby will move from breech to vertex. The procedure works about half the time; the success rate is higher if a woman has had a baby before. Most babies then stay in the head-down position, but some move back into breech. Your doctor's goal is to get your baby head-down and keep her there because your chances of having an uncomplicated vaginal birth are much higher with a head-down baby. Although breech babies are sometimes delivered vaginally, most are born by cesarean delivery.

A version is not recommended for women who have any of the following complications: vaginal bleeding, a placenta that is covering the opening of the uterus, an abnormally small baby, a low level of amniotic fluid, an abnormal fetal heart rate, premature rupture of the membranes, or more than one baby.

Not-so-swell swelling

Swelling occurs even in healthy women with uncomplicated pregnancies. Beginning at week 34 or 35, your body will gradually start to swell. You'll notice your rings are tighter and your feet feel crowded in your shoes. (Take your rings off now, or you may not be able to get them off in a couple of weeks.) Swelling usually worsens throughout the day and is at its worst at night. To alleviate swelling, sit with your feet propped up above the level of your heart at the end of the day. By the next morning, your swelling should be down. During the final weeks of pregnancy, avoid wearing tight clothing or crossing your legs while you sit.

If swelling increases very rapidly or if your face is puffy, call your doctor; it may be a sign that your blood pressure is too high or that you are developing preeclampsia.

Help for aches and pains

Pregnancy places a lot of pressure on your legs, knees, back, and hips. Sometimes that pressure results in aches and pains. It's nothing serious, but is annoying nonetheless. Ice and/or heat can often bring relief. Experiment with heat and ice to see which works better for you.

Heat. Wrap a heating pad, hot-water bottle, or microwaveable heat pack in a towel and apply it to the sore area for 20 minutes several times a day. Microwaveable packs, which are available in most pharmacies, heat up in a minute or two and are very convenient to use. The towel prevents your skin from getting too hot. Soaking in a warm bath or standing under a stream of warm water in the shower may also help.

Ice. To make an ice pack, partly fill a plastic bag with crushed ice. Wrap a thin, wet cloth around the bag and apply it to the sore area. Or wrap a wet paper towel around a bag of frozen peas and use that as an ice pack. Be careful with ice because the cold can damage nerves if it is left in place too long. Remove ice within 20 minutes and wait two to four hours to repeat.

Heat and ice. Alternating heat and ice sometimes relieves pain that neither can take care of alone.

Your Self

Loving a second child

Expectant mothers who already have a child commonly worry that they won't be able to love their second child as much as they love their first. They love their first so very much that they can't even imagine having any love left over for their second. Luckily, mothers have an infinite supply of love, and you'll have enough love for all of your children.

You may not warm up to your second baby right away. You and your first child have had a lot of time together, and your new baby is something of a stranger to you. In time you will form a bond that is as strong as the one you share with your older child.

Wrapping up at work

You'll be leaving work soon. Some women like to work up until the last possible second; others prefer to take a few weeks off before their baby's birth. If you can afford to take some time off during the last few weeks of pregnancy, do it; be sure, however, that the extra time off before delivery doesn't reduce the amount of time your employer will allow you to take for maternity leave. Once your baby is born, you'll have very little time to yourself. Here are a few suggestions to make a smooth exit from work:

Organize your desk. Finish up as much work as possible and make sure all projects are up-to-date. Meet with the person who will be replacing you or, if that's not possible, leave detailed notes. Straighten up your work area and remove any personal belongings and photos; your replacement probably doesn't want to spend 3 months staring at a photo of you and your husband on your Caribbean honeymoon. Return any company-issued items such as laptop computers and cell phones.

Meet with your supervisor to review your maternity leave schedule and to discuss last-minute details regarding the work you are leaving behind. By making your leave-taking as smooth as possible, you reinforce your value in your boss's mind. However, resist the temptation to offer to be on call during your maternity leave. You'll be busy enough taking care of your baby without having to field constant calls from work. Leave your contact information with your supervisor, but make it clear that you want to be called only if absolutely necessary.

Talk with human resources. Make sure that all arrangements have been completed and you've filled out all necessary forms. Let your human resources representative know where to send your paycheck or other important correspondence.

If you're not returning to your job, schedule an exit interview with your human resources department and ask any questions you may have about transferring your pension benefits or 401(k) accounts into a personal account, how long your health insurance coverage will last, and so on. Thank your employer for the opportunities the job provided. Be positive about your job and your company even if you dislike them. You may need a reference someday, and if you burn bridges, you won't get a good one.

Grandparents

Grandparents give children an incredibly important gift as they learn about themselves and the world: unconditional love and acceptance. Parents must set limits and enforce discipline, but the grandparents are free to love without setting limits.

The best grandparent-grandchild relationships come when the parents act as matchmakers: They set the stage for success, bring the two parties together, and then step back and give them the space they need to get to know each other.

Be encouraging. You may need to push your baby's grandparents to take an active role in his life. They may feel concerned that if they try to get involved, they'll be intruding. Some grandparents hold back because they feel uncomfortable handling such a small baby; it may be decades since they held a newborn infant.

Grandfathers in particular may shy away from spending time with your baby; they may have first become fathers in the days when mothers took care of the children and fathers brought home the bacon. The best way to draw grandparents in is to tell them that you value them and then invite them to spend time with your child. Grandparents are so important that if your child doesn't have any, you should adopt some. Older aunts, great-uncles, and retired neighbors can fill in for grandparents.

Recognize that baby-care styles may clash. Of course disagreements are inevitable if your baby's grandparents are heavily involved in her life, particularly if they are caring for her when you return to work. Conflict may arise when the grandparents fail to follow rules that the parents have set for the child or when they push to do things "the old way." Talk with the grandparents about why you set these rules and how important they are. Explain, for example, why you are holding off on solid food until the baby is older or supplementing with formula only

when you think it's the right time. In your parents' generation, babies commonly began eating cereal and other solids within the first month of life. Help the grandparent to understand that ideas about kids' healthy eating have changed since they were parents. Sharing a book or magazine article might help.

Talk openly with your child's grandparents about any disagreements. If you all keep your baby's best interests in mind, you should be able to find solutions.

Coping with distance. If your baby's grandparents live far away, go out of your way to include them in their grandchild's life by sending photos, videotapes, and descriptions of your baby's developmental steps. Call them when your baby is crying and let them hear how strong her lungs are! Small things can help build a relationship between your baby and her grandparents, even if they're living on the other side of the country.

Keeping a baby journal

Even though it may not feel like it when your baby is in the middle of a crying spell, her first few weeks and months will pass by quickly, and before you know it you'll be sending her off to preschool. Since your sleep-deprived brain won't hold on to recollections as well as you'd like it to, writing about your baby helps preserve memories for the future.

Spend a few minutes a day keeping a journal. Jot down notes about what your baby did that day. Don't worry about using a beautiful leather journal or writing with your best handwriting or crafting long, descriptive paragraphs. Put pressure like that on yourself and you'll abandon the journal after a week. Instead, keep a regular notebook someplace where you'll see it every day, such as the kitchen counter next to the coffeepot or in the bathroom beside your toothbrush. If it gets stained with coffee or toothpaste, you can copy it over into a beautiful memory book or type it up on your computer in the future when you have more free time.

Write down quick notes, such as "Heather stretched a lot today" or "Grandma took Thomas for a ride in the stroller today" or "Jasmine seems to be getting a tooth." Notes like these are not particularly telling in and of themselves, but when taken as a whole, a month or a year or five years of little notes will remind you of the small but meaningful details of your baby's life that you might otherwise forget.

Diet & Exercise

Reaching prepregnancy weight

At this point in your pregnancy, you're probably dreaming of returning to your normal weight. Even though your delivery is still weeks away, start making plans now for losing weight after your baby is born. If you have an exercise plan in place, you'll be more likely to follow through on it. Now is a good time to check out health clubs

that have infant care, exercise classes for new mothers (babies are usually welcome), and neighborhood or mall-walking groups. If you gain the recommended 30 pounds during pregnancy, approximately 7 of those pounds will be fat. Your body stores fat while you're pregnant because it needs sufficient fat reserves for milk production during breastfeeding. The additional fat parks on your hips, your buttocks, your arms, your legs—pretty much any place you'd rather not have extra fat.

If you are breastfeeding, losing weight too quickly after delivery is not recommended because it may hamper your body's ability to manufacture milk. Don't even think about weight loss until your milk supply is well established—at least 6 to 8 weeks postpartum.

When you do return to your prepregnancy weight, you may find that clothes don't fit the way they used to. Even if you are the same weight, your body may seem different. You may have a thicker waist, heavier-looking thighs, or a rounder belly. Your fat-to-muscle ratio may have changed. Muscle weighs more than fat, so even if you are the same weight, you may have more fat and less muscle than you used to.

Breastfeeding may help you lose weight. Some women say the extra pounds dropped off while they nursed, although others say their body weight didn't budge an ounce until after they weaned their babies. Losing your baby fat and regaining your prepregnancy body require exercise and a smart eating plan. Exercise builds muscle, burns fat, and tones your body. With hard work, you can have your former body back—or create an even better version of it!

Common Questions

Q. When can we take our baby on an airplane to go see Grandma?

A. An airplane is no place for a newborn. Many planes use recirculated air, which means that if one person has a cold, his germs are broadcast throughout the plane by the ventilation system. That's no problem for adults, whose mature immune systems can fight off germs. But an infant's immune system is no match for some of the viruses and bacteria that float around on airplanes and in airports. If Grandma can't come to you, wait until your baby is at least 2 months old—and preferably 4–6 months old—before taking a flight.

When you do take baby up into the friendly skies, buy her a seat. Airlines allow babies and young children to ride on a parent's lap for no fee, but that's not a safe place for them if the plane hits turbulence or has to make an emergency landing. According to the Federal Aviation Administration (FAA), parents should secure children in an "appropriate restraint." Most car seats fit the bill.

Before you fly, check your car seat for a label that identifies it as certified for use in planes. If there is no label, look at the seat's instructions or contact the manufacturer. A car seat should fit into most

airplane seats if the car seat is no wider than 16 inches. If you have questions about whether your car seat will fit, call the airline and ask.

If you're feeling queasy about the idea of spending a whole lot of money on an airline ticket for a baby, ask your airline for a discounted fare. Many airlines offer discounts of up to 50 percent for children under age 2.

Q. Why does labor hurt?

A. Your uterus has a tremendous job to do when you go into labor. This muscular, elastic organ literally squeezes the baby out of you. Labor commences when the uterus starts to contract and the cervix begins to open. With each contraction, your uterus squeezes your baby deeper into the pelvis and closer to birth.

During a contraction, your muscular uterus flexes so intensely that you can feel it from the outside of your body; your abdomen hardens noticeably during a contraction and softens when the contraction ends. All of this squeezing and flexing and pushing hurts. Imagine how much the muscles in your arms, back, and legs would hurt if you tried to push a car up a hill!

As your labor continues, the contractions will come closer together and last longer, intensifying the pain. During the second stage of labor, you will give your uterus some help. When you feel a contraction, you'll bear down as hard as you can to push the baby through the vagina. Pushing usually isn't painful. In fact, many women experience a feeling of relief when they push. But it is hard work because you're summoning the strength of muscles

week 35

throughout your body to help push your baby out.

Labor does hurt, but women are strong, and you are stronger than you realize. You'll endure the pain, and if it gets to be too much, you can ask for pain medication.

Q. Should I be concerned if I tested positive for strep B?

A. Group B streptococcus (it's also called strep B) is a bacteria that is relatively harmless to adults, but it can threaten the life of a newborn.

Anyone can carry strep B bacteria. In fact, as many as 30 percent of women test positive for it during pregnancy.

Strep B infection usually causes no symptoms, so you don't know you have it. It can cause bladder infections or postpartum uterine infection. (Strep B is not the bacterium that causes strep throat; that's strep A.) Strep B can cause infection of your baby's blood (sepsis), lungs (pneumonia), and the fluid around the brain (meningitis).

Fortunately, most of the time transmission of strep B bacteria to your baby can be prevented. If you test positive, your doctor will treat you with intravenous antibiotics during labor. These medications will greatly reduce the number of strep B bacteria in your vagina or rectum. Antibiotics must be given during labor, rather than during pregnancy; if they are administered during pregnancy, the bacteria may return and infect your baby during birth.

Antibiotics are also administered to any woman who has given birth to a baby with strep B disease in the past and to any woman who had a strep B urinary tract infection during that pregnancy.

If an infected mother is not treated with antibiotics, her baby has a 1 percent chance of becoming infected. Although these babies can be treated with antibiotics, some of them die, and some are left with brain damage.

Week 36

Your Baby

The inside story

As your baby's "rapid growth" period approaches an end, she will top 19 inches and almost reach 6 pounds. However, she will continue to add weight in the form of extra fat until delivery. Those nails are so long, in fact, that she might even scratch herself in utero. The only organ that isn't fully mature yet is her lungs. If she hasn't done so already, this is probably the week that your baby will drop into the birth canal.

You have probably gained 25–30 pounds, and you probably won't gain much more in the final weeks of pregnancy. The placenta's role is coming to an end and producing fewer hormones now that your baby's body is capable of being more independent from yours. Your baby has developed a nicely functioning pair of kidneys, and her liver is processing some of her waste products. You still provide antibodies for your baby through your bloodstream. These antibodies can protect your newborn from whooping cough, mumps, measles, and even mundane coughs and flu.

As your baby has grown inside you, she has developed a sucking reflex. She's tested out that reflex on her own thumbs and fingers. Now she's well equipped to nurse. Her gums are hard and ridged—almost as if teeth are emerging—and those will help her latch on to a nipple to feed herself when the time comes.

Your Body

Delivering more than one baby

The thought of delivering one baby is daunting enough, but two? Or three? Or even four? Yikes! Twins and triplets have become increasingly common, thanks to assisted reproduction techniques and older mothers (age increases your chance of having multiples). Quadruplets and other higher-order multiples are still rare, however. Approximately 3 percent of the babies born in the United States are multiples.

Multiples tend to arrive early: 60 percent of twins, 90 percent of triplets, and virtually all higher-order multiples are born before their due dates. Many twin pregnancies last 36 weeks and triplets 32 weeks.

The type of delivery you have depends on your health, the babies' health, how many babies there are,

week 36

Travel in late pregnancy

Think twice before you hop on a plane to go to your cousin's wedding during these last few weeks of pregnancy. It's best to stay close to home. If you go into labor, you'll be close enough to the hospital to get there in time. Some health insurance companies require you to stay within an hour's drive of your hospital during the last month of pregnancy, and they may not fully cover an emergency delivery far from home. Check with your health insurer to see if it has any such rules.

Airlines may not allow you to fly close to your due date. One U.S. airline requires a doctor's certificate if you want to fly within seven days of your due date, and you will be forbidden to board the plane if you are in labor. Another airline requires any woman in her 9th month of pregnancy to present a certificate from an obstetrician, signed within the previous 72 hours, deeming her to be physically fit for flying. Airlines clearly do not want women giving birth on their planes.

If you must travel, take a copy of your medical record and your doctor's contact information with you in case you do go into labor. Have the name and phone number of a local obstetrician handy and know where the nearest hospital is and how to get there in a hurry.

how much they weigh, and how they are positioned in your uterus. Three or more babies are almost always delivered by cesarean. Twins generally can be born vaginally if they are both vertex, or in the head-down position. If both twins are head-up, or breech, most doctors go right to a cesarean delivery. If one twin is vertex and one is breech, a cesarean isn't always necessary provided twin A (the twin who will be born first because he is closest to the exit, so to speak) is head-down.

When you are admitted to the hospital to deliver your babies vaginally, an ultrasound will be performed to determine the babies' positions. Because of the risk of fetal intolerance to labor, bleeding from the placenta, and the possible need to switch quickly from vaginal delivery to cesarean delivery, you and your babies will be monitored closely throughout labor. An intravenous line may be inserted into your arm so that if you suddenly need a cesarean, time won't be wasted hooking you up to an IV for anesthesia.

When the first twin is delivered, the doctor will hand him over to a pediatric specialist for examination. (Several pediatricians or neonatologists—one for each baby—may attend the delivery, although this varies by hospital.) A trip to the NICU isn't necessary for all twins and triplets, but is more likely for preterm babies or those who need extra help breathing. The second twin may be born anywhere from a few minutes to a few hours later. In years past, doctors believed that the second baby would be in danger if he came out more than 15 minutes after the first baby, but now, with advanced medical equipment, your doctor can monitor the second baby during the time it takes for you to push him out.

If the umbilical cord becomes compressed or the placenta starts to separate too early, the baby or babies may be in danger, and your doctor will perform a prompt cesarean delivery.

If you are having triplets, your doctor will likely want to deliver them by cesarean, and if you're having quads or more, cesarean is the only option. With a cesarean delivery, the babies are delivered one after the other. If they are premature, very small, or have health problems, they'll be taken to the NICU.

Your Self

Predelivery checklist
Even though you may not give birth for another few weeks, it's a good idea to prepare as much as possible now so that you'll be ready if you go into labor early. Here are some things to do now:

- Write down the name, address, and phone number of the hospital where you intend to deliver, along with contact information for your doctor or midwife and your doula, if you're using one. Post a copy of this information, along with the phone number of an ambulance service, next to your telephone. Keep one copy in your purse or wallet (or wherever you can get to it easily) and another in your partner's wallet.
- If you have other children, write down the names and phone numbers of the person/people you've lined up to babysit. (Dog owners should arrange to have someone on call to walk and feed the dog. Give that person keys to your house.)
- Know the best route to the hospital, where to park your car, the best entrance to use (large hospitals may have several entrances), and where to go once you're inside the hospital.
- Check with your health insurer to find out if you need to notify the company when you are admitted to the hospital.
- Make a list of phone numbers (cell, home, office) for the family members or friends you intend to call when labor begins.
- Pack two small bags: one for you and one for your baby. (See "Packing for the hospital," below.)
- Install an infant car seat in the backseat of your car. (See "Common Questions," page 227, for information on choosing and safely installing infant car seats.)

Packing for the hospital
Remember to pack these items in your hospital-bound bag:

Clothing. A nightgown or long T-shirt for labor, pajamas for sleeping, five or six pairs of panties (old ones are best, in case of blood stains), two

week 36

nursing bras, several pairs of socks, slippers, a bathrobe, and an outfit to wear home (think big—even though you won't be pregnant anymore, you'll still have a fairly large belly).

Toiletries. Shampoo, conditioner, a hair dryer, soap, shower shoes, a hairbrush, a comb, lip balm, facial cleansers, body lotion, a toothbrush, toothpaste, floss, and several big, absorbent sanitary napkins.

Comforts. Magazines, books, a CD player, CDs, books about pregnancy and breastfeeding, and a tennis ball for labor massage.

Snacks. Portable nonperishable foods such as granola bars, crackers, cereal bars, travel-size boxes of cereal, and dried fruit.

Necessities. A cell phone or calling card, change for vending machines and telephones, identification for both you and your partner, your insurance card, and your birth plan, if you're using one.

For your baby. Three or four under-shirts and one-pieces, an outfit and cap to wear home, a receiving blanket, and warm outerwear if the weather requires it.

What to leave home. Jewelry, credit cards, and other valuables.

Diet & Exercise

Staying energized

Fatigue visits frequently toward the end of pregnancy. Get as much rest as possible. Sleeping all the way through the night is probably a thing of the past because your bladder can't hold much and you're likely to get up several times to go to the bathroom. If you can fit them into your schedule, take naps in the daytime.

You'll feel less fatigued if you stay well hydrated. Resist the temptation to drink less water in order to decrease trips to the bathroom. Continue to aim for eight glasses of water a day.

Eat lightly and frequently. Snacking throughout the day makes more sense now than eating large meals. Sugary foods give you an immediate burst of energy, but they leave you feeling even more fatigued after the sugar high wears off.

Common Questions

Q. How do I know if there's a problem with my amniotic fluid?

A. The amniotic fluid that your baby swims around in for 9 months plays a crucial role in her health. Your baby needs just the right amount of amniotic fluid to protect her and help her grow; too much fluid or too little can cause trouble. Ultrasounds are used to measure your amniotic fluid.

Having too little amniotic fluid is called oligohydramnios. About 8 percent of women have this condition. It can occur anytime during pregnancy, although it is more common during the late 3rd trimester. During the latter part of pregnancy, severe oligohydramnios may increase the risk of delivery complications, such as umbilical cord compression. Still, most women who develop oligohydramnios at the very end of their pregnancies deliver healthy babies.

If you have too little amniotic fluid, your doctor will monitor your baby's well-being with nonstress tests and biophysical profiles. If the fluid level drops too much, your doctor may recommend an early delivery.

Having too much amniotic fluid is called polyhydramnios. About 2 percent of women have this condition. Mild cases during the latter part of pregnancy usually don't cause much trouble. It is commonly seen with chubby babies. Severe cases of polyhydramnios are rare and are sometimes seen with babies who have blockage along the gastrointestinal tract. Women whose amniotic fluid increases rapidly are at risk for preterm rupture of the membranes, preterm delivery, umbilical cord prolapse, and separation of the placenta from the wall of the uterus.

If you have too much amniotic fluid, your doctor will monitor your fluid level and watch you for signs of preterm labor. What he'll do about the fluid depends on the cause and at what week in your pregnancy the fluid becomes excessive.

Q. My doctor recommended fetal testing because my blood pressure is high. What does that entail?

A. There are several tests that assess the health of a baby; they are used for women whose babies are suspected to be at increased risk for stillbirth. The tests include fetal kick counts, nonstress tests, biophysical profile, contraction stress test or oxytocin-challenge test, and Doppler ultrasound of umbilical artery blood-flow velocity. The tests are sometimes used in combination with each other and may be done once or twice a week depending on the baby's risk factors and condition. Although none of these tests will harm you or your baby, they sometimes can suggest that intervention is needed when in fact your baby is fine. (For a description of each test, see "Prenatal Tests," page 419.)

week 36

Week 37

Your Baby

The inside story

Your baby can benefit from some extra days in the uterus, but he's full-term! He is likely to weigh 6 pounds, and he's probably close to 20 inches long. But even your practitioner can't tell how big your baby will be at birth since some of those 30 pounds or so that you've gained come from increased amniotic fluid, breast size, and placental growth.

In fact, your body weight probably won't tip the scale much higher, but your baby will continue adding ounces. During the few weeks (or days) left before you deliver, your baby may add up to 14 grams of fat each day. At the same time, some of your amniotic fluid is starting to be reabsorbed by your tissues, slightly decreasing the fluid around your baby. This may make it feel as though your baby is moving less, but he's actually just as active as before within his increasingly cramped quarters. As your uterus stretches, more light will permeate your baby's space, and he will move his eyes toward it.

Because placental hormones are now stimulating your breasts to produce milk, those same hormones will cause your baby's mammary glands to swell too. They will shrink back down to size after birth.

At this point, about 3 percent of babies are still breech (positioned with their head up and their feet or buttocks closest to the cervix). Your practitioner may do a pelvic exam to assess the baby's presenting parts. Your baby's feet, hips, head, and buttocks are all fairly easy to distinguish by now.

Your Body

Not just bustier, but busier making milk too

Up until now it may have been possible to think of your breasts as you always have, as a sexy part of your body that gives you and your partner sensual pleasure. Now it's becoming increasingly clear that your breasts have a wonderful function as well as a lovely form: They were designed to nourish your children.

Your breasts are a generous cup size larger than at the start of your pregnancy, and your nipples may have become so sensitive recently that it's painful to pull on clothing or to feel them rub against your terry cloth robe. These are all signs that your

The circumcision decision

If you're having a boy, be prepared to answer this question in the hospital: Do you want to circumcise your baby? The procedure, which is most often performed by OB/GYNs within a day of your child's birth, is a simple one that involves using a clamp or scalpel to remove the foreskin covering the end of your baby's penis.

Is circumcision necessary? That depends on whom you ask. In the United States, circumcision became popular following a study conducted among military personnel in the 1940s. The study showed that men who were not circumcised had higher rates of sexually transmitted diseases than uncircumcised men. This was a flawed study, in that it didn't look at the sexual practices of the men involved; regardless, by 1965, about 80 percent of U.S. boys were being circumcised, supposedly to reduce the risk of infection.

The practice is less common now, with about 65 percent of newborn boys being circumcised. Circumcised males do have a small health advantage: Baby boys are slightly less likely to get urinary tract infections if circumcised, and the rate of penile cancer among circumcised men is lower than among those who are not circumcised. However, both of these conditions are extremely rare and may be more a result of poor hygiene. Another factor to consider is that complications do occur in about 1 in every 1,000 circumcisions; very rarely, there can even be severe damage to the infant's penis during the procedure.

In short, there is no absolute medical reason to circumcise, so it's really up to you. Some couples want their baby to look like his father and make the choice accordingly. Others worry about locker room differences, but researchers say men worry more about penis size than foreskins. In addition, by the time your child plays a sport, the numbers of circumcised versus uncircumcised boys will probably be 50-50.

If you do decide to circumcise your son, talk to your physician about anesthesia. Although substantial clinical research demonstrates that the procedure does cause newborns to feel pain, many physicians still do not use an anesthetic. Safe pain relief is available in the form of a numbing topical cream applied half an hour before the surgery or a local anesthetic medication injected with a needle.

week 37

body is preparing to nurse your baby, whether you plan to or not.

Each breast has about 20–25 branching segments, called "lobes," that separate bunches of fat, connective tissue, nerves, and lymph vessels. Inside each lobe are alveoli that produce milk in response to hormones and your baby's sucking action on the nipple. It's a well-

orchestrated supply-and-demand system in which the more your baby signals your breasts to produce milk, the more milk your body makes.

You may have noticed a yellowish fluid, slightly thicker than milk, already coming out of your nipples. This is colostrum—your baby's first food. Rich in fat and high in protein and antibodies, colostrum is one more example of nature's perfect design. Its nutritional content helps your baby gain weight fast, excrete his first body waste, and fight infection from the very first minutes of life.

A different profile

About 2–3 weeks before labor begins, you may wake up one morning and notice that your baby, who once rode so high in your abdomen that he crowded your lungs and diaphragm (and made it tough to down a sandwich without suffering a heartburn hangover), has dropped in preparation for birth. Usually called "engagement" or "lightening," this downward shift in your baby's position is the result of your uterus thinning and stretching enough to allow your baby to move deeper into your pelvic area. This doesn't always happen before labor, especially in women who have had children before. But when it does, the difference in your profile can be dramatic enough for other people to notice.

The good news about engagement is that you can breathe more easily. The bad news is that you'll have to urinate even more frequently than before because the baby's head is pressing harder against your bladder. You may also experience a low-back ache and constipation as a result of your little one being poised to make his appearance. Take heart. You haven't far to go.

Labor signs (really!)

You may have already noticed prelabor signs. These have probably included an increase in Braxton Hicks contractions, an increased vaginal discharge that might be pink tinged, your baby's head dropping to become engaged in your pelvic area, and sometimes diarrhea.

Now is when you're also most likely to see a "bloody show," that brownish or bloody mucous smear caused by the mucus plug being freed when your cervix dilates enough to let it slip out. (See "Common Questions," page 319). And 10 percent of the time, your water will break just before you go into active labor.

Beyond that, the surest sign that you're really, truly, no kidding, actually in labor is regular contractions that increase in frequency, severity, and duration as time goes on. Before, with Braxton Hicks contractions, you could usually get them to slow down or stop by lying down, changing position, or downing a few glasses of water. This time, the contractions will most likely start in your lower back and radiate around to your abdomen and legs, causing pain that some women describe as "grabbing" or "pulling." They won't go away if you lie down or change position, and they'll get stronger over time. During this first stage of labor, the cervix thins, or effaces, and then dilates about 1 centimeter every hour. The contractions are between 5 and 10 minutes apart. If this is your first baby, it takes lots of contractions to completely thin the cervix.

You may feel euphoric or energetic when you realize that you're in labor at last. You may start washing floors or get three closets cleaned out, top to bottom. You may feel so excited about your baby's arrival that you want to get every last-minute thing done that you can possibly think of, even the grocery shopping, because today is The Day. It would be better to take a leisurely walk. And get some rest too. You need to store up your energy for the active labor to come.

Toward the end of this early labor stage, your contractions will become stronger and you may suddenly feel like curling up in a corner by yourself. When to alert your doctor that it is The Day depends on several things such as whether this is your first baby or your second, the distance from the hospital, whether the baby is known to be head-down, and if there is no bleeding and the baby is moving. Some women follow the 1-5-1 rule. That's when your contractions each last a minute or more, are no more than 5 minutes apart, and have been going on for 1 hour.

Your Self

Older children at delivery?

Childbirth is a time for rejoicing, but it's also a time of enormous physical sensations and equally powerful emotions, much of which won't be within your control. Think very carefully about whether you want older children in the delivery room when your baby is born.

This is a decision that you and your partner must make after considering your own comfort level and the maturity of your children. There are some 4-year-olds who wouldn't be frightened by the potentially scary visual and auditory sensations of a birth, while some 10-year-olds might be terrified by just a glimpse of their mothers bleeding. It's also important to discuss your wishes with your provider; if your midwife or obstetrician is uncomfortable with the idea, your children may need to wait to visit the baby in the nursery.

Most parents who decide to have their older children at the birth want to give them the gift of experiencing that miraculous moment when a baby comes into the world. They may want to introduce the idea of birth as a natural part of life, or they may hope that their children will be closer to their new sibling as a result of having witnessed the arrival. There is very little research, pro or con, on the effect of childbirth on siblings. What you decide is best for your children must therefore be based on your individual upbringing and family culture.

If you do decide to have children present, keep these general guidelines in mind to make the delivery more kid-friendly:

- The sounds and sights of birth might be distressing to some children, so take time to prepare them beforehand. Demonstrate some of the sounds you might make while in labor and let them

week 37

know what's really going on inside your body with the baby. Be sure to use words your children understand and discuss the feelings you and your children might experience. Be prepared, too, for older children to want to know what put your baby inside your body.

- Visit the birth center or hospital and ask your provider or the nurses to give your children a tour of the birthing room. They can explain in advance about the medical instruments and what might happen during the birth. Ask the nurses to explain what's OK to touch and what isn't.

- Ask someone other than your partner to attend the birth—perhaps a grandmother or close family friend—who can take your children somewhere else during the delivery if things get too intense or if your children change their minds about participating.

- Prepare your children for your newborn's appearance because they may be shocked to see that the baby doesn't look like babies on television. It's important for them to know about the umbilical cord and the placenta too.

- Once the baby is born, ask your children if they would like to hold their new brother or sister, but don't force the issue. Some siblings feel more comfortable if the baby is cleaned up first!

Easing through early labor

Early labor typically lasts 5–12 hours,

and it serves to open your cervix to 4 centimeters and thin it out so that your cervix goes from looking like a thick-walled cylinder to a thin cup. The best things you can do for yourself during early labor are to eat a little and rest, preferably on your left side. You may also want to slowly walk about the house, or even in your neighborhood, to help your labor progress and keep things—that is, your baby—moving in the right direction.

As your contractions intensify, you may need some additional support or distractions. This early stage of labor is the longest, and it can start to drag on if you're uncomfortable. You're most likely still at home at this stage, but you can set the mood for a peaceful labor and delivery by using some of the same support techniques you'll rely on once you're at the birth center or hospital. In fact, with most labors, you can remain at home until you're in active labor (see "Labor and Delivery," page 343).

- Start labor on the right foot by setting a peaceful mood. Dim the lights and surround yourself with things you love: favorite photographs, your favorite music, scented candles, audio books.

- If you don't have a doula or labor coach other than your partner, invite a trusted family member or friend to help you through these hours of early labor. Ideally this will be a woman who has had children herself, but the most important thing is that this person be someone you're completely comfortable with. This will offer you support and let your partner take breaks before the real excitement kicks in.

- Even if you're not walking, stay upright during contractions. Lean on your partner, your friend, a chair, or the arm of the couch. Better yet, fold a couple of towels and put them on the kitchen counter or a high table so that you can lean forward and rest your arms on them. You can also use a large exercise ball by kneeling with the ball in front of you and draping yourself over it; rock forward on your knees as your uterus contracts to relieve some of the pain.

- You might think added pressure wouldn't feel good now, but in fact any sort of massage releases those feel-good endorphins and might ease labor pains. Ask your partner or friend to give you a neck rub or foot massage to take your mind off contractions or have him or her press on your tailbone with each contraction. You can also make your own massage tool by stuffing tennis balls into a sport sock and asking your partner or friend to rub it over your back.

- Visualize things that make you happy: holding your baby in your arms, a beach you saw once in Bermuda, your honeymoon picnic in an Italian olive grove.

- Change positions often. (See "Best positions for labor," page 241.) Moving around may help your baby slip farther down into your pelvis; if you get tired of walking, try getting on your hands and knees and rocking back and forth.

- Early in labor, warm water can be the most pleasurable way to take your mind off any discomfort because it makes you feel weightless and soothes your aching back. Sit in a Jacuzzi or stand in a shower and aim the water jets or spray at the small of your back. (If your water has broken, get an OK from your midwife or doctor before sitting in a tub.)

- Keep up your fluids. Drinking water, juices, or sports drinks can keep you hydrated and—as an added benefit—keep you moving because the more you drink, the more you'll have to make that walk to the bathroom. If you start feeling nauseated during early labor, sip fluids between contractions or suck on frozen juice bars.

Diet & Exercise

Planning a breastfeeding diet

A nutritious diet is especially important after delivery if you breastfeed. During breastfeeding, you'll need to consume enough healthy food for you and your baby. Breastfeeding women need about 200 calories a day more than during pregnancy, or 500 calories a day more than before pregnancy. Resist the temptation to go on a diet after delivery. If you don't eat enough, your

week 37

body will make less breast milk. You'll have plenty of time in future months to lose weight.

Healthy ways to increase calorie consumption. The best way to increase your calorie intake during breastfeeding is to add nutritious foods such as fat-free milk and yogurt; lean meats, poultry, fish, and eggs; and whole grains. Some excellent 200-calorie diet additions include half a turkey sandwich on whole wheat bread; a bowl of whole grain cereal with milk; a scrambled egg and a slice of whole wheat toast; and leftover chicken and a glass of milk. Legumes, fruits, and vegetables will continue to serve a crucial role in your diet because they provide a wealth of nutrients for you and your baby.

Getting the right nutrients. While you're nursing, your body requires more of most vitamins and minerals than it needed before or during pregnancy, including vitamin A, vitamin C, vitamin E, riboflavin, folic acid, vitamin B$_6$, vitamin B$_{12}$, pantothenic acid, biotin, choline, chromium, calcium, copper, iodine, manganese, selenium, and zinc, among others.

Your body puts your nursing baby first in line for vitamins and minerals; if you don't get enough nutrients in your diet for both you and your baby, your body's stored nutrients will go into the breast milk, leaving you without them.

Ask your doctor whether you should continue to take your prenatal vitamins; some doctors recommend it, particularly if you're planning on conceiving again within a year or two. Or your doctor may recommend an ordinary multivitamin rather than a prenatal vitamin. Food is the best way to get the nutrients you need, but vitamin supplements serve as a good insurance policy in case you fall short in any areas of your diet.

Plan meals now for the first few weeks postpartum. After you bring your new baby home, you will probably feel too tired to put together nutritious meals. If you can, make some dinners now and freeze them. Better yet, ask family and friends to help out with meals after your baby is born. If someone asks, "How can I help?" tell her you'd love a huge fruit salad or a platter of ready-to-eat vegetables delivered every couple of days for the first few weeks. Washing, peeling, and cutting produce will be the last thing you'll want to do during your baby's first few weeks of life.

Your postpartum body

In a perfect world, you'd come home from the hospital weighing exactly what you weighed the day your pregnancy test turned positive and feeling as good as you felt before conception. Unfortunately, you live in an imperfect world where your postpartum body is shockingly similar to your pregnant body, except for the big belly—and instead of a big belly, you have a medium-size belly.

Your body won't feel like your own during those first couple of weeks postpartum. Your breasts will fill with milk; your vaginal area, episiotomy or not, will ache, as will a cesarean delivery incision; you'll soak a sanitary napkin every hour or two; your eyes will be bloodshot; and you'll feel sore all over. If you had a vaginal delivery you may have trouble urinating, moving your bowels, walking, and sitting. You'll also be shocked to find out that the number that comes up when you step on the bathroom scale will be only about 10 or 12 pounds less than it was before delivery. (If someone tells you she came home from the hospital and slipped right into her prepregnancy jeans, she's lying.)

Hang in there; things will get better fast. Within a week or two your aches and pains will go away, your vaginal discharge will slow down, and you'll grow accustomed to your new milk-producing breasts. Sitting, walking, and using the bathroom will get easier every day. The pounds should gradually start to drop off, particularly if you are nursing and you stick to a healthy diet.

Common Questions

Q. I found a brownish red smear on my underwear. What is this from? Am I going into labor already?

A. You've probably discovered the "bloody show" that your practitioner has told you might indicate the first stages of labor. But don't panic. Throughout your pregnancy, your cervix has produced thick, gooey secretions that formed a "mucus plug" to effectively cork your cervix closed and protect your baby's amniotic sac from infection. This plug sometimes comes out as the cervix gets thinner (effaced) and starts to widen (dilate) in preparation for delivery. That's followed by a thinner mucus. This blood-stained mucous discharge may look brown—from old blood—or pink as the cervix continues to thin and open, causing tiny blood vessels to break along the surface of the cervix and tinge the mucus.

When will labor actually begin? You're still a victim of nature's whims, even now: Some women see a bloody show only minutes before labor begins, while others wait days. Until you're in active labor, there's no need to call your practitioner unless the blood is bright red and heavy like your period, which could be a sign that something's wrong and needs immediate medical attention.

week 37

Your partner: His labor and delivery checklist

Your partner may become even more rattled than you do once labor begins, so it's helpful to have a labor and delivery checklist ready for the Big Day. Consider putting copies of this checklist in your hospital bag and in his wallet; you might want to tape one to the fridge too. Here are some items you may want to include:

- When to call your provider (when contractions are no more than 5 minutes apart, last at least a minute, and have been regular for an hour)
- Names and numbers for babysitters, house sitters, and pet sitters
- What to do in the house before you leave (shut off appliances, lock doors)
- Map to the hospital
- Instructions for parking at the hospital
- Instructions for where to go once you arrive at the hospital
- Name and number of doula, labor coach, or anyone else attending delivery
- Name and number of person to contact at work if you're not on maternity leave yet
- Cell phones and chargers
- Your hospital bag
- His hospital bag
- Your baby's bag
- Infant car seat
- Camera and film
- Phone numbers of people to call when the baby arrives

Week 38

Your Baby

The inside story

Things are really getting crowded now that your baby might weigh more than 6 pounds and stretch beyond 20 inches. The placenta, too, is nearly as large as it will get, probably measuring between 6 and 8 inches in diameter and 1 inch thick. The placenta adds another pound to what's keeping you from tying your shoes.

Your baby is so big that her knees and elbows have to be constantly flexed or even folded. However, she'll still wiggle and bump you, so you should be aware of her movements. Her heart rate will be between 120 and 160 beats per minute during labor and delivery. You'll probably also be very aware of her hiccups now. They're the result of your baby inhaling amniotic fluid as she practices her breathing, and they can be vigorous enough for your partner to see your clothes move. Her lungs are most likely fully mature.

Your baby's umbilical cord is between 12 and 39 inches long but will most likely be about 21 inches. It looks like a moist, white, twisted telephone cord, and it attaches the placenta to your baby.

Your Body

Headaches that don't go away

Pregnant women get headaches for the same reason any person does: fatigue, stress, sinus problems, and a history of migraines. Many expectant moms find that their headaches are worsened during pregnancy because of elevated hormone levels; however, most women find that headaches improve by the 3rd trimester.

If you're continuing to have headaches at this point in your pregnancy, take measures to prevent and treat them. It's bad enough that you're waddling down the hall every 20 minutes to relieve your bladder; it hardly seems fair to have to squint through a headache as well. Keep a "headache log," which can be a simple sheet of paper charting the start, duration, and severity of your headaches. Identifying what causes your headaches will help you sort out what measures to take in preventing and treating them.

For example, you have every reason now to feel stressed and tense. You may not be on maternity leave yet, so you may be frantically putting in extra hours at work to get ready to leave it all behind in good order. You

week 38

may be worrying about an older child and how you'll manage that toddler and a new baby. Or your partner may be withdrawn or physically absent at work, making you feel overwhelmed at home and emotionally abandoned.

To stave off headaches brought on by stressful emotions, turn down the volume on your life. Deal with whatever's worrying you, ask for help, and get enough rest. Find time during the day to retreat to a cool, dark place and do some deep breathing or just stretch out. Get some fresh air, too, and move around. If a tension headache does hit, apply ice to your forehead or the back of your neck to draw blood away from your head. You can also try putting a hot-water bottle or heating pad across your feet to do the same thing.

If your headaches are the result of sinus problems, allergies, or a stuffy head, keep your bedroom cool and run a humidifier in your home. There are treatments for seasonal allergies that are safe in pregnancy. Ask your health care provider.

It's still safe to take a pain reliever containing acetaminophen (the ingredient in Tylenol) during your 3rd trimester. If you are having migraines, turn out the lights, use a cold compress, and try to sleep.

Most important, contact your provider immediately if you experience severe or persistent headaches that won't go away with the measures outlined here or if the headaches reappear often. Persistent headaches can be an indication of preeclampsia,

which should be evaluated immediately. (See "Preeclampsia," page 253.)

Postpartum contraception

There's been so much going on these past months that you probably haven't given contraception a thought. (If anything, you may have been relieved not to have to think about contraception.) And who'd have time for sex with a baby in the house?

It may take weeks, or even months, before your desire returns after childbirth. But when the mood does hit, you don't want to get caught unprepared. Spontaneity will be both more difficult and more necessary after adding a new child to your life! So take some time now to consider your family planning options.

Breastfeeding is not birth control. It's true that nursing your new baby will lower your chance of conceiving. However, if you cut back on breastfeeding at all, you may ovulate even if you haven't had a period yet, so you can't count on nursing hormones to keep you safe from another pregnancy. Use this method only if you really don't mind having your children very close together.

Natural family planning. This is a less reliable contraceptive method that requires you to pay constant attention to your menstrual and ovulation cycles. You also have to be willing to abstain from lovemaking or use another method of birth control during those fertile times. You can keep track of when you ovulate with a basal thermometer: Use it to chart the rise in temperature that accompanies ovulation. Examine changes in your cervical mucus as well. You can also invest in an ovulation predictor kit. This method is about 60 percent effective, so 40 out of 100 couples will conceive in one year.

Condoms. Some patients choose condoms over birth control pills because of a concern about using hormones while breastfeeding. With typical use, condoms are 85 percent effective; they also protect against sexually transmitted diseases.

Diaphragm. If you used a diaphragm before getting pregnant, you might be able to use the same one. Be sure to get refitted by your midwife or obstetrician, though, in case your vagina has changed shape following childbirth. Be aware that even when the diaphragm is used correctly—that means inserting it correctly, using spermicide, and leaving it in for at least 6 hours after intercourse—it isn't a perfect solution. Its effectiveness is 94 percent at the best of times, and for women who use the diaphragm with less attention to detail, that effectiveness rate plummets to 80 percent.

IUD. Worldwide, IUDs (intrauterine devices) are the most popular form of birth control because they're 99 percent effective, never interfere with spontaneous lovemaking, and can be easily removed by a health care provider. They're even safe to use while breastfeeding. Talk with your health care provider about the pros and cons of different IUD brands. There are certain IUDs that can be left in place for 5 years, while others last as long as 10; however, be aware that the IUDs left in place longer may give you a greater risk of increased menstrual bleeding. You are a good candidate for the IUD if you are in a long-term, monogamous relationship and have had no recent STDs. Pelvic inflammatory disease from STDs can be more severe in women with IUDs. The type of IUD your provider will recommend for you will depend on your personal gynecological history.

Birth control pills. Even women who suffered side effects from birth control pills in years past might want to give them another try after having a baby. There are now dozens to choose from, and most have significantly lower hormone levels than pills manufactured in the past. The bottom line is this: If one birth control pill gives you side effects like headaches or breast tenderness, ask your doctor about switching to another. Of course if you're over 35 or a smoker, you'll want to choose another form of contraception since the Pill can heighten the chances of having a stroke.

Many providers suggest a progestin-only pill (the "minipill") while you are breastfeeding because the estrogen in combination pills may decrease your breast milk supply. This minipill is slightly less effective than regular birth control pills, however; for maximum effectiveness, it must be taken at the same time every day. Even then you might have some breakthrough bleeding. If you forget to take a pill, use condoms as a backup.

The Patch and vaginal ring. Like birth control pills, the Patch and vaginal ring rely on combinations of progestin and estrogen to keep you from ovulating and getting pregnant. Because the estrogen might interfere with milk production, these options are usually not prescribed for breast-feeding mothers.

The skin patch is a tiny square of thin plastic that you wear on your upper arm, upper back, hip, or belly. Each patch lasts a week; you wear one patch at a time for 3 weeks in a row, then skip wearing a patch for a week to have your period.

The NuvaRing is a bendable 2-inch ring that you insert in your vagina for 3 weeks, then remove for 1 week; your period typically starts a few days later and lasts for a shorter time than your normal menstrual cycle. Then you insert a new ring and start the process over.

Both of these methods may have fewer side effects than the Pill because they release a slower, steadier stream of hormones. The same women who shouldn't take the Pill—smokers, women with heart conditions, or women over 35—should look to another contraceptive method because they're more prone to strokes, heart attacks, and blood clots on these hormones.

Sterilization. If you and your partner are absolutely certain that this should be your last child, then you may want to consider either a tubal sterilization for you or a vasectomy for your male partner.

A tubal sterilization involves getting your fallopian tubes tied or having tiny, springlike devices inserted into them that trigger scarring and prevent sperm from traveling upward to meet your eggs. Both methods can be done in the delivery room after childbirth. Tubal sterilization typically requires anesthesia and a hospital stay. On occasion, tubal sterilization fails and you are at increased risk for ectopic pregnancy; after your tubes are tied, be sure to get a pregnancy test if your period is more than 2 weeks late. Vasectomies are simpler surgeries than tubal sterilizations because all that's involved is cutting the vas deferens, the tube that supplies sperm to semen. It's an outpatient procedure and your partner can usually go home the same day.

Both of these are considered permanent sterilizations, so it may be best to wait until after the birth of your baby, when your hormones have stabilized and your life has smoothed out somewhat, before making any final decisions.

Eye problems

Those same pregnancy hormones that help your body support your growing baby can wreak havoc with eyesight during the 3rd trimester. Because the hormones cause your tissues to retain more fluid, the very shape of your eyeballs may change. You may become more near- or farsighted than usual, to the point where you might have trouble seeing clearly with your regular prescription lenses.

The rise in estrogen also causes your eyes to be drier because your body is producing fewer tears. This can leave your eyes feeling irritated and looking red. "Dry eye syndrome" can even cause your eyesight to be blurred, damage your cornea, or increase your sensitivity to sunlight.

With so few weeks to go, you needn't do anything drastic. You might not be able to wear hard contact lenses—switch to soft ones or wear glasses—but you can usually relieve any discomfort with "artificial tears" available at most pharmacies. Wear sunglasses to protect your extra-sensitive eyes in strong light. You can certainly get new prescription lenses, but don't do this if it's too costly or if you can make do without them. Your eyesight will return to normal after delivery. For this reason, you should also wait to have laser surgery until your hormones stabilize—at least 6 months after your baby is born—to avoid overcorrecting your vision.

However, if you experience any drastic or sudden changes in your eyesight, like blurred vision, dimming eyesight, double vision, or spots that aren't just the temporary ones you get from standing up too fast, contact your health care provider immediately. Sudden, significant changes in vision like these during pregnancy can signal preeclampsia, especially if accompanied by headaches.

Your Self

Your nesting instincts

You may be the sort of person who has always tossed things into a junk drawer in your kitchen or disregarded the growing piles of clean laundry crowding every horizontal surface in your bedroom. If you're like most women, you may be seized by a sudden burst of energy late in pregnancy and become a human dirt devil, scaring your partner and friends with your obsessive new devotion to organizing closets and scrubbing bathroom tiles with a toothbrush.

Making a safe, warm, comfortable place for your baby is probably instinctual, brought on by that cascade of hormones, as well as an emotional response to feeling your baby move inside you and growing more attached every day.

Make the most of these last weeks or days before your baby arrives. Go ahead and refold those baby clothes. Get rid of the recycled newspapers that have been taking up space in your garage too. But choose low-key activities instead of rearranging the furniture or climbing ladders. Remember that you're clumsier than usual, and there's no need to get tired or achy when you'll need every ounce of your stamina and strength for delivering your baby.

A need for solitude

By this time, you can actually see your due date on the calendar

week 38

hanging in your kitchen, and you may be increasingly reluctant to leave the house. This is only natural. Why would you want to be caught in a shopping mall when your water breaks or suffer through an action-packed movie when your nerve endings seem raw? You may also long to stay near familiar things because your nerves are frayed and sitting on your own couch, surrounded by your favorite pillows, is comforting.

There's nothing wrong with staying home. However, be sure that you're seeing friends so that you don't feel too isolated and grow increasingly anxious as a result. Ask your girl-friends over for a pasta supper. (They can bring the sauces, and all you have to do is boil the pasta.) Have your partner arrange a take-out dinner party with couples you're especially close to or enjoy romantic dinners at home with your partner. A good laugh and an understanding look can go a long way toward helping you stay calm and happy during these final weeks. And remember, if you're feeling less agitated and more content, your baby may too.

Diet & Exercise

Snacks during labor

While laboring at home, keep up your energy with very light snacks such as fruit, toast, crackers, or soup. Once you get to the hospital you may not be permitted to eat. You probably won't want to anyway because labor can make you nauseous. You may even vomit, which is reason enough to keep snacks on the light side at home. Continue to drink fluids when you are laboring at home.

Late-pregnancy exercise

If you've continued to exercise throughout your pregnancy, congratulations! During these last few weeks, keep going as long as your doctor permits. If you're having a healthy pregnancy, there's no reason to quit exercising. Continue to stay hydrated. Listen to your body, and if you feel fatigued, take a break. Several short bouts of exercise make more sense than one long one. As always, stop working out immediately if you experience any warning signs (see "Are you exercising too hard?" page 27).

Common Questions

Q. How should I prepare "down there" when it gets closer to my due date?

A. If you're talking about shaving or waxing your pubic hair, don't bother unless that's your personal preference anyway. Your mom or grandmother might have had her pubic area shaved for delivery (though she might not have mentioned that little detail) because medical practitioners were once concerned that a baby could be infected by bacteria in the vaginal area during delivery. The current thinking is that you're actually more likely to transmit bacteria to your baby if you are shaved because little nicks and cuts make a handy breeding ground for that sort of thing. For this reason, you might want to switch to waxing your bikini line or just leave it alone until after delivery, though with the anti-septic wash commonly used in birth centers or hospitals, there's really very little cause for concern. At most, your practitioner might trim a little hair around the site of any tearing or an episiotomy, if you need stitches in that region after the birth.

Q. Do I have to have an enema before delivery or is that optional?

A. Enemas are no longer routinely given to birthing mothers. Practitioners once adopted this practice to empty a woman's bowels before her baby made his way through the birth canal, believing that with less crowding, the baby would emerge more easily and into a more sterile environ-ment. Mothers didn't protest because everyone is embarrassed by the possibility of having a bowel movement as well as a baby in the delivery room. But since most labors are hailed by loose bowel movements before contractions even get going, you don't have much waste stored up anyway. There's very little evidence that giving you an enema will make birth any easier or cleaner.

Q. I have a golden retriever who's like a child to me. Now my mother is warning me that the dog won't adapt to our having a baby, and I'm wondering if I have to get rid of him. Is it safe to have a dog around a newborn?

A. Whether your family includes a golden retriever or a black cat, you certainly don't need to get rid of beloved pets to make room for baby. However, no matter how unlikely you think it is that your trusted pet would hurt your infant, keep them apart. Most pets wouldn't harm a baby intention-ally, but why take the risk of an accidental injury? Don't leave your baby lying on a blanket on the floor unattended, for instance, and be sure not to shut your cat in the baby's room. Starting now, train your pets to stay out of the nursery and off the furniture.

You should be aware that household pets can communicate viruses, bacteria, and parasites. The common belief that a pet's mouth is cleaner than a human's is just a myth; the reality is that a dog or cat bite can become infected quickly. Even minor nips or cat scratches need to be thor-oughly cleansed with soap and water and possibly treated. Check with your pediatri-cian if your baby is bitten or scratched.

Your baby will probably be delighted by doggy and kitty kisses, but don't make that a habit. Cats and dogs often sniff or lick other animals, tasty tidbits in the neighbor's trash, and feces. It's also important to keep your pets free of fleas and ticks.

Q. Should I play Mozart for my baby?

A. Some child development experts believe that playing classical music to your baby before he is born will stimulate your baby, boost his IQ, enhance his creativity later in life, and improve his ability to speak, see, and hear. Advocates recommend playing music to your baby anytime after the 4th month of pregnancy because it can stimulate the development of complex neural pathways that allow the brain to process information.

Will Mozart really make your baby smarter and more creative? Maybe. In animal studies, rats who listened to Mozart before and after birth were able to find their way to the end of a maze more quickly than those that didn't. Human studies have found that babies' heart rates increase and they stay awake longer when music is played before birth.

If you think classical music will give your baby an intellectual boost, and if you enjoy it, go ahead and listen. If you can't stand Mozart or you don't have time to play music for the baby, that's fine. If classical music does make a difference in a baby's IQ, it's probably a very slight difference.

Week 39

Your Baby

The inside story

At last your baby is ready for the world. He's better-looking than ever, now that his facial features are fully formed, his eyes are open, and his ears stick out from his head. (Not like his grandfather's, you hope, but there's not much you can do about that now.) He may have a full head of hair, but don't be surprised if it's an unexpected color; many blond couples have dark-haired babies, while parents with dark hair may produce babies with nothing more than pale peach fuzz on their heads.

Your baby's body has grown enough to catch up with his head, which is now just one-fourth the size of his body instead of nearly as big as the rest of him as it was in your early weeks of pregnancy. One odd fact: Your baby's head and abdomen have the same circumference now, which makes it easier to understand why it's so tough sometimes to pull an article of clothing over a newborn's head.

In any case, your baby can forget the water ballets. He's so tightly packed inside your womb that he's literally shoving and kicking your organs to make space for himself.

Luckily, it usually doesn't matter how big your baby is because his head can elongate and mold to your birth canal. This may make him a bit cone-headed and comical looking at birth, but never mind. His head will soon shape up to be just as lovely as the rest of him approximately 24 hours after delivery.

Predicting baby's birthweight

How much will your baby weigh? At birth a full-term infant of "average" size generally weighs anywhere from 6 to 8 pounds. Most babies are right in the middle, weighing somewhere around 7⅓ pounds. Boys average about 3½ ounces more than girls. Your baby will continue to gain weight for as long as you carry him. Research has taught us that an optimal birthweight is setting the stage not only for a healthier baby and an easier delivery but also for a healthier child and adult. Babies born at less than 5½ pounds are at risk for various health problems, both upon delivery and as children. It turns out that babies born weighing more than 9½ pounds are also at risk because they might be more likely to be over-weight as a child and as an adult too.

week 39

Forceps and vacuum extraction

Despite the scary look of forceps and vacuum extractors, these instruments—which are used to assist vaginal deliveries about 10–15 percent of the time—pose no greater risk to your health or your baby's well-being than a cesarean delivery. Some births go much more smoothly because these instruments help things along. Talk to your provider about circumstances where she might use these instruments, and have her explain them in detail now so that you won't feel nervous if she needs one of these tools during your delivery.

Reasons for use. Typically, forceps or vacuum extraction is used if there is a prolonged second stage of labor—perhaps 2–3 hours of pushing with little progress due to maternal exhaustion. These tools might also be required if the baby is about to come out but her heart rate drops and she needs to make a quick exit. Neither instrument is used unless your cervix is fully dilated with the baby's head positioned no more than 2 inches above your vaginal opening.

Choosing the instrument. Whether your practitioner chooses forceps or vacuum extraction will probably depend on her training. Both have been around a long time. Forceps have been used in assisted births since the 16th century. They resemble a large pair of curved salad tongs. The most primitive form of vacuum extractor—a device that even today looks like a plunger—was first used in 1705. Now that the instruments have soft, synthetic rubber cups instead of the metal cups originally used, vacuum extractors have become increasingly popular in the United States.

If your practitioner opts to use forceps, you will be anesthetized around the perineal area and have your bladder emptied with a catheter. Each side of the forceps must slide into your birth canal around the baby's head. Forceps can help remove the baby; they are also used to rotate the baby's head to a better position for delivery. You may need an episiotomy to make more room.

If your practitioner opts for a vacuum extraction, you may also get perineal anesthesia and have your bladder emptied. Then the cup is placed on the crown of the baby's head. Pressure is generated by your provider using a handheld pump or by a nurse pumping from an external source. Traction is applied only during contractions, and you will be encouraged to continue bearing down as much as possible. Vacuum extraction is usually abandoned if the suction cup slips off more than 3 time, or if the procedure lasts more than 20 minutes. In that case, your provider will perform a cesarean delivery. You are less likely to need an episiotomy with the vacuum because the cup does not take up space in the vagina.

Your Body

Labor day surprises

You've read all the baby books and diligently taken notes as your childbirth instructor gave you information on riding labor contractions with a combination of breathing, massage, position changes, and, possibly, pain medications. Despite all your preparation, your baby may still deliver some surprises on labor day, since classes, books, and even your dearest friends might not be willing to share some of the grittier realities of childbirth. Even some of the most common labor scenarios can come as a complete shock if you've never heard anyone mention them, so it is helpful to have some insider knowledge beforehand.

For starters you can expect to forget every single thing they showed you in childbirth class. In the throes of labor, your mind may go blank. Breathing? Labor positions? Huh? You might find yourself suddenly lying on your back and gripping the bed—the last thing you ever imagined yourself doing during labor. To prepare for this, confirm that your labor partner knows the breathing techniques, has photos of the birthing positions you've talked about, and is armed with a list of your birth wishes in both best- and worst-case scenarios.

At some point during labor, your teeth might chatter. About half of women in labor complain of shivering and chattering teeth, even though their body temperatures are actually higher than normal. This is normal and nothing to worry about.

You may vomit. The nausea is normal; digestion slows when you're in labor, and you may still have food sitting in your stomach when you start having active contractions.

Occasionally, you may vomit if you have an epidural because epidurals can cause your blood pressure to drop.

In the movies, women growl or grunt and then cry when they have babies. You may already know that making these noises really can help you give birth; giving voice to your effort makes you feel more energetic and powerful as you ride a contraction or push your baby out during the second stage of labor. However, be prepared to rant and rave and perhaps even scream at your practitioner and swear at your partner. This is especially true if you haven't had any pain medication since you'll be exhausted and hurting and wanting it all to end. Don't be embarrassed; your practitioner has heard it all before, although your partner may be shocked.

You may make other, less cinematic noises too. For instance, the motion of your baby through your birth canal may cause you to pass gas, especially if you've had an epidural. You may be too busy to notice. But if you do notice, it's important for you to know that this is a normal sound and there's no need to be embarrassed about it.

You may also have a bowel movement during the delivery because your muscles are working to squeeze out your baby—and

week 39

everything else is bound to come out too—especially since the baby is squeezing your rectum as his head moves through the birth canal. Again you may be too engaged in riding out your contractions to notice, but if you do, don't worry. Your practitioner has seen it before.

Your partner may be as stunned by the process of labor as you are, and you may be secretly (or not so secretly) fretting that he'll be put off by seeing you in the physically and emotionally chaotic stages of labor. Give him some credit: Your partner will be as awed by the process as you are, and his overwhelming reaction will be one of pride in how strong you are and joy at seeing the baby you've both created.

Your Self

Involving your partner

You've said your final good-byes at work. You've outfitted the nursery. You've had your baby shower. Now you're intently focused on those little Morse code taps on your belly.

When you're so intently focused, you may forget that your partner might be making his own emotional odyssey as your due date draws ever nearer. While you're fending off well-meaning comments from friends or sidestepping nosy strangers who want to pat your belly for good luck, he might be withdrawing, scared by his own rocky moods as he sees your body become unrecognizable. He may be

feeling anxious or ambivalent about your new attachment to a person who seems extremely abstract to him at the moment or terrified of what you've both gotten yourselves into.

Get him involved by talking to him about how he can best support you during delivery. Here are some important tasks he can tackle:

- Keep you company during early labor when you'll likely still be at home. Take a walk, rent a movie to watch together, or take a nap.
- Rub your lower back.
- Help you get into and out of the shower or tub.
- Feed you ice chips and frozen fruit treats.
- Give you a massage.
- Time your contractions and talk soothingly to you during the rest between contractions.

Diet & Exercise

Why hydration is so important

No matter how swollen you feel, how often you have to urinate, or how full your stomach is, keep drinking water. Staying hydrated is vitally important at the end of pregnancy. You could go into labor at any time, and if you're fully hydrated when labor starts, you'll have far more energy and stamina than you will if you're dehydrated. Also if you're hydrated, you may be less likely to need intravenous fluids.

Drink water, milk, decaffeinated tea or coffee, fruit juice, seltzer, or sports drinks; suck on ice chips; or eat frozen fruit treats and water-drenched fruits such as watermelon and grapes—whatever helps you get your 8 glasses of fluids a day.

Walking late in pregnancy

If you've walked your way through to week 39, there's no reason to stop now. Keep walking right up into labor if you can. It will continue to tone your muscles, help stabilize blood sugar, strengthen your heart and lungs, improve your mood, and give you a fabulous sense of accomplishment. Continue to drink plenty of fluids and plan walking routes that give you ample opportunities to stop for bathroom breaks. If you tire easily, avoid hills and take several shorter walks rather than one long walk.

Common Questions

Q. I'm terrified that I'll have a fast labor like my mother did with me and that I'll end up delivering my baby at home or in the car on the way to the hospital. What do I do if I end up in that situation?

A. First of all, you probably won't end up in that situation. You're already aware of your genetic predisposition to birth your baby faster than most, so you'll probably be timing those contractions from the moment labor begins and already on your way to the hospital in plenty of time because you're anxious. However, if you've been in labor only a little while when you

suddenly are overcome by an urgent need to push, stay calm. Whether they appear in hospitals, taxis, kitchens, cars, elevators, or log cabins, babies usually do a fine job of coming into the world all by themselves. However, being prepared for an emergency delivery at home may help ease your anxiety and give you confidence that you'll be able to handle the situation, in the rare case it should arise.

The American College of Nurse-Midwives (ACNM) launched a campaign several years ago called "Giving Birth in Place" to educate people about emergency delivery preparation. For a detailed guide, including a list of supplies and step-by-step directions that you can print out and save, see the ACNM website (www.midwife.org).

According to ACNM, if you go into labor at home and don't think you can get to a hospital or a birth center in time, you should stay where you are; it's better to have your baby at home than in the backseat of a car. Call your practitioner immediately. If she's there, she might be able to instruct you over the phone until emergency help arrives. If you can't reach your practitioner, call 911. Ask for emergency assistance with the birth and ask the 911 operator to contact both your practitioner and the hospital.

The ACNM recommends that pregnant women put together a supply kit that can be used during an emergency delivery. The supplies should be kept in a waterproof bag away from children and pets. The kit should contain the following:

- A bag of large-size underpads with plastic backing to protect sheets from messy fluids
- Baby-size bulb syringe (made of soft

plastic, often called an ear syringe; should not be a nasal syringe, because the plastic tip does not fit into a baby-size nose)
- A small bottle of isopropyl alcohol
- A package of large cotton balls
- A box of disposable plastic or latex gloves
- White shoelaces (to tie umbilical cord)
- Sharp scissors (to cut umbilical cord)
- Twelve large sanitary pads
- A chemical cold pack (the kind you squeeze to get it cold)
- A hot-water bottle (to help keep baby warm)
- Six disposable diapers
- Pain pills such as acetaminophen or ibuprofen
- A small bar of antibacterial soap or liquid antibacterial hand sanitizer

Q. I just came back from my prenatal visit, and my midwife says I'm already 3 centimeters dilated and 50 percent effaced! Does that mean I'll go into labor today?

A. In simplest terms, labor is the process of your cervix thinning out (effacement) and opening up (dilation). Thanks to those marvelous Braxton Hicks contractions, by the final weeks of pregnancy your practitioner may pronounce you to be 50 percent effaced or more. A cervix that is 100 percent effaced has gone from the shape of a thick-walled cone to that of a flat, thin cup beneath the baby's head. If you're 50 percent effaced, that means you're halfway there.

Your labor contractions will gradually open your cervix to that magical dilation measurement of 10 centimeters. When your cervix has dilated to that point (about the width of your hand), your midwife or obstetrician will tell you that it's all right to push during your contractions and deliver your baby. The fact that you're 3 centimeters dilated right now means that your cervix is already starting to open up. That's a great sign. However, when you'll actually go into the active labor phase is still a mystery. In general, though, once active labor begins, the average progress is about 1 centimeter dilation per hour for your first baby and 1½ centimeters per hour for a second baby.

Week 40

Your Baby

The inside story

Your baby is plump now; a full 15 percent of her body is made up of fat that will help her regulate her body temperature. She probably weighs between 7 and 8 pounds and is about 21 inches long if she's an average-size baby. Most of her body hair has disappeared, but she still wears nature's wet suit—a thin layer of that greasy white stuff called vernix caseosa that will provide additional protection against the first cool air on her skin.

Her body has been processing bilirubin—the breakdown product of red blood cells—by moving it across the placenta into your body where it is flushed out along with other waste products. Once your baby is born and her umbilical cord is clamped and cut, she will have to rid her own body of bilirubin. This may take a few days after birth; if levels of bilirubin build up in her body, she may become jaundiced. The classic symptoms of jaundice are a yellowish tinge to the

Babies more than 9 pounds

Having a baby whose weight falls beneath the average range of 6–9 pounds poses some potential health risks. Birthing a baby who weighs more than 9 pounds can cause problems too, for both baby and mother. Women who gain large amounts of weight during pregnancy or have diabetes are more likely to give birth to high-birthweight babies. Although most of these babies are born healthy—women around the world have vaginally delivered babies of 9, 10, and 11 pounds without problems—birth-related complications can include a prolonged labor, intolerance to labor, shoulder dystocia, and neonatal low blood sugar.

If your provider suspects a large baby, she may suggest an ultrasound. An ultrasound will allow your provider to measure the diameter and circumference of your baby's head—the biggest part of him—and to estimate your baby's birthweight within half a pound. However, unless you or your baby seems to be suffering a medical complication, your provider probably won't do anything to induce your labor if your cervix isn't ready. That's because ultrasound measurements only offer estimates of a baby's size; labor is the only true test of whether your baby is too big to move safely through your birth canal. Many petite women give birth to 9-pound babies (or larger) vaginally. Likewise, some large women have pelvises too narrow to accommodate even a 7-pound baby.

skin and whites of the eyes. Usually, this is nothing to worry about. Exposure to light generally takes care of things.

At week 40 your baby recognizes your voice better than anyone else's. At long last she's ready to meet you.

Your Body

Home remedies for inducing your labor

If your due date is history, you may be longing to jump-start your labor, even if your practitioner seems to think it's fine to wait another couple of weeks. Is there anything you can do to induce labor yourself?

Most methods that expecting moms have tried don't work. However, most of these methods are harmless, so if you want to give them a whirl, go ahead. Be forewarned that some of the results may be uncomfortable, if not downright unpleasant. For instance, some moms consume spicy foods or chocolate, thinking that the spices and caffeine might act as laxatives and start contractions. All you'll probably induce with this kind of behavior is heartburn and puffy ankles because the food taxes your digestive system. Others swear that walking is the way to the delivery room because gravity will lower the baby and put enough pressure on your cervix to prompt it to open. Although walking extra-long distances can start contractions by irritating the uterus, it won't do much to bring on

labor unless your cervix is already effaced; the contractions generally stop after you stop moving. It's the same story with sex: Orgasms can cause your uterus to contract, and semen contains prostaglandin—a natural fatty acid that helps soften and dilate your cervix—but sex won't bring on labor unless your baby is ready to arrive. Frustrated pregnant moms have also tried taking a single dose of castor oil to stimulate the production of contraction-inducing prostaglandins. However, the most likely thing to follow castor oil is terrible diarrhea because castor oil is a laxative.

Although using herbs or herbal teas to induce labor seems like a great idea, there is little evidence that they work—and some evidence that certain herbs may be harmful.

In some studies, acupuncture has shown promise, but other studies link it to prolonged pregnancy.

About the only thing research has definitively linked to self-induced labor is nipple stimulation. Ask your provider about this method before trying it. The reason nipple stimulation sometimes starts contractions is because rubbing your nipples in late pregnancy can help your body release oxytocin; oxytocin is a hormone similar to Pitocin, which is the drug most practitioners use to cause contractions in pregnancies where labor needs to be induced or helped along. Unfortunately, for nipple stimulation to be effective in bringing on labor, you have to tweak and twiddle your breasts for an hour at a time, three times a day. Who has time for that? Nipple stimulation has another downside: It can cause very strong contractions that may affect your baby's heart rate, so your practitioner might have you try this method only at the birth center or hospital, where the heart rate can be monitored.

Overall, getting labor started is something that's probably best left up to your baby, even if you're overdue.

Mending the muscle gap

Like most expecting mothers, you're probably spending a lot of time with your hands on your belly right now, either patting your unborn child or begging him to stop testing his soccer moves on your rib cage. In doing so, you may have noticed a gap along the middle of your abdomen where the skin bulges out in an odd way. If this gap is unusually large—say the width of two fingers—it's called diastasis recti, a condition that occurs in about a third of all pregnancies. There is no other noticeable symptom and there is no pain.

What it means is that those two long, parallel bands of muscle running between your rib cage and pubic bone have separated. This is caused by a combination of factors: pressure from your enlarged uterus, your own genetic predisposition, the hormonal softening of the fibrous connection between the muscles, and poor muscle tone. The only one of these factors that you can control is muscle tone. Although your muscles will

probably move back together on their own a few months after you deliver your baby, it's important to keep them as strong as possible both now and after you give birth. Strong abdominal muscles mean fewer backaches during and after pregnancy and will help prevent diastasis recti in subsequent pregnancies.

There are many abdominal-strengthening exercises you can do after pregnancy (see "Abdominal exercises," page 393). You may want to avoid ab busters like stomach crunches or leg lifts after the 1st trimester. Consider working the following ab tighteners into your late-pregnancy regimen:

- Abdominal breathing. Inhale deeply. As you exhale, tighten your abdominal muscles.
- Pelvic tilt. Stand with your back against a wall. Press the small of your back against this vertical support, inhale, and then tighten your abdominal muscles and buttocks as you breathe out. You can also do this exercise lying on your back or kneeling on all fours.

Your Self

When you're overdue

The first question to consider, of course, is whether your due date is accurate. Often what appears to be a late baby is really only a mistake in calculations; having a baby 9 days "late" is fairly common. The calendar wheel doctors use to calculate your due date is based on counting back 3 months from the first day of your last menstrual period, then adding 7 days. However, these calculations are based on a perfect 28-day menstrual cycle, and very few women have periods that perfect. The reality is that 80 percent of babies arrive between 38 and 42 weeks of pregnancy, so your due date window is much bigger than you might think.

Only about 1 out of every 10 babies is officially overdue, which means that the baby is born after 42 weeks of pregnancy. No one really knows why some babies come early and others come late. Of the many factors that possibly influence pregnancy duration, researchers have found that ethnicity and the number of babies you have play the most important roles. African-American women generally have shorter pregnancies— by three days—than Caucasian women. How many babies a woman has had can also influence gestation time; pregnancies tend to be shorter with each subsequent pregnancy.

If your pregnancy lasts more than 41 weeks, your practitioner will start monitoring your baby's health more closely. She'll probably ask you to do a kick count every day, which means keeping track of your baby's movements. A decline in activity can signal that your baby is ready to exit. Your provider may also do nonstress tests (NST) a couple of times each week to be sure that your baby's heart rate accelerates when he moves. An NST is a painless way of ensuring

your baby's health. You'll go to the doctor's office, have a belt with a transmitter placed around your abdomen, and sit comfortably while the fetal heart rate is measured for 20–30 minutes. You may also have an ultrasound to measure amniotic fluid volume or a biophysical profile. The combination of the NST and the ultrasound can provide a host of information on your baby's well-being.

Other than that, the best thing you can do if you're overdue is relax and have fun. Take a walk on the beach, see a funny movie, make love with your partner if your water hasn't broken and your practitioner says it's OK, visit friends, read a book, and store up your energy for delivery day. Most of the time labor happens when it's going to happen. If something you do seems to induce labor, it's probably only a coincidence.

Inducing labor

If you've reached this point in your pregnancy without going into labor, then you may be champing at the bit and ready to leap at any suggestion to speed things up. By 42 weeks, your practitioner may suggest inducing labor artificially. Many providers will consider this even earlier, at 41–42 weeks, especially if your cervix is open already. About 15 percent of all labors are artificially induced in the United States, and there are certainly many situations where inducing labor seems like the best choice for both mom and her baby.

If you're overdue, your practitioner

may want to induce labor before your placenta ages too much—an aging placenta can deprive your baby of essential nutrients and oxygen. One of the first signs that the placenta is not working well is a decrease in the amount of amniotic fluid. You may notice that the baby is less active. At that point, the baby may be better off out than in. Induction jump-starts a labor that may not have naturally begun until several days in the future; it also increases the risk of ending up with a cesarean delivery. However, babies who are not thriving anymore in utero may be much happier in your arms, even if the induction fails and the baby is delivered by cesarean.

After 42 weeks, there's a greater risk of your baby inhaling meconium—his first bowel movement—or suffering from dysmaturity syndrome. Hallmarks of dysmaturity syndrome include a thin face, overly long limbs, prominent eyes, and skin as thin as parchment paper. Babies with dysmaturity syndrome are less likely to tolerate the stress of labor. It's also possible that incubating your baby too long will result in a baby too large to fit through your pelvis—that's another situation where the risk of cesarean delivery is possibly higher.

There are many other circumstances that would prompt your provider to offer you induction. If you are full-term, for example, and have been struggling with mild preeclampsia, you may be induced to cure your preeclampsia. You also may be induced if your baby seems very small and you are full-term.

If your provider suggests inducing labor, gather all of the information you can in the time allowed. An induced labor is generally longer than a natural labor. The contractions are as strong as those you'd experience in natural labor, but there may be no gradual increase in their intensity. If prolonging your pregnancy carries a significant health risk for you or your baby, however, an induced vaginal delivery is generally considered better for both you and the baby than a cesarean delivery.

Getting labor started

Doctors have several methods of inducing labor. The one your practitioner uses will depend on a number of factors, such as the readiness of your cervix and your baby's health.

Membrane stripping. Your health care provider will do a cervical exam, and with her finger, she will separate the amniotic sac from the wall of the uterus. Many women have cramping and spotting after this is done. When the membrane is separated, prostaglandins are released, and these ripen the cervix by causing contractions. Membrane stripping can be done only if your cervix is dilated.

Ripening the cervix. Before inducing labor, your practitioner may use a point system called a "Bishop Score" to determine whether your cervix is ready for labor. She will examine your cervix to see how effaced and dilated it is and will check to see if your baby has descended into your pelvis. Studies show that induced labors are most effective in women whose cervices are ready for labor, so if yours isn't, your health care practitioner may help things along by using one of several ripening agents. These include prostaglandin E suppositories, a prostaglandin-laced gel, prostaglandin on a vaginal device, or a prostaglandin tablet. Some women who go this route go into labor within 24 hours without needing to have any other intervention.

Other tricks used to open your cervix include laminaria (seaweed sticks, which absorb water from the cervix and slowly open it) or a urine catheter bulb (which gets blown up in the cervix and gradually opens it).

Rupturing the membranes. Your practitioner may insert an obstetric tool that looks a little like a crochet hook through your cervix to tear a small hole in your amniotic sac. (This technique is also called an "amniotomy.") It mimics what sometimes happens in nature when your water breaks before labor begins. This procedure can be uncomfortable if you're less than a centimeter dilated, but otherwise it doesn't hurt at all. If labor doesn't begin within 24 hours after your water is broken, your practitioner may then induce you with Pitocin or another method to decrease the risk of infection.

Pitocin drip. Pitocin is a synthetic form of oxytocin, which is your body's contraction-inducing hormone. It's one of the most commonly used drugs in the United States. For most pregnant women, labor begins in part as a result of higher levels of oxytocin in the blood; your practitioner is aiming to mimic this natural process by administering Pitocin.

If your labor is induced with Pitocin, you will be admitted to the hospital where you will have an IV needle inserted into your arm. It usually takes at least 30 minutes for the Pitocin to kick in, and your practitioner will probably start slowly and monitor your reactions and your baby's response to the drug as it builds in your system. There is no guarantee of rapid labor with Pitocin; still the uterine contractions may be strong, and each contraction may last 1 minute or more. Many women find that the breathing exercises they've practiced for labor help them a good deal during an induced labor as well.

Labor induction is a process, and if this is your first baby, you may have one or more interventions. For example, cervical ripening followed by Pitocin is an everyday occurrence. Ask your provider for an overview of what you can expect and then sit back and be patient.

Diet & Exercise

Postpartum exercise

You may be excited about the fact that you'll soon be able to lace up your sneakers (and see your feet again) and head outside for a run or to your favorite step class. Though you'll need to wait until your doctor gives you the OK to start to exercise again, you can start planning your post-pregnancy workouts now.

Start with walking. Take a 5-minute walk and then come home and see how you feel. If nothing bleeds, pulls, or aches, take a 6-minute walk tomorrow and a 7-minute walk the next day. During these first few forays out into the world, don't carry your baby in a frontpack or push him in a stroller because the strain may be too much. Ask your partner to take care of the baby while you go out or have your partner push or carry the baby.

Let your body tell you how much activity to do during the first few weeks. After you've walked comfort-ably and safely for a week or two, build up from there, adding some gentle upper-body stretching or a postpartum exercise class.

If you're breastfeeding, forget about weight loss until a couple of weeks postpartum when your milk supply is firmly established. Some weight will come off automatically during the first few days as your body relinquishes the stored fluids it needed during pregnancy. The rest will come off gradually as you become more active. If you're nursing, your body needs 500 calories a day more than it needed before you conceived, so eat enough and eat healthfully.

Postpartum fitness classes

If your hospital or community center offers postpartum exercise classes, consider signing up. These classes are designed for women who have just had babies; the instructors know what moves a new mom should be doing and what moves she should be avoiding. If you take a postpartum exercise class, check that the instruc-tor is qualified. As you exercise, slow down if any of the moves feel too rigorous, even if you feel as if you should be able to do them. A good instructor will explain how various exercises can be modified so that they're less taxing. Now is not the time to push yourself to exhaustion.

What's great about postpartum exercise classes is that you can take your baby with you to class and keep her next to you either in her car seat or on a blanket. If she needs to eat or be comforted or have a new diaper, you can stop and attend to her. Nobody in a postpartum fitness class bats an eye when you pull up your T-shirt and start breastfeeding. These classes are a great place to meet other mothers with babies about the same age as yours. Many new moms build lasting friendships with the women they meet in their postpartum exercise classes.

Common Questions

Q. My doctor says I'll probably need to have a cesarean delivery because I'm in my 40th week of pregnancy and my baby is still breech. I've never had any kind of surgery before, so I'm really scared. Do I really need a cesarean?

A. According to the National Center for Health Statistics, about 85 percent of breech babies are born by cesarean delivery. Your baby's head is the largest part of his body, so if he descends headfirst, the birth canal is stretched enough for the rest of his body to follow easily. However, if his feet, buttocks, or legs emerge first, there is a higher risk of your baby's head getting stuck in the birth canal, or the baby's buttocks and legs may squeeze the umbilical cord, cutting off your baby's oxygen supply. Although there are some practitioners who are experienced in delivering breech babies vaginally, most now opt for a cesarean. Some practitioners may wait to see if the baby turns on his own when labor begins rather than schedule the surgery. (For more information on cesareans, see "Planned cesarean delivery," "Elective cesarean delivery," and Performing a cesarean delivery," pages 234-236.)

Q. I'm pregnant with my second child, and I'm really nervous about delivery because I had such a difficult labor with my first baby. Is this one likely to be the same?

A. Every labor and delivery is unique, so there's no way to predict what will happen. However, if this isn't your first baby, you'll most likely have an easier time of childbirth than you did with your first pregnancy.

Why? Your body already knows what to do. This time around, your cervix is more likely to dilate quickly and shorten your labor. The fact that your vaginal muscles are already stretched from your first birth will also speed things along because they'll give more easily this time. Of course if you had a cesarean delivery without labor the first time around, none of this applies unless the cesarean was performed after you entered the pushing stage.

labor and delivery

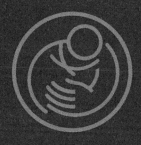

For several weeks before your baby's arrival, those Braxton Hicks contractions may occasionally become so rhythmic that you feel convinced your baby is coming soon—maybe even this minute! In fact, although some might call these contractions "false" labor, they are an important warm-up for the real thing, thinning out and softening your cervix. At last, you're about to really, truly be in labor. It won't be long before your beautiful baby is sleeping peacefully in your arms and you're faced with another big decision: What name is going to be written on the birth certificate?

Labor and Delivery

Stages of labor

Most health care providers divide labor into three distinct stages. Stage 1 involves the dilation of the cervix, which allows your baby to pass through the birth canal, and includes the early phase (the cervix is dilated from 0–4 centimeters), active phase (4–8 centimeters), and transition phase (8–10 centimeters). Stage 2 is the birth of the baby. Stage 3 is the delivery of the placenta. (Stage 4 is recovery!) During the course of the three labor stages, your uterus goes from being shaped like an upside-down pear to being shaped like a tube as the lower muscles soften and relax to open up while the upper muscle groups contract.

Stage 1: Early phase

During the early phase of stage 1 labor, your uterine contractions will thin your cervix and open it up to 4 centimeters. This early phase of labor is the longest, lasting between 12 hours and 18 hours if this is your first baby. You'll notice a gradual increase in the strength, duration, and frequency of your contractions.

During the early phase of stage 1 labor, the contractions themselves probably won't feel worse than very strong menstrual cramps, and you should be able to move around and rest between them. During this part of labor, many women prefer to stay home, where they can rest more comfortably. Eat small amounts of food and drink fluids or suck on icepops to stay hydrated. Your amniotic sac may or may not break during early labor.

When the water breaks, some women describe a "pop" followed by a gush of clear fluid. Other women's experiences are less dramatic: They feel a continuous leak of warm, clear fluid from the vagina.

Call your provider when your contractions are consistently 5 minutes apart, are lasting 1 minute apiece, and have been going on for 1 hour. (Another good clue that it's time to call is that you are no longer walking or talking through the contractions but have to stop whatever you're doing.) Your provider will help you decide when to go to the hospital. That decision will be based in part on whether your pregnancy is considered high-risk, whether your water has broken, how much pain you're in, and how nervous you are.

If you're feeling extremely anxious, by all means go to your birth center or hospital and ask to be examined. If it's a false alarm, they'll send you home again with more information about what to expect over the next few hours and with reassurances that your baby is fine.

Stage 1: Active phase

When you're admitted to the hospital or the birth center, your cervix will probably be dilated at least 3–4 centimeters, and you will be in active labor. The nurse or doctor will do an internal exam to check your progress. He or she will place one electronic monitor around your belly to measure your baby's heart rate; a second belt will monitor your uterine contractions. If your baby is fine, there is no reason you have to wear the fetal monitor constantly. Intermittent monitoring is just as safe for you and your baby, and it allows you to move around more freely. If the sound from a fetal monitor worries or annoys you, ask the nurse to turn down the volume.

Most women will have either intermittent or continuous external monitoring. However, sometimes external devices do not provide your doctor with enough information, particularly if the baby is active or your belly is large. Your doctor may suggest an internal monitor called a fetal scalp electrode, which clips onto the top of the baby's scalp.

If you are having your baby in a hospital, the nurse may hook you up to an IV when you arrive. If your pregnancy is low-risk and you're fairly certain you don't want medication, there may be no need to have an IV. However, if you're dehydrated, or if

you feel fairly certain that you will have an epidural during labor, the nurses may insist. If that's the case, ask for a portable IV stand that will allow you to keep changing positions during labor. If it is hospital policy to have every pregnant woman on an IV, but there is no medical reason for you to have one, you can ask for a heparin lock, which is an IV needle with a cap on it. That way if you need medication or fluids delivered by IV at any point while you deliver your baby, the needle is already securely in place and will make these interventions easier while still granting you freedom to move around.

During the active phase, which typically lasts 3–4 hours, your contractions will be moving your baby downward, so his head is putting pressure on the cervix. Your contractions will become more intense and come every 3–5 minutes; they will be rhythmic and usually regular enough that you can focus your breathing. You'll start to feel an intense pressure on your perineum and rectal area as your cervix dilates between 4 and 8 centimeters. You may have an intense backache or feel a pulling and stretching above your pubic bone. Though you won't want to eat anything now, it's still important to stay hydrated by sipping fluids or sucking ice chips. Move around to let gravity do some of the work for you, and pull out every relaxation, breathing, and pain management trick you've gleaned from your childbirth classes and reading.

labor and delivery

Empty your bladder every hour during labor. This will make you feel slightly more comfortable, and the act of walking to the toilet and squatting over it will help move your baby downward and open your pelvis. Try different labor positions—kneeling, leaning, squatting, lying on your side—to see what feels most comfortable for you (see "Best positions for labor," page 241). Go for a dip in the labor tub if your facility has one or stand in the shower with warm water aimed at your lower back. Drape a towel over your shoulders under the shower to really feel warm. Ask your labor staff for a birthing ball if you didn't bring one and sit on it to help open up your pelvis while you keep up your breathing techniques (see "Practicing for labor," page 266). You may feel "zoned out" at times, and that's fine. That's the endorphins kicking in to naturally ease your pain.

Your nurses and coach will be making suggestions and fulfilling your requests for massages, music, ice chips, and hot or cool compresses; they'll also support you in your various breathing and position changes. This is not a time to be shy about asking for what you need or asking questions about what's happening. And don't worry, even the shyest women—the sort too timid to introduce themselves at parties—have no problem being vocal during labor. (For what your partner can expect to do during your labor, see "Your partner: Preparing him for delivery," page 262.)

Stage 1: Transition phase

As your contractions start coming harder, your provider or coach may tell you that you're entering the "transition phase" of labor. This is when the contractions open your cervix from 8 centimeters to 10 centimeters. Transition can be the toughest time for some women: They may already be exhausted, and now the contractions might come faster and harder. The contractions may also be erratic with much less time between them to rest. Luckily, this phase of labor is the shortest, lasting from 15 minutes to an hour for a total of perhaps 20 contractions. Just at the point when you're vomiting, trembling, or shouting, "I can't do it anymore!" it will be over and you will be ready to push your baby out. However, if you're not quite fully dilated, it's essential to use your breathing techniques to hold back from pushing your baby down too soon; otherwise you risk having a swollen cervix.

Stage 2: Delivering the baby

Once you're fully dilated, you are in stage 2 labor, which is when you will deliver your baby. There may be a 20-minute lull between transition and the urge to push. Then, when the urge to push hits, work with your contractions to move your baby through the pelvis and—at long last—through the birth canal and cervix.

How long you push will depend on your baby's size and position. Many women imagine they'll push their babies out all at once, but in fact it can take anywhere from several minutes to several hours (the average is 2 hours) from the time the baby's head is at the top of the vagina to delivery. Take deep breaths, lean into each contraction, and bear down, tightening your abdominal muscles. Then rest and regroup between the contractions. You also may feel an intense backache.

You may want to start watching your labor now, using a mirror placed at the foot of your bed—it's a great time to see your baby emerge. This is also prime time for creative positioning to get yourself upright for the homestretch. Use a birthing ball to lean and rock, get up on all fours, hang from a squatting bar attached to your bed, or lean on your partner. If you've had an epidural, your legs will probably still be wobbly, so the easiest way for you to push will probably be lying on your side or in a half-sitting position with your birthing bed cranked up behind you. Your coach and the labor nurse can support your legs or feet as you push. Although this is hard work, you probably won't mind it as much as the other parts of labor because the end is in sight (so to speak) and you're actively engaged in bringing your baby into the world. The contractions may feel less painful, and they'll probably be more widely spaced apart, perhaps every 3–5 minutes or so. Use short, frequent pushes— maybe 3 per contraction—to conserve your energy.

When your baby's head crowns, your provider will let you know that the top of the head is visible. The baby's head will stretch your perineum and you may tear. You'll feel an intense burning sensation; however, the pressure of your baby's head will quickly numb the nerve endings in your perineum. Then you'll feel as if you're straining hard to have a bowel movement. All the while, your body will be manufacturing more oxytocin, stimulating more contractions so that your abdominal and pelvic muscles get into the act and begin exerting even more pressure on your uterus. Finally, your baby's head will emerge, followed by one shoulder, then the other. The rest of his body will slip out easily, and your baby's birth will be complete.

Stage 3: Delivering the placenta

While your baby is taking his first breaths, your childbirth marathon will continue. After your newborn has his umbilical cord clamped and cut (see "Your baby's first day," page 353), you will feel more contractions. These will be less intense, and you may not even be aware of them after all that's gone on, especially with your baby now wonderfully present and occupying every bit of your attention. This third stage of labor lasts a short time—only 5–30 minutes—as the uterus expels the placenta and a final gush of blood. You may be given Pitocin if your uterus needs help contracting enough to expel the placenta;

the Pitocin can be administered by a shot or through your IV. Your provider may massage your uterus to help it clamp down on blood vessels to ease the bleeding. Afterward your provider will stitch up your tear or episiotomy, if necessary, as your uterus contracts and the bleeding decreases.

Reconsidering pain relief

It is during active labor that many women, even those who entered their pregnancies determined to birth their babies with no medical intervention, request an epidural or IV opioids for pain relief. Should you? That's an impossible decision to make until you're actually in active labor. You can't predict what's going to happen while delivering your baby, so your best bet is to stay open-minded.

How a woman copes with the pain she experiences during labor depends on many things, including stress, fatigue, fear, how long her labor lasts, and what position her baby is in. You may surprise yourself. Labor pain is very different from the sort of pain you feel when you're injured. This is pain with real gain at the end. One part of you will be thinking, "This hurts!" At the same time you will be excited because you're finally going to meet your child.

You may be encouraged and reenergized if you are checked periodically to see if your labor is progressing. For instance, if you hear that you're 8 centimeters dilated, that may inspire you to keep going without any pain medication.

If you're exhausted or hurting badly, it's OK—really it is—to ask for pain relief. Most women do. There's no medal for She Who Can Withstand the Most Pain. Anesthesia techniques pose very few risks to you or your baby. Your health care provider will help you decide whether an epidural or opioids will make you more comfortable; then he or she will tell you when the medications should be administered.

Common labor and delivery complications

When complications occur during labor, it can be frightening. However, knowing about the most common childbirth complications—and how providers address them—before you go into the delivery room can ease your fears.

Your baby doesn't tolerate labor. If the fetal heart monitor shows your baby's heart is racing or has an erratic pattern, your practitioner may announce that your baby isn't tolerating labor. What does this mean? Unfortunately, the fetal heart monitor is not a very sensitive—or specific—test of a baby's condition. Doctors know what healthy labor patterns look like on a fetal heart monitor. However, if there's a chaotic pattern, they don't necessarily know what's going on until the baby is born (and perhaps not even then).

The most common reasons for a baby to be unable to tolerate labor include problems with the placenta, the baby being too small, or cord compression because the cord is wrapped too tightly around the baby's neck or the baby is sitting on it. To further assess your baby's well-being, your provider may do a fetal scalp pH test, which involves taking about 10 drops of blood from the baby's scalp. The blood is analyzed to determine whether your baby is getting enough oxygen. If the baby seems fine, your provider may decide to let you labor a while longer, monitoring your baby's heartbeat constantly as labor progresses. If not, she may opt to deliver your baby by cesarean (see "Emergency cesarean deliveries," page 276).

Labor doesn't progress. If your cervix isn't dilating despite your contractions, or if the contractions aren't strong enough to move the baby downward, your provider may tell you that your labor has "stalled" or "isn't progressing." You might be exhausted if this has been going on for hours.

At this point, your provider might measure the intensity of your contractions by putting her hand on your belly or by using an intrauterine pressure catheter (IUPC). An IUPC is a tiny tube that's thinner than IV tubing and that slides between the baby's head and your uterus. If the contractions aren't strong enough, she may hook you up to an IV and administer Pitocin—a synthetic oxytocin—to strengthen your contractions or make them more frequent. If your labor still does not progress, she may then do a cesarean delivery.

There are many reasons why labor doesn't progress, including a baby that's too large for your pelvis, the baby's head position, and a uterus that can't coordinate contractions.

Back labor. You may have heard friends describe "back labor" in dire terms. Ordinarily if you are lying on your back during delivery, your baby will be facing down toward the floor in what's called the occiput anterior position. Some babies face up toward the ceiling (occiput posterior position); see the illustration below. Laboring with a faceup baby is called back labor, and it means your pain won't let up between contractions, because the baby's head is pressing against your tailbone or spine.

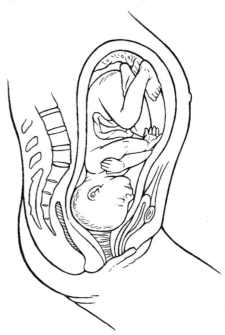

Fetal position during back labor (occiput posterior)

Intraamniotic infection (IAI). During labor, if you have a fever with uterine tenderness or your amniotic fluid smells, you may have an intraamniotic infection. You are more likely to get this infection if you have a lot of vaginal exams, have a long labor, or rupture your membranes a long time before you go into labor.

The intraamniotic infection can make you very ill and can cause your baby to get an infection also. If your doctor diagnoses you with IAI, you will receive antibiotics until you deliver (and in some cases, after birth). Your baby may need blood tests in the nursery, and she also may get antibiotics.

About 15 percent of women who have regional anesthesia for labor get a fever, but many of them do not have an infection. The problem is that there are no quick tests available to tell doctors who has an infection and who doesn't, so you are likely to get antibiotics as a precaution.

Shoulder dystocia. Shoulder dystocia is one of the most difficult obstetric situations: The baby's head emerges, but because of the baby's positioning or size, the shoulders are stuck in the birth canal. This rare complication is more likely to happen with larger babies, but it can happen with an infant of any size. Unfortunately there's no way to predict it ahead of time. Your provider may have to perform a bigger episiotomy to help the baby emerge. She may also push your knees up toward your abdomen to change the angle of your pelvis, or she may rotate the baby's shoulders into a better position for birth. In worst-case scenarios, she may have to break the baby's collarbone or tuck the baby's head back in and perform a cesarean delivery.

Forceps or vacuum delivery. If your baby has crowned, or is low in your birth canal, and you are too exhausted to continue pushing or the fetal heart rate has dropped, your practitioner may use forceps or a vacuum extractor to deliver your baby (see "Forceps and vacuum extraction," page 330). This method may be faster and more efficient in these situations than a cesarean delivery, and there's minimal risk to your baby.

Is labor good for your baby?

As you're having contractions and listening to your baby's heartbeat on the fetal monitor, or panting to keep from pushing your baby out into the world too soon, you may worry that all of the pain you're feeling is harming your baby. The truth is that labor is actually good for babies because it causes their adrenal glands to secrete high levels of stress hormones. These hormones get their systems geared up for a real fight for life, upping blood flow to vital organs and raising the number of infection-fighting white blood cells in your baby's blood. As the baby travels through the birth canal, amniotic fluid is squeezed out of his lungs, and he may gurgle less and breathe easier at birth.

A guide to your newborn's appearance

You know those babies on television, the ones with the big eyes and soft, peaches-and-cream skin? Yours won't look like that. In fact, many infants are alien-looking in the beginning. They can come out with cone-shape heads, bruises, rashes, and pimples. Most of these things are merely side effects of birth and soon disappear; within days your baby will look better, and people will be stopping your stroller on the street to admire your little one. Meanwhile, here are some of the temporary conditions that might affect your newborn:

Lanugo. Most of this fine body hair will disappear before your baby is born. However, your infant might still have a fine covering of soft fur, especially across his back and shoulders. It should disappear within a week or so.

Vernix caseosa. That gooey white wet suit your baby has been wearing might still cling to his skin, especially in the creases behind his knees and elbows. It washes right off in your baby's first bath.

Caput succedaneum. If you had a vaginal delivery, your baby's head will probably be molded into a cone shape by his journey through the birth canal. It should pop back into shape within a day or so.

Cephalohematoma. If your baby experienced any pressure on his head during delivery—as most do—he might have a benign bump beneath his skin on one side of his head caused by bleeding under the scalp. It will disappear in a matter of days or weeks.

Erythema toxicum. This whole-body rash looks like little pimples with red rims. There may be a lot of these pimples, but they'll all be gone in a few days.

Cyanosis. A bluish tinge in the hands, feet, and lips, this common condition is the result of poor blood circulation and shouldn't last more than two days.

Milia. Many babies are born with these white or yellow pimples on their faces. The pustules usually disappear within a month.

Breech delivery. About 3 percent of babies are breech. A breech baby is one whose bottom or feet are positioned to emerge first instead of his head. Your provider probably will have realized your baby is breech during one of your prenatal visits and may have even made an attempt to manually turn the baby around before your due date (see "Singleton breech babies and version," page 300). Not all breech babies are detected ahead of time: Surprise turns can happen, and sometimes doctors think that the baby's bottom is her head. If you arrive in labor and your baby presents as breech, your provider will most likely do a cesarean, unless your labor has progressed to the point where it makes more sense to deliver the baby vaginally or your provider feels comfortable with vaginal breech deliveries. Vaginal deliveries for breech babies are safest when the babies are in a "frank breech" position (the buttocks presenting first,

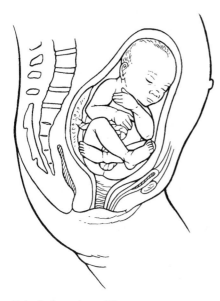

Baby in breech position

with the heels up around the ears) or a "complete breech" (buttocks and feet presenting first; see illustration left). (See "Babies in the breech position," page 240.)

Uterine rupture. If you had a previous scar on your uterus, you may suffer a uterine rupture or tear. This happens in fewer than 1 percent of women who attempt labor after a low uterine scar. (See "Once a cesarean delivery, always a cesarean?" page 178.) For women with other deep scars on the uterus, such as from a high vertical cesarean delivery or a surgery to remove fibroids, labor is not recommended because the risk of rupture is higher. The first sign that your uterus has torn is usually a searing pain in your abdomen. You may feel as if something has actually ripped, but there might not be any bleeding. If this happens while your

Apgar scoring system

When your baby is born, a nurse or doctor will measure five components of your newborn's health after 1 minute of life. After 5 minutes, these same components will be measured again. For a healthy Apgar score, your baby should pass these quickie measures:
- Skin color that is more pink than blue
- Heart rate greater than 100 beats per minute
- Strong breathing and a good, strong cry
- Active flexing of arms and legs to show good muscle tone
- Reflex responses (sneezes, coughs, grimaces)

From these five vital signs, your baby will get a score ranging from 0 if she's unresponsive to 10 if she's healthy and requires no special medical attention. Two scores of 7 or higher indicate good health; if your baby scores under 7 on anything at the 1-minute testing point, your caregivers will try to improve whatever needs attention to raise that score. For instance, your baby's poor reflexes might be improved if your caregiver rubs her back. The doctor will keep trying to improve your baby's Apgar score, testing every 5 minutes if necessary, until your baby looks healthy and stable.

baby is being monitored, your doctor may notice abnormalities in your baby's heartbeat; in this case, your health care provider will most likely perform a cesarean delivery and repair your uterus.

Postpartum hemorrhage. After a vaginal delivery, you may lose 200–400 cc (cubic centimeters) of blood; during a cesarean delivery, you may lose two to three times that amount. Rarely, a woman experiences severe bleeding, or hemorrhaging, after delivery; this is the leading cause of maternal mortality.

If you experience postpartum hemorrhage, you may feel very light-headed and dizzy. It may happen if your labor was very long, your baby is big, or you had an intraamniotic infection (see page 350) and the uterus is too tired to contract (uterine atony). It can also happen if you had placenta previa or placental abruption. Excessive bleeding can also occur if fragments or pieces of afterbirth stay attached to the uterus. In this instance, the bleeding may occur immediately after delivery or as long as 2 weeks after delivery. The treatment will depend on the cause of bleeding and the amount. Sometimes all you need is IV fluid and medicines to make your uterus contract. In any case, the odds are good that you'll recover fully and rapidly.

Your baby's first day

You give one last push, and there she is: the baby you've been so eagerly awaiting for 9 months. For you it's a moment of joy, as the pain of labor suddenly diminishes and you finally have a chance to see and hold the life you've created. It is such an amazing moment that it cannot be put into words. For your baby, though, the first 48 hours are filled with stimulation, excitement, and new challenges as she tries to regulate her body temperature and adjust to her body's new sensations. The passage through the birth canal has changed her from an aquatic being, safely surrounded in a warm, dark, sterile bag of fluid, to an oxygen-breathing person who must feed herself.

As soon as your baby's head emerges, your provider will suction amniotic fluid out of your newborn's nose and mouth with a small rubber bulb. Then the remainder of her body will be delivered, and the umbilical cord will be clamped and cut. (Dad might step in to do the honors and cut the cord.) The cord has no nerve endings, so your baby won't feel the moment when she stops receiving oxygen from your blood. If your baby doesn't cry, whimper, or cough once she's fully out in the world, your provider will dry her off, rub her back or hand to stimulate her, and then— once she makes her first cry or cough—hand her to you or to a nurse. Soon after that, you'll deliver the placenta. This process may be hastened if your baby manages to latch on to your breast and suck; the sucking will cause your body to produce another rush of oxytocin to help your uterus finish contracting.

While you deliver the placenta, a physician or nurse will perform a series of routine checks to see if your baby is healthy (see "Apgar scoring system," page 352). They will also examine her to check that her ears, feet, and skin show signs of maturity and to determine whether she has birth defects. She'll have a shot of vitamin K to help her blood clot normally. Your provider may then give you some time to cuddle with your baby before anything else happens, or a nurse will weigh the baby, measure her length and head circumference, and take her temperature before diapering and swaddling her. The nurse will put erythromycin ointment in your baby's eyes to prevent infection, put a cap on her head (newborns lose a lot of heat through their scalps), and then hand her over to you.

Newborns are amazingly alert in the first hour of life, and your baby might be awake enough to suck. If you're breastfeeding, she'll nourish herself on colostrum, the thin yellow fluid that precedes your breast milk. She may stay in your room if she's healthy, or she might stay in the nursery and visit you to feed every 3 or 4 hours. Most babies sleep deeply after birth, though, and it's difficult to wake them; you may have to keep tickling her cheek or tapping her foot to get her to eat. As she

sleeps, nurses will keep an eye on her temperature, breathing, muscle tone, and activity level.

Your baby's second day

By the second day, your baby may establish a pattern of sleeping for a couple of hours, then waking and crying to be fed. She should be wetting her diaper within 24 hours after birth and passing her initial bowel movement. This is called meconium, and it looks like a smear of greenish black tar. Tell your doctor or nurse if you don't see any signs of urine or meconium in your baby's diaper within this time.

The second day brings plenty of surprising experiences for your newborn, so be prepared to comfort her. Although newborn tests vary depending on your state laws, she'll be subjected to a series of tests for diseases that can be effectively treated if diagnosed early. Some hospitals also test newborn hearing, and you may choose to have your baby receive her first hepatitis B vaccine while she's in the hospital. In addition, if your baby is a boy, he may be circumcised within his first 24 hours of life if you request it. After such a full day, your baby may be cranky and need extra cuddling. And there's much more ahead: the challenge of breastfeeding, sitting in a car seat for the first time, weight checks, jaundice checks, and a full newborn exam. For now, all your baby wants is to be wrapped up and held.

Mom's first two days after delivery

The first two days postpartum will be a complete emotional and physical whirlwind. There are many things still happening to your body that may bring you anxiety; however, most are nothing to worry about. The good news is that because you'll still be in the hospital or birth center, your nurses will be around to field your questions and help you start breast-feeding, if you choose to do so. If you had a cesarean delivery, you will likely stay in the hospital at least 3 days after delivery; most women who have cesareans stay for 4 days. Believe it or not, each day you will feel a little better, although the rate of recovery is different for each woman.

Day 1. Be prepared for extreme fatigue on your first day as a new mom. You'll have sore muscles all over your body, mostly from pushing. You may even have a patch of numbness on your upper outer thighs, which is likely the result of pulling your legs back while pushing; this will resolve with time.

If you had pain medication, you may experience low-back pain or soreness at the anesthetic site; that will resolve within a couple of days.

Expect some swelling in the perineum from pushing the baby's head through, whether you had an episiotomy or not. The swelling should go down within 1–2 days; in the meantime, you may get relief by applying ice to the area.

Finally, don't despair if your legs are so swollen that you can't see your ankles. You were given a lot of fluids during labor, and your body will take 7 days or so to naturally lose those fluids. It is not necessary to take water pills.

Day 2. On day 2 of your baby's new life outside your belly, you'll find that your own belly is still bloated. Most of the bloating is due to air, but the uterus itself is still much larger than it was prepregnancy.

You may have intense cramps, especially while you are breastfeeding. Vaginal discharge called lochia is still heavy, and you'll be using quite a few sanitary pads to absorb it. The flow will decrease over the next few days.

Perhaps most unnerving is the pelvic pressure you'll feel. You may feel as if your uterus is falling out of your body. This pressure is normal, and your uterus will not fall out. It may take a couple of weeks for your pelvic tissue to return to normal.

When to bring your baby home

A federal law requires insurance companies to cover at least two days of hospitalization if you have a vaginal delivery and four days of hospitalization after a cesarean delivery. Those are important days for both you and your baby, allowing you both to rest and be examined by your health care providers, who will watch for and treat any postpartum problems. Take this opportunity to ask questions about new skills such as bathing or feeding your baby. Most important of all, use this time to lie with your little

one, holding her and talking to her.
That way she'll know that even
though the world might look and feel
different, her mom is still with her.

feeding your baby

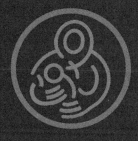

If you can't imagine anything better than spending hours gazing at your baby's sweet eyelashes and darling dimples, you'll have plenty of time to do just that: During the first few months of your baby's life, you'll spend more time on feeding than on any other kind of baby care. Newborn babies eat up to 12 times a day, and each feeding session can last anywhere from a few minutes to half an hour. Your baby will eat frequently to help fuel all the growth you'll see in the next few months. Choosing whether to feed by breast or bottle— or some of each—is a personal decision based on many factors. Use this guide to help you make the decision that's right for your family.

Feeding Your Baby

Making the right choices

Your baby will eat frequently because her body needs fats, protein, carbohydrates, vitamins, minerals, and other nutrients in order to grow—and she's got a lot of growing to do during the next few months. When she lived inside you, she received a constant stream of nutrients from your body. Even though she's living outside your body now, she still needs that stream of nutrients so that her brain, organs, muscles, bones, nerves, and other body parts and systems will develop and grow in a healthy way.

You have a choice of breastfeeding, bottle-feeding, or doing some of each. All of the major medical and nutritional organizations recommend breastfeeding as the better choice. The American Dietetic Association calls breastfeeding "the gold standard of infant feeding." The American Academy of Pediatrics considers itself to be "a staunch advocate of breastfeeding as the optimal form of nutrients for infants." The March of Dimes calls breast milk "the best food for most babies." And according to the American College of Obstetricians and Gynecologists, "research in the United States and throughout the world indicates that breastfeeding and human milk provide benefits to infants, women, families, and society."

Experts recommend breastfeeding for the first year of your baby's life. That means breast milk exclusively for the first 6 months and breast milk accompanied by solid foods during the second 6 months.

But rest comfortably knowing that whether you feed by breast or bottle, your baby will be well nourished.

Reasons to breastfeed

"Breast is best" for many reasons: Breast milk benefits a baby's health, immune system, development, and intelligence. For example, breast milk provides antibodies that reduce your baby's risk of colds, ear infections, bacterial meningitis, urinary tract infections, diarrhea, and other infections. Babies who breastfeed are less likely than formula-fed babies to develop food allergies and eczema; they have less colic and constipation too. Human milk protects babies from sudden infant death syndrome, childhood cancers, insulin-dependent diabetes mellitus, Crohn's disease, ulcerative colitis, and other chronic digestive diseases. On average, breastfed babies have higher IQs than formula-fed babies. And breastfed babies are less likely to become overweight or obese during childhood and adulthood.

Mom benefits too. Right after birth, breastfeeding causes the release of hormones that increase uterine contractions, which cut down on blood loss. Breastfeeding may help you return to your prepregnancy weight more easily because your body uses more calories when you are lactating. Breastfeeding offers some cancer protection too: It reduces your risk of ovarian cancer and premenopausal breast cancer.

Breastfeeding also offers mother and baby time to get to know each other, to bond, and to cuddle. During breastfeeding, the mother's body releases hormones that contribute to feelings of relaxation and attachment. Breastfeeding saves money and time because you don't have to buy formula or sterilize bottles and nipples. It also delays the return of your period; however, you shouldn't count on it as birth control because you may ovulate without knowing.

Breastfeeding is a major commitment. Unless you pump breast milk for a bottle, you can't ask your partner to do the 2 a.m. feeding. If you go back to work, you can pump during the workday and store it for your baby's use another time. However, spending 10 or 15 minutes pumping two or three times daily can be inconvenient for some women. And although most women nurse successfully without any problems, some develop breast infections and other painful breast ailments.

Reasons to bottle-feed

Bottle-feeding may be the right choice for many families. Nutrition scientists work continuously to find ways to improve infant formula so that it is as close as possible to breast milk. The amount and types of nutrients in infant formula are regulated by the U.S. Food and Drug Administration (FDA). The FDA also regulates how infant formulas are manufactured, labeled, and, if necessary, recalled. Bottle-feeding is a convenient way to feed your baby, especially if others are involved in his care. Bottle-feeding is easier to fit into a busy schedule than breastfeeding, particularly for working mothers whose employers do not support pumping during work hours. It also allows you to keep track of how much your baby is eating.

Some women simply don't want to breastfeed. They are concerned it will hurt, or they dislike the possibility of exposing their breasts while nursing. They may not like the idea of using their breasts, which they think of in a sexual way, to feed a baby; or they may fear that their partners will not be attracted to them if they nurse. They may feel that other responsibilities in their lives—other children, aging parents, and so on—take so much out of them that breastfeeding would overwhelm them.

Family members sometimes encourage women not to breastfeed. They may believe that formula is better for babies than breast milk or that babies who nurse don't get

Breast or bottle? The impact of medical conditions

Certain women should not breastfeed for medical reasons or for the safety of their babies. Do not breastfeed if you:

- Are infected with HIV.
- Have tuberculosis that has not been treated.
- Are receiving certain cancer treatments.
- Abuse alcohol or use street drugs.
- Are taking certain medications that can pass into your breast milk and harm your baby.
- Have a baby with galactosemia, a rare genetic disorder of carbohydrate metabolism.
- Have a baby with phenylketonuria (PKU), a rare genetic disorder of protein metabolism.

Women with other health problems can often breastfeed despite their medical condition or that of their baby. You may be able to breastfeed if you:

- Are being treated with antibiotics for endometritis or a breast infection.
- Have hepatitis A, B, or C.
- Have an active herpes simplex virus infection, provided there are no vesicular lesions in the breast area and you wash your hands carefully.
- Have had breast surgery (breast reduction, breast augmentation with implants, and biopsies), depending on whether the surgery severed milk ducts.
- Have a baby with a cleft lip or palate, depending on whether the baby can latch on.

enough to eat. These are myths; regarding the latter, with rare exceptions a woman's breasts produce as much milk as her baby needs.

Some women have complicated medical conditions that may make bottle-feeding a better choice for them. This may be true even if the medications that they're taking won't harm the baby. Talk to your pediatrician about your concerns.

Bottle-feeding Basics

Stopping your milk

Hormones released by your body during delivery tell your breasts to start producing milk. If you choose bottle-feeding, you'll need to "shut off" your breasts. Believe it or not, you can do this with cabbage leaves, of all things. Buy some fresh cabbage and remove two large leaves. Crush them a little; then put one over each breast inside your bra (wear a sports bra or other tight bra that will bind your breasts). Replace them with fresh leaves when they wilt and wear them continuously for at least 48 hours. Why cabbage leaves? Nobody knows for sure, but the leaves probably contain some kind of natural anti-inflammatory chemical.

Within a week or so your breasts will return to their normal size. If your breasts hurt during this time, apply cold compresses and take acetaminophen. Don't pump or stimulate the nipples because that will signal your breasts to make more milk.

Choosing formula

The formula aisle of your grocery store, pharmacy, or discount store may overwhelm you at first. However, the dizzying selection is easier to navigate than you might expect. There are three main types of infant formula:

Cow's milk formula is, as its name says, made from cow's milk. However, the milk has been modified to make it as close to human milk as possible. Most doctors recommend cow's milk formula as their first choice for bottle-fed babies; 80 percent of the formula sold in the United States has a cow's milk base.

Soy-base formula is good for babies who are allergic to cow's milk or who are lactose intolerant. Signs of lactose intolerance include watery diarrhea and cramps. (A baby with cramps will pull his knees to his chest as he fusses and cries.) If your baby has any intolerance symptoms, talk with his pediatrician.

Protein hydrolysate formula is the least likely of the three to cause allergies because its proteins have been broken down into smaller parts called amino acids, which are easier to digest. It is more expensive than other formula but is the only formula that some allergic babies can tolerate. It may be recommended for babies with a strong family history of milk

allergies. Specialized formulas for premature babies and infants with certain diseases or disorders are also available.

Formula comes in three forms: powder, concentrated liquid, and ready-to-feed. Formulas that must be mixed with water are less expensive than ready-to-feed. Some formula is iron-fortified because some babies require extra iron; talk with your pediatrician about what your baby needs. There are many brands of formula, but they are all about the same because the FDA regulates what ingredients formula manufacturers can use.

Some formula manufacturers add fatty acids known as DHA and ARA to their products. In breast milk, these fatty acids appear to promote brain development; whether formula with added fatty acids delivers the same benefit hasn't been determined.

If your baby develops an allergy to formula, call your pediatrician immediately. The signs may include bloody, mucousy stools; persistent vomiting that is increasingly forceful; an eczema-like rash; or unusual tiredness or weakness.

Selecting nipples and bottles

There is no "best" bottle style. In the baby products aisle, you'll see glass bottles, plastic (polyethylene or polycarbonate) bottles, disposable bottles, bottles that attach to breast pumps, and bottles with an array of options: disposable liners, angled bottoms, built-in burpers, easy-grip handles,

feeding your baby

and internal vents. The same is true with nipples—there is no "right" kind among the many you'll see: latex, silicone, rubber, anti-vacuum, slow-flow, flat-top, round-top, orthodontic, and on and on. Some bottle and nipple "systems" cost a lot and are sold in pricey baby specialty stores; inexpensive bottles and nipples can be found at discount stores.

Ultimately the best bottle and nipple for your baby is the one he prefers. Buy a few different kinds of bottles and nipples and give them a try. If your baby does well with the inexpensive kind, save yourself some money and use them. If he is gassy or has trouble feeding, try the more expensive ones. Either way, always use infant-size nipples. Nipples designed for older babies have larger holes that allow milk to pass through more quickly than an infant needs.

Breastfeeding Basics

How to begin

Start to nurse your baby as soon as possible after delivery. Hold your baby in one arm with your hand under his bottom and his head in the crook of your arm. With your free hand, put your thumb on top of your breast and your other fingers below. Try not to touch the areola (the dark skin around the nipple). Touch your baby's lips with your nipple until he opens his mouth wide, as if he is yawning. When his mouth is open, put your nipple all the way into his mouth while pulling him toward you. His entire body should be facing you, not the ceiling; he shouldn't have to crane his neck to get to the nipple.

When your baby "latches on," his mouth will feel kind of like a suction cup on your breast. His lips should pout out and cover nearly all of the areola. When he starts to eat, his jaw will move up and down and you'll hear swallowing noises. If it hurts when he nurses, he's not latched on correctly. Reposition him and try again. Don't feel frustrated if it takes a few tries to get him to latch on—that's normal. If you need help, ask for a lactation consultant to be sent to your room; many hospitals have them on staff.

You can hold your baby in three different positions while nursing:

In the cradle position, you support your baby's back and bottom with your forearm and hand and his head with the crook of your arm.

In the football position, you tuck your baby under your arm like a football with his head resting on your hand and his body on your forearm. This is a good position to use after a cesarean.

In the side position, you lie on your side facing your baby, who is also lying on his side, facing you. This is a good position to use in the middle of the night because you can doze off while nursing.

Alternate which breast you use first. The nursing positions—particularly football and side—may initially feel awkward. It commonly takes mothers a few weeks to feel comfortable with the various nursing positions. Using pillows to prop up your arms or your baby's body sometimes helps too. Again, keep in mind that although you may need several carefully arranged pillows to breastfeed at first, it will get easier and the need for props will disappear.

First feedings

The first fluid your breasts will produce is colostrum, which contains ingredients that help the baby's body fight infection. Two or three days after delivery, your breasts will become full—they will look surprisingly large and feel hard. This is a (sometimes painful) sign that your breasts are producing milk. You can relieve engorgement by frequent nursing. If your baby doesn't drink enough to ease the soreness, use an ice pack or a frozen bag of peas or corn to get relief and reduce swelling: Hold the pack to your breasts for 20 minutes; then leave it off for 20 minutes and repeat.

Feed your baby whenever he seems hungry, usually 8–12 times a day. Allow him to nurse until he is satisfied; usually a satiated baby falls asleep and unlatches from the breast. In a newborn, this can take 10–15 minutes per breast. As your baby gets older and becomes more of a breastfeeding expert, he'll drain the breasts in as little as 5 minutes each, but he'll continue to nurse for comfort and to ensure a continuing milk supply. Until he's 6 months old, all he needs

is breast milk. He won't need supplemental bottles of juice or water or formula unless you have chosen to combine breastfeeding with formula feeding. For as long as you nurse, the composition of your breast milk will adjust to match your baby's nutritional requirements.

Your baby will show you that he's hungry by giving you feeding cues such as opening his mouth in search of the nipple (an action known as rooting), sticking out his tongue, sucking on his hands and fists, and becoming more alert and active. Don't wait until he cries to feed him because crying means he's very hungry. A hungry baby can be so impatient to feed that he has trouble latching on—a situation that's frustrating for both mother and baby.

If he is a heavy sleeper, wake him every 4 hours to feed; tickling his feet, rubbing his back, or undressing him down to his diaper will help wake him up.

Many women breastfeed without any trouble; others develop sore or cracked nipples, clogged milk ducts, and breast infections. If breastfeeding isn't going smoothly, talk to a lactation consultant before you decide to quit.

A satisfied baby

You know your baby is getting enough to eat if he has 6–8 wet diapers and four or more bowel movements a day from day 4 through week 4. Some of the more absorbent diapers feel dry even when they're wet. If you have trouble determining

Supply and demand

Most babies experience growth spurts at 2 weeks and 6 weeks of age. During a growth spurt, your baby will be extra hungry, nurse more often, and appear dissatisfied with the amount of milk he is receiving. Don't give up on breastfeeding when this happens. Nurse your baby frequently, and within about 24 hours your body will increase its milk production to match your baby's needs. Breastfeeding works on a supply-and-demand basis—the more your baby eats, the more milk your body makes.

whether his diaper is wet, put a piece of toilet tissue inside your baby's diaper. It's a clear, quick indicator of whether your baby has urinated. His weight is another good indicator of whether he's getting enough to eat. Your baby's pediatrician will weigh him at each visit to ensure that he's gaining the proper amount of weight.

You may notice a sudden feeling of fullness in your breasts, either shortly before or shortly after you start to nurse. This is called "let-down," and it is caused by the milk glands literally letting down milk through the ducts into the nipples. You will feel this every time you nurse. It may feel a little strange at first, but you'll get used to it within a few weeks. If you wait too long to nurse, your milk may let down even if you're not feeding your baby. Sometimes looking at a picture of a baby or hearing a baby cry—even if it's not your baby—will set off your let-down.

Your breastfeeding diet

While you're nursing, eat a nutritious diet that contains plenty of fruits and vegetables, whole grains, lean protein, and fat-free dairy products. Dairy is especially important for nursing mothers because your baby needs calcium; if your diet lacks a sufficient amount, the calcium will come from your bones. Your doctor may recommend that you continue to take your prenatal vitamins for as long as you breastfeed. If your iron stores are low, your doctor may advise you to take a vitamin supplement.

Drink lots of water every day while you're breastfeeding. A good rule of thumb is to drink a tall glass of water during every nursing session and more if you're thirsty. Some caffeine while breastfeeding is fine, but it will get into your milk. Check with your doctor before taking any medications while breastfeeding.

Pumping milk

Mothers who go back to work can continue to feed their babies breast milk by expressing, or pumping, their breasts. This can be done manually, although it's far easier with a breast pump. Pumping with a breast pump takes about 10 minutes on each breast—20 minutes total, or 10 minutes if you use a double pump, which expresses both breasts at the same time. Your milk is pumped directly into bottles or milk collection bags that can be stored in the refrigerator for up to 48 hours. (Ice packs can keep milk cold at work if no refrigerator is available.) Breast milk can also be frozen for up to 3 months. Defrost it by placing it in a cup of warm (not hot) water. Never microwave it; doing so can destroy proteins in the milk. Once the milk is thawed, use it within 24 hours; never refreeze it.

Pumps can be manually operated, battery operated, or electric. Most women prefer electric pumps because they are faster than the others. They are expensive, however, costing $60–$300 and up. Breast pumps can also be rented; the parts that come in contact with your breasts and your milk are replaceable to prevent contamination. Whether you buy or rent depends on how long you intend to breastfeed and how many more children you plan to have.

If you intend to pump your breasts at work, start practicing a couple of weeks before you return to your job. Pump after your baby feeds or between feedings. Most likely you'll collect only an ounce or two, but after about a week of regular pumping, your breasts will produce more milk.

Start your baby on bottles a few weeks before you go back to work. Some babies take to them easily and have no trouble switching from breast to bottle to breast; others struggle with the transition. This is called nipple confusion. To avoid nipple confusion, wait until your baby is 3–4 weeks old before introducing a bottle.

If you're lucky, your workplace has a lactation room set aside for nursing mothers. Most workplaces don't. You can set up your own lactation space in any room with a door and a chair—and an electrical outlet if your pump is electric. Talk with your employer if there is no obvious place to pump.

Nursing an older baby

Some women choose to continue breastfeeding their babies after they reach their first birthdays. Nursing a toddler is different from nursing a baby. Toddlers receive most of their nutrients from solid food, so breastfeeding becomes more emotional than nutritional. Toddlers feel comforted and secure while nursing, and mothers feel extra close to their children. Breastfeeding can provide a welcome, loving break for both mother and child. Nursing a toddler is not for everyone, however, and American society is not very receptive to the idea of breastfeeding toddlers.

If you do decide to nurse past age 1, you'll benefit from the advice and support of other mothers who have made the same choice. Consider attending a La Leche League meeting—La Leche highly recommends nursing through toddlerhood. For more information, consult the book *Mothering Your Nursing Toddler* by Norma Jane Bumgarner.

Nursing privately

One of the roadblocks to breastfeeding is modesty: Mothers don't relish the idea of exposing their breasts for the world to see. You can nurse discreetly using specially designed nursing shirts with flaps and hidden slits. For further coverage, drape a receiving blanket over your shoulder. At first you may have trouble getting your baby to latch on discreetly, but after a couple of weeks it will become much easier. If you're concerned about what shows while you're nursing, practice in front of a mirror.

Breastfeeding support

Many individuals and organizations can provide information and support for nursing mothers.

Your delivery hospital. Many obstetric services have on-staff lactation consultants who can help you get started in the hospital. When you are discharged, ask for a list of lactation consultants in your area and a list of breast pump rental sites.

Your pediatrician's office may employ a nurse who specializes in lactation issues. If not, your pediatrician can refer you to local lactation consultants. Or contact the International Lactation Consultant Association (919-861-5577 or www.ilca.org).

La Leche League is probably the most well-known breastfeeding-support organization. This nonprofit, nonsectarian organization provides education, information, support, and encouragement to women who want to breastfeed. All women are welcome to attend chapter meetings or to call a group leader for breastfeeding help. Contact www.lalecheleague.org or 800-LALECHE or 847-519-7730.

The African-American Breastfeeding Alliance is committed to raising the number of African-American women who breastfeed; the alliance offers support and education about the benefits of breastfeeding. Contact www.aabaonline.com or 410-225-2006.

Websites. Good sources of information are the American College of Nurse-Midwives breastfeeding website (www.gotmom.org) and the National Women's Health Information Center, which is part of the U.S. Department of Health and Human Services (www.4woman.gov/breastfeeding).

Books. Check out these informative books:
- *The Womanly Art of Breastfeeding* by La Leche League
- *The Breastfeeding Book* by Martha Sears and William Sears
- *The American Academy of Pediatrics New Mother's Guide to Breastfeeding* by Joan Younger Meek
- *The Nursing Mother's Companion* by Kathleen Huggins
- *So That's What They're For: Breastfeeding Basics* by Janet Tamaro

postpartum and
baby care

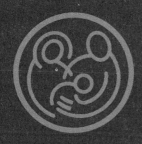

Remember your first weeks of high school? You were excited because you couldn't wait to try new things. But you couldn't open your locker, you kept getting lost, you got no sleep, and you kept worrying that you'd do something wrong. In the first weeks at home, you and your baby will feel as dazed and confused as you did in high school. However, you'll soon be at ease. Most babies are born without complications, and they are remarkably resilient. You and your baby will learn a lot about each other in the coming weeks, and you'll quickly begin to relax and enjoy each other. Here's a no-worries guide to help ease your way.

Week 1

Bringing baby home

In your first weeks after delivery, you'll be thrilled to finally be at home with your baby—until you realize that your baby doesn't have an instruction manual or a switch to turn her off when you need a break. Your body feels as if it's been hit by a steam-roller, and things at home seem so overwhelming that you may sometimes find yourself weeping in the shower. You might worry that your body won't ever be the same, that you don't have the energy to be a mother, or that you'll somehow hurt your baby. If you have older children, you may wonder if you'll ever again feel like running with them at the play-ground or even coloring.

Your baby is stressed out too. Instead of feeling warm and safe, she's now constantly bombarded by new sensations. The shrill ring of a telephone assaults her ears, the bright light makes it hard for her to open her eyes, she's suddenly put down to sleep on a hard surface surrounded by bars, and every few hours somebody thinks it's a good idea to bare her bottom to the cold air.

At this point, you and your partner may gaze down at your baby with equal parts adoration and terror. What do you do now?

Be assured: You'll quickly learn everything you need to know. This practical guide will help ease your mind so you can focus on growing your happy family.

Your Body

The first week of your baby's life will be a recuperation week for you. Going through labor and delivery takes a toll on your body, whether you delivered vaginally or by cesarean. Arrange for household help if possible, either by hiring someone or asking family to lend a hand.

Here are some things you may be experiencing this week:

Uterine contractions. During the first few days after delivery, your uterus will contract as it returns to its normal size. Contractions may intensify during breastfeeding. Usually they feel like menstrual cramps and disappear by the end of the first week.

Soreness at the incision site. If you've had a cesarean delivery, the incision site may be quite sore. If it feels itchy, don't scratch it. Take sponge baths or showers and watch the incision site for signs of infection (redness and drainage). Follow your doctor's recommendations regarding keeping the site clean, changing dressings, and so on. Avoid lifting, stairs, and driving until you've healed. If your doctor prescribed pain medications, take them as you need them; as long as you use them as they are prescribed, they'll help you feel better and will not harm you or your baby even if you are breastfeeding. Acetaminophen and ibuprofen are also safe for you to take.

Excess weight. During delivery you lose 10–15 pounds; the rest hangs on for a while. You may need to wear maternity clothes during the first couple of weeks after delivery.

Vaginal discharge. Blood and fluid called lochia flow from your uterus for several weeks. During the first few days after delivery, lochia is bright red and is made up primarily of blood and shreds of the disintegrating uterine lining. It may also contain blood clots that are surprisingly big; don't be shocked if you pass a clot that's as big as a golf ball. However, after 2 or 3 days the flow slows down and becomes pink rather than red. At about day 14 postpartum, it turns yellowish brown. The flow will continue for up to 5 weeks. Use sanitary napkins to absorb the flow. Don't use tampons, which could cause infection.

Constipation. Your first bowel movement may be delayed until the third or fourth day after delivery. Passing it can be painful, especially if you've had an episiotomy, even more so if you are constipated and the stool is hard. Talk with your doctor about using stool-softening medication for several days starting shortly after delivery. You should also drink plenty of water.

Episiotomy soreness. If your vaginal area tore or was cut during delivery, it will feel tender this week as it begins to heal. Apply ice to ease soreness and swelling in the first 24 hours and keep the area clean to speed healing and prevent infection. Use a squirt bottle with warm water to gently cleanse the area several times a day and after you urinate. Taking a warm (not hot) sitz bath a few times a day can help too. Keep walking to a minimum and consider using a donut cushion when sitting.

Breast swelling. Two or three days after delivery, your breasts will become engorged with milk. This can be quite painful. Tame the pain with frequent nursing. If your baby doesn't eat enough to ease soreness, express a small amount of milk or apply ice packs to your breasts. If you do not plan to breastfeed, use cabbage leaves to reduce swelling (see "Stopping your milk," page 360). During the most intense engorgement—which occurs the day your milk comes in— put on a supportive bra and keep it on for 24–48 hours.

Hemorrhoids. Soothe the pain of these swollen anal tissues with sitz baths, ice, witch hazel pads, and over-the-counter hemorrhoid creams. The hemorrhoids should shrink and disappear within several weeks. Using a stool softener and getting enough fiber in your diet will also help.

Your Baby

A baby's days

You can probably list 10 things already that have surprised you about your baby. Perhaps he has red hair instead of blond, or maybe he has fingernails longer than yours. Now that you're home together, you'll be tuned to your personal Baby Channel 24/7. Does he need his diaper changed? Why is he sleeping so much? (Or so little?) Does he really need to eat this often?

Of course your baby's typical day will depend somewhat on his individual personality. However, you'll have an easier time getting through this first tense, joyful, scary week of caring for your baby if you know some basics about an average newborn's day.

Eating. If your baby is breastfed, she'll eat up to every 2 hours over a 24-hour period. Formula-fed babies need to eat about every 3 hours. In other words, there's a reason you're not getting the laundry done: You may have to sit down for 4–6 hours a day to feed your baby! It's OK: Let the house go. Holding and feeding your baby are among the most important things you can do. Your baby's tiny stomach can hold only about 3 ounces of milk at a time, and she's growing so fast—an ounce a day—that her metabolism burns it off in a few hours. Then she's ready for

more. Use your feeding times to talk or sing to your baby. By becoming attached to you, your baby will become a more confident, resilient child and adult later on.

Crying. No matter how hard you work to satisfy your baby's every need, you can expect her to whimper, sob, or even howl for up to 3 hours a day. Colicky babies may cry even more than this (see "Could it be colic?" page 384). Crying is your baby's way of getting her needs met. She needs you to know that she's wet, tired, or hungry; sometimes she may be irritable because she isn't sure what the heck she wants. The best thing you can do to get through her crying spells is to hold her and talk to her so that she knows you're responding to her needs. You can't spoil a new baby by holding her too much.

Diaper changes. All that milk your baby is consuming will mean lots of diaper changes. A newborn baby wets his diapers 6–8 times a day, and it'll probably take you a total of an hour a day to change his diapers. In the first few days, your baby should also pass meconium, that black sticky stuff that filled his intestines in the womb. After that his stools will be yellow with small seeds.

Within a week, these weird stools should become soft and light yellow if you nurse your baby; if you give him formula, they'll be firmer and tan in color. It's normal for a newborn to need his diaper changed every time you feed him because babies are born with a "gastrocolic reflex." As soon as they eat, their intestines are stimulated to have a bowel movement. This process should slow down after 4–6 weeks.

Sleeping. Your baby should sleep 16–20 hours a day. Up to 80 percent of her zzz-time is spent in active, or REM, sleep rather than deeper, dreamless sleep because her nervous system is still immature. You may wonder why you're so tired if your baby is sleeping so many hours a day. The answer is simple: Your newborn is probably sleeping only 3–5 hours at a stretch, and you're not used to having your sleep interrupted. Your baby doesn't know the difference between day and night; it will take her at least a month to start sleeping more after dark than she does during daylight hours.

Your baby's first doctor visit

Your baby should have had his first checkup no more than 24 hours after his birth, and his doctor should also have visited you in the hospital or birth center to tell you what to expect over the next few weeks.

At your baby's next doctor visit—which will take place within 1 week of his birth—the pediatrician will weigh him. Don't be surprised if he actually weighs up to 10 percent less than at birth! He will gain the weight back (and more) by his second week of life. Your doctor will also measure your baby's length and head circumference. He'll check your baby's reflexes to assess his motor development, listen to his heart and lungs, and feel his belly for obstructions.

Your doctor will want to know how the baby is eating and sleeping, and he'll ask how you're doing too. Be prepared with a list of your own questions about car seats, smoking, crying, and more. You'll get a chance to ask these questions both now and at your baby's 1-month checkup. In fact, you'll have lots of opportunities to chat with your pediatrician; most babies see their doctors at least five times in the first year of life.

Jaundice

Nearly all newborns get jaundice, which is the result of their immature livers being unable to cope with processing bilirubin, a natural by-product of their red blood cells. If your baby's skin or eyes look yellow, he may have jaundice. It typically clears up without treatment. However, if the skin or whites of his eyes become an intense yellow, or if he acts lethargic, see your pediatrician.

Newborns' belly buttons

Your newborn's umbilical cord stump should shrivel within a week of your arrival home. It will take 1–2 weeks to fall off completely. Meanwhile, although your mom may have told you to dab the umbilical cord stump with alcohol, the latest research shows that alcohol doesn't do much to prevent infection. In fact, using alcohol on your newborn's belly button might even extend the time it takes for the cord to fall off. Hospital staffs typically recommend letting the

When to call your obstetrician

During the weeks after delivery, call the doctor if you experience any of the following symptoms:

- Unexplained fever of 100.4 degrees Fahrenheit or above
- Increased vaginal bleeding or a flow that is so heavy it saturates a sanitary napkin in less than an hour
- Redness, swelling, pus, or drainage around the site of an episiotomy or cesarean incision
- Painful urination
- Unexplained pain, tenderness, or swelling in your legs
- Foul-smelling vaginal discharge
- Increasing pain in your vaginal area
- Unexplained coughing, nausea, vomiting, or chest pain
- Inability to control your bowel movements
- Feelings of depression
- Thoughts of hurting yourself or your baby
- Hallucinations
- Breasts that are red, painful, or hot to the touch

umbilical cord air-dry. You don't have to worry about getting the stump wet if you bathe your baby either; gently pat it dry when the bath is over.

During the time your baby has this little reminder of his connection to you, secure his diaper so that it doesn't rub on the stump and irritate it: Fold the top of the diaper over so that it rests an inch below the stump. If, after a few weeks, the stump is still there but is dangling by a thread, your doctor can painlessly snip off the remains during your baby's 1-month checkup. It's normal for your baby's belly button to have a little brown pigment inside it, even after the cord falls off completely.

Umbilical cord stumps rarely become infected. However, if you notice swelling, pus, redness, or a strong odor around the navel, see your baby's pediatrician. She can treat the area with a silver nitrate antiseptic to dry it out.

Week 2

Your Self

If you had a cesarean delivery, you're probably still feeling sore. It is, after all, major surgery. Continue to take pain medication if you need it (prescription pain medication, acetaminophen, or ibuprofen). How long you need pain medication varies; if you underwent a cesarean delivery or a vaginal delivery with tearing or an episiotomy, you'll probably need prescription pain medication for 2 weeks or so, followed by acetaminophen or ibuprofen for a few more weeks. If you had a relatively easy vaginal birth without tearing or an episiotomy, you may do fine with a week or so of over-the-counter medications. Avoid aspirin though; it is not as effective at relieving uterine pain as acetaminophen and ibuprofen are, and aspirin can increase bleeding.

This week try to get up and walk around because moving will increase circulation and decrease your risk of developing blood clots. Ask family or friends to help with housework.

By the end of this week you should start feeling better. Take short walks, but don't do too much. If your vaginal bleeding increases, you may be doing too much too soon. Vaginal pressure can be intense and you may wonder if your uterus is going to fall out of your body. Be assured, your uterus will not fall out, but it may take a couple of weeks for stretched and swollen pelvic tissue to bounce back to normal. Try to rest when the baby is sleeping, even if it means you have to let the dirty dishes stack up in the sink. Your health is more important!

Vaginal discharge. This will continue whether you delivered vaginally or by cesarean. This week it may turn from pink to yellowish brown and will decrease in volume, although you'll still need to replace your sanitary napkin every couple of hours. As your body loses some of the fluids it added during pregnancy, you may find it easier to fit into non-maternity clothes.

Sore nipples. If you're nursing, your nipples may be getting sore. This happens to most breastfeeding mothers, and it usually goes away within a couple of weeks as the nipples toughen up. Nipple soreness can often be corrected with small changes, such as alternating nursing positions and making sure your baby latches on correctly (with the whole areola in his mouth, not just the nipple). Treat sore nipples by spreading some expressed milk onto them after feeding. When you're showering, avoid using soap on your breasts because it can dry the skin. Wear cotton bras that wick moisture away from the skin. After nursing, allow your nipples to air-dry.

Keep in mind that most babies have a growth spurt around week 2; for a day or two they'll nurse more frequently and seem less satisfied with what they're getting. Within a day or so, your milk supply will catch up and your baby will be more satiated, although more-frequent feedings will continue for a couple of days.

Your Baby

Bathing basics

Now that you're on your own, the prospect of dunking your slippery, squirmy newborn in water may make you cringe. Once you've mastered a few simple techniques for hanging on to your little tadpole, however, you'll find that bath time can be one of the best times of day for both of you.

Frequency. How often you bathe your baby is up to you; twice a week should be plenty. Between baths, sponge off her chin and diaper area.

Supplies. Check that the temperature in the room is at least 75 degrees and gather everything you'll need beforehand: towel, washcloth, mild baby soap, baby shampoo, cotton balls, and a cup for rinsing. Put a few inches of warm water in the sink or infant bath. Test the water temperature on the inside of your wrist.

Washing your baby. After you've undressed your baby, slide her into the bath feet first while supporting her head and neck on your forearm and wrist. Wet the washcloth with your free hand and gently wet her head; then work your way down her body and finish up around her genitals and bottom. You don't have to use much soap, and you can wipe your baby's sensitive spots—such as her ears and face—with cotton balls.

Never clean the inside of your baby's ears; just swab the outsides with cotton balls or a soft washcloth. Wax inside her ears will come out by itself. To wash her face, moisten it with plain water and wipe around her eyes, starting from the inside corner and moving outward. Her hair (if she has any) requires only a tiny drop of shampoo. Use a cup to rinse the shampoo off her head.

When you've finished bathing your little bundle, wrap her in the towel. Keep eye contact and talk to her gently all through her bath, and she'll soon look forward to these private times with you.

Baby manicure

Your baby's nails may already be long; infant nails grow fast. Trim her nails right after bath time, when they're at their softest. Many parents also like to trim their infant's nails during nap time to prevent squirming. To trim, hold each finger and cut the nail along the shape of the fingertip. Use baby-size clippers.

Reducing the risk of SIDS

Almost 5,000 babies die of SIDS (sudden infant death syndrome) each year. SIDS describes the death of a healthy infant during sleep, for no apparent reason. It is the major cause of death in babies from 1 month to 1 year old. Although the cause of SIDS is unknown, the American Academy of Pediatrics recommends that you take these steps to decrease the risk of your baby dying in her sleep:

- Put your baby to sleep on a firm, flat mattress (no waterbeds or soft bedding).
- Have your baby sleep on her back, not her stomach or side.
- Don't overdress your baby (you'll avoid overheating her).
- Don't let anyone smoke around your baby.
- Breastfeed your baby.

Week 3

Your Self

Postpartum emotions

So many things are going on in your
life right now. Your body is continuing
to heal. You're taking care of an
infant, perhaps for the first time, and
that can be very stressful. You and
your partner are relating to each other
in a different way. And, of course,
you're tired. Sleep deprivation goes
hand in hand with new motherhood.

This is an incredibly emotional
time. You may feel happy one
moment and sad the next—and then
happy again a few minutes later.
Tears flow easily during these first
few weeks, and feelings of depression
are common. About 80 percent of new
mothers experience some kind of
sadness or anxiety during the first
2 weeks after delivery. In most cases,
these blue feelings go away quickly.
However, 10–20 percent of women
develop a more serious condition
called postpartum depression.

Postpartum depression

Postpartum depression can affect any
woman, no matter what her age,
economic status, or cultural background. Symptoms include sadness,
irritability, apathy, intense anxiety,

lack of appetite, insomnia, crying
spells, irrational behavior, feelings of
worthlessness, and an inability to
make decisions or to concentrate. It
can begin anytime during the first
few days, weeks, or months after
delivery. Nobody knows for sure what
causes it, but fluctuating hormone
levels, exhaustion, and stress may
trigger it.

In extreme cases, women may
suffer from delusions or hallucinations, and they may become suicidal
or have thoughts of hurting their
baby. Severe postpartum depression
is referred to as postpartum psychosis.
It is rare, affecting only about 1 in
1,000 new mothers.

Women with postpartum depression
sometimes fail to seek help because
they are ashamed of how they feel,
but postpartum depression should not
cause embarrassment. It is a medical
condition, not a character flaw. If you
are depressed, talk with your doctor.
Postpartum depression is very
treatable with counseling and/or anti-
depressant medications that are safe
for nursing mothers.

If you're feeling blue, take good
care of yourself. Nap when your baby
naps. Ask friends and family for help
with household chores and caring for
your other children. Eat nutritious

food. Lower your expectations of yourself—your job is to take care of you and your baby, not to be the perfect housekeeper. Take a shower and get dressed every day and don't spend too much time alone. Join a new mothers' group or sign up for a postpartum exercise class or anything else that will get you out of the house and into the company of other new mothers.

Your Baby

A get-to-know-your-baby guide

By now you're moving around more easily, and you may feel less socked in by fatigue. Consequently you may notice some things about your baby that escaped your notice before, and you may be worrying about your newborn's health as a result. Here's a head-to-toe baby guide that will help you know what's normal, and what's not, about your newborn:

Breathing. It's normal for a newborn to breathe heavily because her heart is beating fast. She should breathe more quietly by 6 months of age. You may be frightened if you notice that your baby stops breathing for several seconds at a time, but this sort of periodic breathing is actually quite normal for newborns. It happens because your baby's brain still isn't fully in control of her breathing. There's no link between periodic breathing and sudden infant death syndrome (SIDS).

Head. The top of your baby's head has a fontanel (soft spot) where the skull bones haven't yet joined together. Your baby's brain is still well protected, though, by cerebrospinal fluid and tough layers of skin. That conelike look, which was caused by the head molding to fit through the birth canal, should disappear within a few weeks. You can treat red, scaly patches of cradle cap with gentle brushing and shampooing or let it go away on its own. However, if any area on your baby's head ever becomes scabby or pussy, your baby might have an infection. Call your pediatrician immediately.

Mouth. Your baby's constant need to nurse may cause her to develop tiny blisters on her lips, or she might have tiny white bumps on the roof of her mouth. These are both normal. If you see white patches on her mouth, try gently rubbing them off with a damp cloth; if they don't go away, call your doctor. These white patches can signal thrush—a common yeast infection in babies.

Neck. Support your baby's head whenever you lift or hold him because his neck muscles are still immature and his head is heavy in relation to the rest of his body. He'll be holding his head up on his own by 4 months. Meanwhile, if you notice red, flaky patches on his neck or behind his ears, it's probably cradle cap that spread. It should disappear on its own.

Eyes. Those beautiful blue eyes may stay blue, or they may change within a year. Usually the eyes of a darker-skinned infant are brown from birth. If your baby seems to be constantly winking at you, don't worry: His eyes may open one at a time initially or move randomly and look in different directions. However, his eyes should be focused by 2 months of age, even though his eye muscles are still immature. If you see green or yellow discharge, gently wipe your baby's eyes with a warm, damp cloth. This is probably from a blocked tear duct. Call your doctor if the whites of your baby's eyes are red because they might be infected.

Nose. Does it sound like your baby has a cold? She's probably fine. Most newborns sound as though they have a stuffy nose because the nasal passages are swollen. Don't try to clear her nose with a bulb syringe unless you're positive she has a cold because this can cause her passages to swell more.

Legs and feet. You may think your little guy is pigeon-toed like his athletic dad. He might be. But the feet of most babies rotate inward as a result of having been curled up so long in their mothers' wombs. Your baby may also look bowlegged, but when he starts walking, his bones will get stronger and his legs should straighten out.

Bottom. Diaper rash looks like red bumps or raw patches on the buttocks or thighs. Although diaper rash is common in babies, it is not typical in newborns who are under a month old. Talk to your doctor if your baby's rash seems severe.

Skin. It's normal for newborns to break out in pinhead-size pimples called erythema toxicum. They'll probably look white on a red base, and most often babies get this newborn acne on their faces, chests, bellies, or backs. This is usually caused by your baby's skin reacting to maternal hormones and to the change from amniotic fluid to air. There's no need to do anything about it. However, if the pimples are bigger than a pinhead, or if they blister or crust over, check with your doctor to make sure your baby doesn't have a bacterial or fungus infection.

Week 4

Your Self

By week 4 your body should be healing well. If you haven't started to exercise, now's a good time to begin. Gentle exercise will help increase circulation, reduce any remaining swelling, improve your mood, and tone your muscles. It can even help you feel less fatigued.

How much exercise you do depends on how you are healing and how fit you were before delivery. Walking is the best choice for women at all fitness levels because it delivers the benefits of exercise without the risk of muscle strain or pulling of incision sites. If you are of average fitness and had a routine delivery, begin with 5–10 minutes of walking a day; if that feels right, walk 7–12 minutes next week and 10–15 minutes the following week. Subtract from those times if you're sedentary and add to them if you're at an above-average fitness level. If anything feels sore, slow down. Four weeks postpartum is not the time to adopt a no-pain, no-gain attitude toward exercise.

Doing Kegel exercises will help strengthen your pelvic floor muscles. Kegels are especially important if urine is leaking from your bladder when you cough, laugh, or sneeze. (See "Kegel exercises," page 98.)

Nursing problems

If you're breastfeeding, you and your baby have probably established a routine by now. Unfortunately that routine may be interrupted by several breast problems that can occur in nursing mothers. All of them are treatable, and with a little time and patience you'll feel better.

Plugged milk duct. Milk is produced in glands deep in the breasts, and it is transported to the nipple through a collection of milk ducts. Occasionally a duct can become blocked. Blocked ducts are caused by several things: wearing a too-tight bra, not nursing frequently enough, or not emptying the breasts fully during feedings. A plugged milk duct causes discomfort and tenderness in one area of the breast, sometimes accompanied by a small lump. To clear the blockage, apply warm, wet washcloths to your breast and take warm showers before nursing. Massage the lump while you nurse your baby and offer that side first. The problem should clear in a couple of days.

Burning nipples. Your nipples may or may not be cracked and itchy, but if your skin burns or you feel shooting pains while nursing, it may be yeast. Check your baby's mouth for thrush and call your provider for ointment to treat it.

Mastitis. A plugged milk duct can become infected, causing a breast infection (mastitis). Symptoms of mastitis are the same as those of a plugged milk duct, but you'll also have a fever, redness, and possibly flulike symptoms. Mastitis is treated with oral antibiotics or, if it's severe, IV antibiotics. It's fine to continue nursing through the infection and the antibiotics; neither will harm your baby. In fact, frequent nursing is good because it can help clear the blocked milk duct.

Your Baby

What your baby sees, hears, smells, and tastes

Your baby's skin is his largest and most highly developed sensory organ at birth. Within hours of birth, your baby's other senses are helping him become acquainted with the world and the most important people in it— his parents. His senses will continue developing throughout the first years, but he'll begin integrating them after the first few weeks of life. Soon he'll be able to stay calmer and pay better attention to his surroundings.

Each baby's sensory development is highly individual, and it depends on genetics, physique, and temperament. Some hardy babies are readily

adaptable and easygoing in different surroundings, while others are so hypersensitive that loud noises or sudden sensations on their skin can make them jumpy and irritable. You can help your baby adapt to the world by closely observing how he responds to sensory input.

Eyes. At birth your baby is near-sighted. His vision is so blurry that he may not be able to see anything more than 6–18 inches away from him. (Nature knows what she's doing: This is the perfect distance for gazing at your face while he nurses.) It's not his eyes that need developing, however, but his brain. Right now he doesn't care about much besides eating and sleeping. By 3 months, however, your baby will want to look at everything around him. Meanwhile, forget pastels. Your newborn will be best able to see things with sharp contrasts, such as black and white pictures or bright colors.

Ears. Your baby's hearing is even less advanced than his vision. Although he can hear muffled sounds before birth, his middle ear still needs to develop, and so do the sound processing centers in his brain. He can't distinguish sounds the way you can; in fact, his hearing probably won't be fully developed until he's in elementary school. Newborns are equipped to hear low-frequency sounds such as the human voice, though, and by 3 weeks they seem to recognize lip movements used to make "ooo" and "eee" sounds. Talking to your baby as you feed, change, and soothe him is a

Hearing and vision tests for infants

Your baby will be screened for potential hearing problems. Most infants are given a hearing test that involves either listening for an inner-ear echo or recording electrical activity in the brain in response to noise. This is often done before your baby leaves the hospital; if not, it should definitely be done by your pediatrician by age 3 months. Babies most at risk for hearing problems include those who were premature, those whose mothers had infections while pregnant, and those whose families have a history of hearing loss.

Shortly after birth, your baby's eyes will also be checked. If you discover a problem with your baby's eyes, or if you have a history of eye abnormality in your family, your pediatrician might refer you to an ophthalmologist. Your baby will also have her vision checked if she was premature and required prolonged oxygen as a newborn.

great way to introduce him to the wonders of language.

Nose. Studies show that within hours of birth babies can use their noses to find their mother's nipples. This means their sense of smell is functioning from the start. They're already tasting different flavors too; scientists have shown that newborns prefer sweet-tasting substances over bitter ones. This makes sense because breast milk tends to be sweet, while bitter-tasting substances are more likely to be poisonous.

Week 5

Your Self

Week 5 brings further healing. Your vaginal area or cesarean incision feels better, although it will continue to feel different from how it felt before pregnancy. Your vaginal area may feel tighter or looser than before. Over time it will return to normal.

During the past 5 weeks you've been immersed in helping your body heal, taking care of your baby, getting into a good feeding pattern, and trying to get some sleep. All of those tasks leave little time for you, but having time to yourself is important. This week, ask someone you trust to take care of your baby for an hour or two. Do something pleasurable (and not baby-related): Go out for a walk, visit a friend, have lunch with your sister. It may be hard for you to be apart from your baby, but having time to yourself is important for your emotional health. The healthier you are, both mentally and physically, the better able you will be to take care of your baby.

Make time for yourself every day, even if it's only 15 minutes. Read a trashy novel, listen to music, lounge in the backyard. Focus on you.

Your period's return

Not having periods is one of the great conveniences of pregnancy and new motherhood. But like many things, it must come to an end.

If you began bottle-feeding immediately after delivery, menstruation will resume 1–3 months later. For nursing mothers, the range is wider. Your period may start up again while you're nursing—particularly if you supplement with formula or if your baby is eating solids and nursing less—or it may wait until you wean your baby. You may not have a period again for several months after weaning, particularly if you are breast-feeding exclusively. If you think you should be menstruating and you're not, call your doctor.

Your bladder and bowels

Passing a bowel movement may still hurt sometimes if you gave birth vaginally. If your stool is hard or you are constipated, increase your water intake and eat extra high-fiber foods such as whole grain cereals, fruits, and vegetables. Use an over-the-counter stool softener. Sometimes even half a dose can help move things along. Don't use laxatives or suppositories without your doctor's approval. If you have blood in your stool or intense pain with bowel movements, call your doctor.

Slight urinary incontinence may continue to occur for several more weeks, although it should improve steadily. (If it doesn't, mention it to your obstetrician during your week 6 visit.) Urinary tract infections sometimes develop postpartum. Call your doctor if you feel the need to urinate frequently, if you notice blood in your urine, or if you experience pain or burning while urinating.

Your Baby

The crying game

By now you're becoming a pro at feeding and diapering your baby. You've even taken him outside in the stroller, perhaps, or to the grocery store. However, you may still feel shattered every time your baby cries. Why, you wonder, isn't he happier?

Crying is your newborn's way of communicating, and how you react to it sets the tone for your relationship with your newborn. If you come when he cries, your baby learns that the world is a place where good things can happen.

How much your baby actually cries each day will naturally depend on his temperament and how quickly you learn to read his signals and distinguish hunger cries, for instance, from general 5 o'clock crabbiness. Most often, a newborn's crying jags begin after a week or two of life. They peak at 6 weeks, when babies cry for nearly

3 hours a day. That's because their nervous systems are still too undeveloped to allow these little people to calm themselves once they get all worked up.

You can, however, soothe your baby—and make life easier on yourself—with the following baby-calming strategies:

Swaddling. Your baby feels safer in your arms than anywhere else. However, you can soothe a crying newborn and still get dinner made by swaddling him to make him feel secure. Lay a lightweight cotton or flannel receiving blanket down like a diamond. Fold down the top corner and place your baby on the blanket, faceup, with his head on the fold. Wrap the left corner over your baby's body and tuck it beneath him, over his arm. Bring the bottom corner of the blanket up over his feet and pull it up to his chest; then wrap the right corner around your baby. Tuck the right corner under his side; there's no need to pin it. You may feel as if you're making a burrito, but hey, if it eases your baby's cries, do it! (Note: Never put a swaddled baby down to sleep on his tummy because he might have trouble breathing if he can't turn his head. It's also important not to keep him swaddled all day because he needs to move his limbs and work his muscles.)

Motion. When you carried your baby inside you, he grew accustomed to your motion. Use motion to keep your baby calm now by rocking him in a chair, strapping him into an infant swing, going for a ride in the car, wearing him in a frontpack, or taking him for a walk in his carriage.

Sucking. Babies suck instinctively. They use this motion to comfort themselves as well as to eat. You can help your baby stop crying by giving him a pacifier or help him find his wrist or fingers to suck on. You can also wash your hands and let him suck on one of your fingers.

White noise. Run the vacuum cleaner, play soft music, or sing to your baby to distract and soothe him.

Could it be colic?

Almost every new mother of a wailing baby is convinced at some point that her baby has colic. Pediatricians used to diagnose a baby with colic if the baby cried for more than 3 hours at a stretch in one day, 3 days a week, for 3 consecutive weeks—a condition that affects about 25 percent of all infants. New research demonstrates that only about 8 percent of infants have "true" colic, a condition defined as bouts of inconsolable crying accompanied by a physical characteristic such as your baby arching his back or pulling his legs up. And even these babies are probably just at the high end of the spectrum of normal crying. A baby with colic is not in any pain.

If your baby cries excessively, see your pediatrician, who will first rule out any medical reason for your baby's noisy distress, such as an ear infection, urinary tract infection, or reflux, which occurs when stomach acid rises into the esophagus and causes stomach pain.

If your pediatrician does diagnose colic, you may feel reassured that at least there is no other medical concern. However, that doesn't mean the constant wailing is any easier to take. Try to remember that colic isn't a reflection on your parenting skills. Nor is your baby in pain. Studies show that colicky babies experience no greater increase in stress hormones than those without colic.

There's no need to give up breastfeeding if your baby has colic. Breastfeeding is never a cause. Most dietary changes, including avoiding dairy products, don't make any difference. Don't bother with anti-gas drops either; these medications have been shown to be ineffective. Never give your baby alcohol or herbal tea as a treatment; both of these can be harmful.

What can you do for colic? Talk to other parents about survival strategies, test out the baby-calming methods in "The crying game" (page 383) and take care of yourself during this trying time. The best thing you can say about colic is that it seldom lasts more than 4 months.

Week 6

Your Self

This week you'll see your obstetrician for a postpartum checkup. Here are some of the things that may happen during the visit:

A pelvic exam. Your doctor will examine your vaginal area, cervix, and uterus, and your abdomen if you had a cesarean delivery.

A conversation about postpartum depression. Your doctor will ask you how you're feeling emotionally. Tell her if you've been feeling sad or anxious or have been crying frequently.

Advice about birth control. Breastfeeding offers some protection against pregnancy, but not enough that you can count on it as a form of birth control. Unless you plan on conceiving again soon, talk with your doctor about what kind of birth control to use. Some women start back on the Pill or contraceptive injections at this time; others prefer to use condoms or a diaphragm. If you used a diaphragm before pregnancy and would like to use it again, take it with you to your appointment so your doctor can verify that it still fits properly. If it doesn't fit correctly, it will be less effective at keeping sperm out of your cervix.

Suggestions about exercise, diet, and vitamin supplements. Your doctor will let you know when you can resume your prepregnancy exercise regimen of walking, jogging, swimming, weight lifting, or playing sports. She may give you suggestions about losing weight, particularly if you gained a lot during pregnancy. She will also talk with you about vitamin supplements.

If you plan to conceive again within the next year or two, she may suggest that you continue taking your prenatal vitamins to ensure that you get adequate amounts of folic acid and build up levels of fat-soluble vitamins that are stored in the body and depleted during pregnancy and breastfeeding.

Answers to questions about your next pregnancy. If you have questions about how this pregnancy will affect future pregnancies, discuss them now. For example, if you developed a complication such as high blood pressure or gestational diabetes during pregnancy, talk about what you can do between now and your next pregnancy to reduce the risk of developing those complications again.

An OK to start having sex again. Most doctors recommend waiting about 6 weeks after delivery to have intercourse; this helps reduce your risk of infection or bleeding. You may not feel ready physically or emotionally; if so, share your feelings with your partner. Go slowly the first time because intercourse may hurt. If you are breastfeeding, the low levels of estrogen decrease vaginal lubrication. Water-base vaginal lubricants can come in handy for the next few weeks; they're sold in pharmacies. If lubricants do not work, your doctor can prescribe an estrogen cream.

Answers to any other questions. During the week or two before your appointment, write down any questions you think of and bring your list with you to the visit. (Use the form on the next page.) Your sleep-deprived brain is unlikely to remember anything that isn't written down.

Your Baby

Surviving spit-up
One thing that becomes abundantly clear in the first weeks of parenting is that dry-clean-only clothes should stay in your closet. No sooner have you fed your baby than he might spit up, to the point where you may worry how he could possibly be getting enough nourishment.

Spitting up after eating is perfectly normal. Baby tummies are structured differently from those of adults. The valve that keeps the stomach shut, which is called the esophageal sphincter, doesn't mature until your baby's first birthday. That's why burping and jostling your baby can cause some of the contents of his stomach to leak right out. This should happen less as your baby gets older, and it generally stops around 6 months.

Meanwhile, your baby is fine as long as he's gaining an ounce a day for the first few months and growing normally. You may perceive that he's spitting up all of his formula or breast milk, but it's probably only a teaspoon of liquid. Test this theory by filling a teaspoon with water or milk and pouring it on a towel to see how widely it soaks the fabric.

Gastroesophageal reflux (GERD)
It's rarely the case, but sometimes spitting up is a sign that your baby has gastroesophageal reflux disease (GERD). If your baby has GERD, she may cry and scream as soon as she starts to eat, and she may constantly spit up her food. GERD is a condition in which your baby's stomach acids, normally in the stomach to digest food, might enter the esophagus and erode it. This can be uncomfortable for your baby and might lead to more serious problems such as sleep apnea, in which your child stops breathing, or closure of your baby's larynx when stomach contents come up the esophagus and down the windpipe. If you suspect GERD, your pediatrician can usually prescribe a baby-safe antacid. It's also possible for babies to have surgery to create an artificial sphincter from stomach tissue; it's a strategy that cures reflux in more than 90 percent of otherwise healthy children.

To help your baby keep more food down, feed him more often and give him smaller amounts. Burp him at regular intervals. If you're using a bottle, angle it so that your baby gets only milk (and no air) from the nipple. Gulping air can cause your baby's stomach contents to move back up the esophagus.

It may help if you feed him in a quiet place and keep him upright in your lap or in an infant seat for 20 minutes after feeding. Spit-up can also be the result of overfeeding. Don't force the issue if your child turns his head away.

Postpartum Doctor Visit

6–8 weeks after delivery

Date _____   **Blood Pressure** _____

Weight _____

Can I use birth control pills while I am breastfeeding?

_____

_____

I am still leaking urine. Will this get better? When?

_____

_____

I have not gotten back to my prepregnancy weight yet. When will that happen?

_____

_____

_____

When do I need to schedule my next primary care visit? My next gynecological exam?

_____

_____

When can I get pregnant again?

_____

_____

Other:

_____

_____

Week 7

Your Self

Lovemaking after baby

When your doctor gave you the OK to start having sex again, your partner may have leapt with joy. You may have had a very different reaction. You're exhausted, your breasts are sore, you feel fat, and you're anxious about whether your vaginal area is ready for intercourse, even though your doctor says it is. Making love may be the last thing on your mind.

Communicate with each other about sex in an open, loving way. Tell your partner if you feel less sexy because of the changes your body has undergone or that you're nervous about activity in your vaginal area. Ask him to be patient with you if sleep seems more attractive than sex. At the same time, stay in touch with your sexuality and don't think of yourself exclusively as a mother. Don't focus too much on how you look; it probably bothers you more than your partner. He sees you cuddling and hugging your baby, and he wants to be close to you too.

Connecting with your partner

Having a baby—especially your first baby—changes your relationship with your partner. Once you focused your love and attention on each other; now you're focusing it on your baby. You may not have anticipated this. New parents often find that although they've spent months preparing for a new baby, they haven't spent any time preparing for a new relationship.

The stresses of a new baby, from sleepless nights to increased financial pressures, can disrupt the balance of a marriage. Marital conflicts often arise when the husband feels he's being pushed aside. He may feel envious. Suddenly the affection that was once bestowed on him is going to the baby. This can be particularly true if you breastfeed because you and your baby are an intimate unit that doesn't include him.

Including your partner in everything from diaper changes to settling the baby down for a nap can help dispel feelings of displacement. It also takes some of the burden away from you, which, in the long run, can help your relationship. If you're doing all the baby care, you're going to be resentful, and you'll have no energy. When you have no energy, you have no interest in romance. Then your partner gets resentful. He gets mad at you, you get mad at him, and before you know it, you've got a marital crisis.

It doesn't have to be that way,

provided you are both willing to work on redefining your relationship. Start by making it a priority to spend time alone as a couple. Schedule a standing appointment with a sitter for Saturday nights, plan "home dates" midweek, or make it a daily ritual to sit down to dinner together each night after the baby is asleep. These special times give you a chance to reconnect and to focus on each other. If you both make an effort, your relationship will weather the transition into parenthood.

Your Baby

Out and about in the world

A month into parenthood, you may feel less like an actress in a play as you care for this new little person in your life. You're getting to know what your baby's cries mean, your body is healing, some of your energy has returned, and your baby's sleep-and-wake cycles are more predictable.

It's time to start exploring the world together. Walk your baby in a stroller or baby carrier. This will keep you both in a better mood and help you sleep better. You'll also be stimulating your baby's senses and offering him valuable lessons about the world. What does the color green look like? What sound does a dog make? Talking and singing to your baby, or having him near you as you make conversation with other people on your outings, is a great way to socialize your child as he learns about the world. If you don't have the energy to move around, put a quilt on the ground beneath a shade tree and lie down on it next to your baby. Talk to your baby about the leaves, the weather, the birds—or play with his hands and feet and smile at him. In the next few weeks, he'll be able to smile in response.

Don't worry about your baby getting too cold or too hot. A general guide to dressing your baby for the outdoors is to dress him in one layer more than you're wearing or add a blanket.

Sunshine is healthy for all humans. It activates the body's production of vitamin D and therefore helps build strong bones and teeth. Remember, however, that your baby has never been exposed to sunlight, and his skin will burn easily.

Try not to expose your baby to direct sunlight; he'll still reap the

postpartum and baby care

Don't feel bad when you're too busy

Sure, it's fun to watch your baby, talk to her, or play with her. But there are lots of things you have to do in a day, especially if you have older children. Letting babies learn to amuse themselves is just as important as interacting with them. (Remember: At this point your baby is stimulated just by breathing.) Even a very young infant can entertain himself with a mobile or by gazing at the shifting patterns of light on the kitchen curtains. Keep your baby nearby in a carrier or infant swing, or lay him on a blanket on the floor, but go about your business. Moving him to a new place with fresh visuals is usually enough to stop the whimpering.

benefits of sun exposure and fresh air if you keep him in the shade or keep him covered with lightweight clothing, one of those cute hats you got at the baby shower, and a sunscreen with an SPF of at least 15. He might burn in the sun even when the weather is cool, so minimize his exposure to the early morning or late afternoon hours as he builds up some sun tolerance.

Protecting your baby against the sun now may also protect him against skin cancer later in life.

Is that a smile?

You bet! That first social smile shows up between 6 and 8 weeks, and oh, what a sweet sight it is! (Especially at that 2 a.m. feeding.)

Week 8

Your Self

Fighting fatigue

Sleep deprivation is one of the hardest parts of new parenthood. During your baby's first few months she needs to eat frequently, and, if you're breastfeeding, you may go weeks or months without getting more than a few hours of uninterrupted sleep. By week 8 you may be feeling quite exhausted, particularly if you've got other children, if you've gone back to work, or if your baby has day and night confused and is wide awake after nighttime feedings.

Full nights of undisturbed sleep are still several months away, but in the meantime, make use of these postpartum fatigue busters:

Eat smart. Junk food and sweets may give you a temporary rush, but it doesn't last long. Keep blood sugar and energy levels even by eating healthfully and regularly.

Go for variety. Select a wide variety of foods to ensure you get all of the vitamins and minerals you need. Being low on certain nutrients can cause fatigue.

Exercise. You might think that exercise will tire you out more, but in fact, moderate exercise energizes you.

Drink water. Dehydration causes feelings of fatigue.

Take naps. Even a 20-minute snooze on the couch can make a difference.

Get out of the house. Fresh air and a change in routine can help wake you up.

Ask for help. If you are breastfeeding and the nighttime feedings are wearing you out, ask your partner to help. He can't do the nursing, but he can bring the baby to you and change her diaper afterwards.

Rest while you feed. Stop multitasking and start resting while feeding your baby. Instead of talking on the phone, watching TV, reading a book, or writing thank-you notes (or doing all of those things at once), lie down and feed your baby in bed. Afterward, you'll probably both drift off to sleep.

Don't rely on caffeine to wake you up. Caffeine can pass into breast milk and keep your baby from sleeping.

Cut down on cooking. Who says a nutritious meal requires an hour at the stove? You and your partner can get all the nutrients you need from cereal, milk, fruit, yogurt, scrambled eggs, sandwiches, bread and cheese, and other easy-to-prepare foods.

Don't be a hero. If you're really, really tired, call your mother, sister, mother-in-law, neighbor, or friend and ask her to spend the night and take care of the baby while you sleep. Pump milk or prepare a formula bottle for the middle-of-the-night feeding, put in earplugs, and get a solid 5 or 6 hours of sleep. You'll be amazed at how refreshed you'll feel.

Your Baby

Increasing muscle control

Right now, your baby's arms and legs may seem to be thrashing about at random, or she may clutch onto your finger or the edge of the blanket and not let go. Her muscles are developing, and her brain is learning how to tell them what to do, a process that takes a year or two.

Newborns have little or no muscle coordination. Most of her early movements will be jerky, sporadic, and random. At most, she might wave her arms and legs simultaneously when she's excited by something she sees or hears. As her brain matures, though, billions of nerve cells will start connecting in more intricate pathways, allowing her brain and muscles to send signals back and forth.

Your baby will gain control of her head first, and her muscle control will develop downward to her toes. For instance, by 3 months she'll have no problem holding up her head or turning it to see what you're up to in the kitchen. By 5 months, she'll start sitting up, though she won't be able to stop herself from falling over. She'll also learn how to roll in either direction as she coordinates her upper- and lower-body muscles. She'll be able to sit up straighter and even catch herself on one arm by 7 months or so as she simultaneously reaches out to grasp that rattle you're waving in front of her.

What your baby's head size tells his doctor

At every visit for the first 24 months, your pediatrician will measure the circumference of your baby's head. A baby's head grows rapidly; it will increase to three times its original size just in the first year. Measuring that growth reveals a lot about your baby's health. For instance, a small head at birth might indicate a chromosomal abnormality. A head that suddenly gets larger could signal a rare condition called hydrocephalus (water on the brain). Don't worry too much if your baby's head looks smaller or larger than the heads of other babies. Heads come in all sizes, and it's the rate of growth that matters most.

Week 9

Your Self

Congratulations! You've survived the first 2 months postpartum. Most mothers agree that the first 2 months are the most difficult and that life with baby starts getting more manageable around now.

Your body continues to get back to normal, although now that you've had a baby, you probably have to alter your definition of normal. Your belly is probably still larger than you would like. It takes time for your abdominal muscles to tighten up, but abdominal exercises can help.

Your weight is probably still higher than you would like. Although some women lose their baby weight quickly, most hold on to it for several months or longer. Continue to exercise and eat smart, and the weight will come off eventually. Remind yourself that it took 9 months to gain the weight, and it takes a while to lose it.

Fatigue is probably still an issue, whether you are breastfeeding or bottle-feeding. Most babies don't sleep through the night at 9 weeks (and won't for a couple of months) and still need to feed once or twice a night. If he hasn't already, your baby may drop a night feeding session soon; you can help that along by feeding him just before bedtime.

If you're breastfeeding, you and your baby have probably established a pattern, if not a schedule. As your baby gets older, he should need to feed less often; as his stomach grows, he is able to take in more milk at one time than he could as a newborn.

Abdominal exercises

As your baby's stomach grows bigger, you want yours to grow smaller. Here are some abdominal exercises that can help move you toward that goal:

Knee to chest. Lie on your back with your knees bent and your feet hip distance apart and flat on the floor. Keep your arms by your side. Inhale and then, as you exhale, press your low back toward the floor, tilting your pelvis. Inhale, then exhale as you lift your left leg off the floor and bring your left knee to your chest. Inhale, and exhale as you return your left foot to the floor. Repeat with your right leg. Be sure to keep your low back pressed toward the floor the entire time. Do 5–10 repetitions. Next do a second set, but this time bring your left knee to your chest, then your right knee (so that both knees are at the chest), then lower

postpartum and baby care

your left foot to the floor and then your right. Coordinate your breathing so that you're always exhaling when shifting positions and inhaling while between movements.

Hip roll bridge. Lie on your back with your knees bent and your feet hip distance apart and flat on the floor. Keep your arms by your side. Inhale, and then as you exhale, use your abdominal muscles to press your low back toward the floor. In a smooth motion, lift your hips up off the mat into a bridge position. (The upper part of your spine and shoulder blades should stay on the floor.) Hold for 3–5 seconds, squeezing the butt muscles as you hold. Then, starting from your upper back, roll your spine back down onto the floor. Do 5–10 repetitions.

Spine twist. Sit upright on the floor with your knees bent and together and your arms reaching out to your sides, palms facing the floor. Inhale. As you exhale, rotate your body from the waist up as far to the left as possible while keeping your hips stable and facing forward. (Use the abdominal muscles to twist from the waist, not the hips.) Take three breaths and twist a little bit farther with each exhale. Then inhale and return to the start position. Repeat, twisting to the right. Do 3–5 repetitions.

Oblique. Lie on your back with your knees bent and your feet hip distance apart and flat on the floor. Place your hands behind your head. Inhale. As you exhale, curve your spine off the floor, bringing your whole torso up and your nose toward the outside of your right knee. (Be sure to rotate your whole body, not just your head.) Inhale and return to start position. Exhale and rotate to the left side. Do 8–10 repetitions on each side.

Your Baby

When will he sleep all night?
As the novelty of watching CNN at 2 a.m. wears off, you may be wondering when your baby will ever sleep through the night. Babies usually change their sleep routines every 2 or 3 days in their first few weeks, so it's no wonder you're feeling like a zombie.

During the first 2 months of your

Is it OK to nurse or rock your baby to sleep?
In the first weeks of your newborn's adjustment to the big, bright world, she'll need a lot of comforting. It's fine to rock or nurse your baby until she falls asleep. However, as she gets older—between 8 and 12 weeks—you might have to adjust your routine to help her learn to fall asleep. Instead of rocking or nursing her to sleep, put her in her crib while she's still awake and give her a chance to fall asleep on her own. If she doesn't, comfort her until she's groggy, then pick her up and soothe her before putting her down again. Try this a few times. If she continues to cry, give up and try this routine again in a week.

Bedtime for baby

Your baby will sleep better through the night if you help him associate bedtime with a certain routine. For instance:

- 6 to 7 p.m. Give your baby a calming bath, massage him gently, dress him for bed.
- 7 p.m. Feed him in a quiet, dim room.
- 8 p.m. Put him to bed in a dark, quiet room with a night-light. If he cries, check him every few minutes to see that he's all right. Stroke him gently if he's clearly upset, or pick him up to soothe him, but keep visits short and distractions to a minimum to help establish a bedtime routine.

baby's life, almost any sleep routine can be considered normal, and you can't force a schedule on a newborn. By your baby's 2nd month, however, you can certainly encourage better sleep habits. Consider whether you're inadvertently preventing your baby from sleeping for longer amounts of time by jumping to pick him up as soon as he makes a squeak. Babies are notoriously active sleepers, often whimpering, groaning, and moving, so wait a few minutes after your baby stirs before picking him up. He might go back to sleep on his own, and then he'll become more accustomed to sleeping for longer stretches of time.

If your baby is a night owl or seems to have days and nights mixed up, you can start teaching him the difference. During the day, give your baby lots of stimulation. Keep the lights and radio on and do your chores while he's nearby in an infant seat or playpen. Keep talking to him or take him outside. (Back off if your baby fusses or withdraws and let him fall asleep.) Then, when it starts to get dark, give your baby signals that it's time to settle down and be quiet. Change his diaper and his clothes, then put him to sleep in his bed. Keep the room dim when you feed him and don't play or sing to him when you get him up at night. Your baby soon will shift his sleeping pattern when he learns that daytime is fun time!

Week 10

Your Self

How long should I breastfeed?

The American Academy of Pediatricians recommends that infants be fed only breast milk (no formula, water, juice, other liquids, or any solid foods) for the first 6 months of life. Breastfeeding should continue for the next 6 months while solids are introduced. Not all mothers follow those guidelines, however. Some wean earlier, after a month or two, and some continue nursing past age 1.

Weaning an infant

Stopping all breastfeeding suddenly can be painful for you and your baby. Your breasts will engorge, and you might develop a breast infection, and your baby may protest a total switch from breast to bottle. Weaning gradually makes the most sense for both of you. Start by dropping one feeding and replacing it with a bottle or a cup. If your baby doesn't accept a bottle from you—after all, he associates you with nursing—have your partner or someone else feed him. After a few days, drop another feeding, then wait a few days and drop another feeding, and so on until he is weaned.

Usually within 3–4 days of dropping

a feeding, your breast milk will not "let down" after that feed. If after 3–4 days, however, your milk still "lets down" at the dropped feed, wait a few more days before dropping the next one or you will be very uncomfortable.

Nursing strikes

No, your baby won't be marching around with a banner, but after the age of about 3 months, he may suddenly refuse to nurse. This is called a nursing strike, and it can happen for several reasons, such as illness, teething, a change in the taste of the milk, frequent use of bottles or pacifier, low milk supply, a change in the way you smell (because of a new perfume or deodorant), a condition that makes nursing uncomfortable (such as a stuffy nose or sores in the baby's mouth), or a change in the baby's life, such as a new babysitter, a move to a new house, or your returning to work.

To help your baby through a nursing strike, spend extra time cuddling him. Try nursing in a different place, changing positions, dimming the lights to minimize distractions, and feeding him when he's drowsy. To feed him, express your milk and offer it via a bottle or, if you prefer not to bottle-feed, a cup or spoon. (If you do bottle-feed during a nursing strike, don't cuddle your baby as you would while breastfeeding to discourage him from becoming so fond of the bottle that he doesn't want to start breast-feeding again.) Nursing strikes usually last no more than a few days, and most babies return to the breast. If your baby is underweight when he goes on strike, talk with his pediatrician about feeding alternatives.

Your Baby

Boosting your baby's IQ
Your baby's intelligence is a mix of genetics and environment. However, the care you give your baby is crucial to her development. You can help stimulate her brain with these ideas:

Talk to her. Research shows a correlation between the number of words a baby hears and her verbal IQ.

Give her private time. If you bombard your baby with stimulation every time she's awake, she'll be worn out in minutes. Even babies need to learn how to amuse themselves.

Read to her. Even as an infant, your baby can grasp the basics of story-telling and vocabulary if you read to her; she'll soon observe that books have letters on the pages and that you read them from left to right. Picture books will show her things she might not otherwise see—like jungles and elephants—and teach her new words. When you reach the end of a book, read it again to help your baby sharpen her memory.

Cuddle. Make plenty of eye contact with your infant and hold her often. The biggest learning motivator for most kids is the desire to connect with people and form bonds as they explore the world. You want your baby to be attached to you.

Learning by mouth
Putting objects in their mouths—nipples, fingers, toys, thumbs, blankets—helps babies learn about different tastes and textures and prepares them for eating solid food.

Best games for babies
Get down to your baby's eye level a few times a day, especially during feeding, changing, and bath time, and linger long enough to play. Here are some activities that will take you beyond peekaboo:

Going Up. Lift your baby's arms up and down over his head, then in and out over his chest, reciting a rhyme.

Sitting Pretty. Grasp your hands around your baby's chest and back (not her arms, or you could dislocate them). Pull your baby up to a sitting position and let her down again gently, singing or talking to her as you go. Say her name and tickle her toes at the end.

Whoopsie Daisy. Begin with your baby's thumb and say "daisy" as you gently touch the tip of each finger. When you get to her pinkie, say, "Whoopsie daisy!" and slide your finger down the side of her hand and back up to her thumb, where you start over.

Week 11

Your Self

Having another child

Despite the vows you may have made during labor that you would never have another baby, you and your partner may be thinking about conceiving again. You may want your children to be close in age so they can play together and be on the same soccer teams; if you're an older mother, you may want to conceive again soon because you know fertility declines with age.

There is no perfect age-spacing, but research shows that having babies at least 18 months apart is associated with the fewest number of pregnancy complications. There are pros and cons to every age arrangement, and it ultimately comes down to personal choice. There are some health factors to consider, however:

Birthweight. A study of more than 560,000 infants in Michigan found that second babies who were conceived 18–23 months after the birth of the first baby had the best chance of being born at a healthy weight. The risk of low birthweight and preterm birth increased with babies conceived before 18 months and after 23 months postpartum.

Your weight. If you gained excess weight while you were pregnant and you haven't lost it yet, you might want to shed some of those extra pounds before conceiving. It's best to start pregnancy at a healthy weight because overweight mothers have a higher risk of high blood pressure, gestational diabetes, back pain in pregnancy, prolonged labor, complications during childbirth, and cesarean deliveries. Their babies are at increased risk of being born with high birthweight, and they are more likely to be overweight later in life. Plus, the more you weigh when you start your pregnancy, the more you have to lose afterward.

Sibling rivalry. Research suggests that sibling rivalry is least likely to occur in children who are less than 1 year or more than 4 years old when a sibling is born.

Nutrient needs. Your stores of iron, vitamin K, and other nutrients may have been depleted during your pregnancy and breastfeeding. If you plan to conceive again soon, talk with your health care provider about whether you need to build up nutrient stores before conception.

Folic acid. Taking 400 micrograms of folic acid a day, before and during early pregnancy, greatly reduces your risk of having a baby with neural tube defects, so if you're even thinking about conceiving, be sure you're getting enough folic acid. If you have already had a baby with a neural tube defect, the March of Dimes recommends that you begin taking 4,000 micrograms of folic acid every day for one month before conceiving and continue taking the folic acid throughout pregnancy.

Prepregnancy exam. To maximize your next baby's chances of being born healthy, see your doctor for a checkup before you conceive. This is especially important if you have a preexisting health problem such as diabetes, high blood pressure, or epilepsy, or if you take any medications that might impact pregnancy.

Your Baby

Communicating with your baby

Learning to respond to your baby's nonverbal cues is a great way to let your baby know that the world is a good place where people understand him. It's easy to tell when your baby is happy now because he'll give you that big, drooling grin. Knowing when your baby is dissatisfied is easy too. Watch for a pouting face, a grimace, or a cry. More subtle signals: If your baby is tired of a game you're playing, or if you're holding him too tightly, he might put his hand to his mouth or ear or push you away with his hand. Or he might sneeze or cough if he's worn out, overstimulated, or unhappy.

If this happens, stop whatever you're doing and watch your baby. When he seeks your gaze again or reaches toward you, lower the stimulation factor by talking more softly or playing a different, quieter game. If he withdraws by pulling in his arms and legs like a turtle or by turning his head away, he's all tuckered out.

To improve your baby's communication skills, talk to your baby and watch his face and limbs. Studies show that even the youngest babies move their arms and legs in time to their mothers' voices. They also make facial expressions to indicate their pleasure or displeasure: They raise their eyebrows and open their mouths when surprised and happy, they frown when they're angry, they look away and touch their faces when they've had enough, and they focus their eyes on your face when they want to play.

These give-and-take dialogues are a way that your infant develops a sense of self. She is no longer physically connected and completely dependent on you; she is showing signs of her own personality and becoming increasingly separate from your body, even if she's breastfeeding. She is literally learning "This is me, and this is my mom."

As your baby explores and gains more control over her muscles, she will use her hands to explore her body even before she knows these hands are hers. She may just watch her own hands for weeks, then suddenly seem to "get it" that she can make the fingers open and close

Safety tips for letting your baby play alone

Always stay within hearing range of your baby even if he's out of sight. In addition, follow these safety tips:

Remove mobiles or crib gyms as soon as your baby can push himself up onto his hands and knees and make sure these toys have no strings or small, detachable parts.

Don't put cribs near radiators, windows, or heating vents.

Remove tags and loose thread from playpens and don't put large toys in the playpen that could fall over on your baby. Be sure not to use a playpen that has any torn or large mesh weave that might pose a strangulation risk.

Don't string toys across the top of a playpen that might fall on your baby and strangle him.

Keep electrical cords, lamps, and lighting fixtures out of reach of the crib or playpen.

If your baby is on the floor, keep him in sight at all times. Before putting your baby down, scan the floor and coffee table to be sure there are no objects that might pose a choking or strangulation hazard; your baby isn't moving now, but he will be soon.

around an object. This usually happens between 2 and 4 months.

Once she has found her hands, your baby will use them as tools for exploring the rest of her, patting her chest, touching her knees, and pinching her belly to learn how her skin feels different from that flannel blanket you've put over her in the stroller or the stuffed giraffe her grandmother gave her. Don't be surprised if she explores her own genitals with the same enthusiasm she brings to touching everything else; this is all a natural part of human development.

Blanket time for baby

By the time your baby is 3 months old, you can place him near you on a blanket on the floor for a little play time. Put him on his back sometimes and on his stomach at other times so that he can practice rolling over and can look at the world from different angles. (Be sure there aren't any older children or pets around who might find him in their paths.) He will use his blanket time to explore his body with his hands and practice reaching for a mobile or toys placed around him. Or he may just watch the changing shadows on the wall across from your sun-filled kitchen window. Don't worry that you're ignoring your baby; the ability to entertain himself is an essential skill, and you're helping him hone that ability.

Week 12

Your Self

The end of maternity leave

Your maternity leave is over, and it may be time to go back to an outside-the-home job. Whether you take off for 6 weeks, 3 months, or longer, transitioning from full-time mother back to employee is not easy.

The emotional roller coaster. Leaving your baby and spending so much time away from her can be heartbreaking. While you're at work you may worry about her and feel anxious about her childcare provider. Did you make the right choice? Is your baby in the right hands? You may envision terrible things happening to your baby. All of these feelings are normal. As you adjust to being back at work, the anxious feelings should subside.

Returning to the world of work may feel disorienting. Your company kept going while you were at home, and the work you return to may be different from the work you left. So, in addition to adjusting to being away from your baby, you may have to master new skills or catch up on ongoing projects.

You may also feel that you have to make up for your absence by working extra hard. Working late is not an attractive option because you want to get home to your baby, so you have to focus on getting everything done during work hours. Of course, it can be difficult to focus on your work when you're exhausted, worrying about your baby, and perhaps taking breaks two or three times a day to pump your breasts.

The upside of a job. Getting up, feeding the baby, dressing yourself (What to wear? Your old work clothes don't fit!), gathering the supplies that your baby needs for the day, taking your baby to the sitter or the daycare center, then doing your morning commute. By the time you get to work, you're exhausted.

Despite all that, going back to work can be satisfying in a way that baby care isn't. At work you may be relieved to spend time with adults who talk about topics other than babies. You may relish the intellectual stimulation of the workplace. Once you get back into the groove, doing a job that you like and doing it well can be tremendously rewarding, particularly if you didn't warm up to the idea of being a stay-at-home mom during your maternity leave.

When you return to work, remember that the first few weeks

can be very difficult (remember the first few weeks of your baby's life?), but before long you'll hammer out a routine and start feeling less stressed by the transition. It helps if you are comfortable with your childcare choice—if not, try to find new childcare because you'll struggle to settle down at work if you're worried about your baby.

Enlisting help. Arrange with your partner to share duties such as taking the baby to the sitter. Lower your expectation of a clean house and divide up chores with your partner. If you can afford it, hire someone to clean, cook, or run errands, even just for the first few months.

When work isn't working. If after a month or two at work you feel torn and guilty about leaving your baby, reevaluate. Even if you have to work for financial reasons, you may have options, such as cutting additional expenses at home and working part-time for a while, working from home a few days a week, retraining for another job that will fit in better with your new role as a mother, or leaving your job and finding one with a shorter commute, less responsibility, a more family-friendly culture, or on-site daycare. Or perhaps your partner has options. Can he work part-time, work from home, or leave his job? If you think creatively, you may be able to put together an alternative solution that will give you more time with your baby. If the problem is childcare, spend the extra time getting comfortable with your baby's daycare

provider. It is almost impossible to work if you are worried about your baby's safety.

Your Baby

What to do if your baby is sick

Once again, Mother Nature is looking out for us: Babies come into the world protected against illness by antibodies from their mothers' wombs. If you breastfeed, your baby will probably be even healthier because there are antibodies in your breast milk too. However, your baby is only human, and she's bound to get sick at some point in the first year of her life. Here is a guide to the most common baby ailments and how to take care of your baby if she gets them:

Colds. Babies get between 6 and 10 viral colds a year. (If they're in daycare, they might get even more.) Your baby will most likely catch her first cold between 1 and 3 months after birth, and she'll react much the way you do—with a stuffy or runny nose, sore throat, and perhaps a raspy cough. Help your baby breathe more easily with a cool-mist humidifier in her room; you can also use saline drops in her nose if she's too stuffy to nurse. Warm baths or sitting her in an infant seat in the bathroom while you take a hot shower can also help loosen things in her chest. Talk with your pediatrician before giving your baby over-the-counter cold medicines. Do call your doctor if your baby is younger than 12 weeks since young infants are more likely to get complications like pneumonia.

Croup. Some babies commonly develop an infection of the windpipe and voice box after having a cold. This is called "croup." Symptoms include a dry cough that sounds like a seal or a dog barking, plus scary, noisy breathing. It's usually worse at night. Steam can help ease the symptoms, so hold your baby on your lap and sit in the bathroom with the shower running. Cold air can help too; take your baby outside for a few minutes. Be sure to keep him hydrated. If he strains to breathe even after those measures and if his lips turn bluish or grayish, call the doctor. You may even want to go to the emergency room if your baby is laboring for breath.

Diarrhea. Mild diarrhea—a few loose stools over the course of 2 to 3 days—is common in babies. As long as your baby acts like he feels good and continues to wet his diaper regularly, there's no need to worry. Just continue to feed your baby breast milk or formula. Don't use any over-the-counter antidiarrheal medications. If the diarrhea persists more than

3 days or if your baby begins to act listless or urinates less often (classic signs of dehydration), contact your doctor immediately.

Ear infections. When a virus or bacteria infects a child's eustachian tube in his ear, it can cause swelling and pain behind the eardrum. Young babies and preschoolers—from 3 months to 3 years—are most apt to get ear infections because their tubes are small; most children have at least one ear infection before age 2. Talk to your pediatrician about treating the ear infection first with just acetaminophen or ibuprofen to bring down the swelling and ease pressure and pain. You can also apply warm compresses for pain relief. If the pain continues, see your doctor for an antibiotic.

Eczema. The most common type of skin problem in babies is eczema (atopic dermatitis). It looks like a red, itchy rash and usually appears on your baby's face and head, most often between 2 and 6 months. Use moisturizing lotion. If the rash oozes, ask your pediatrician about steroid creams or a prescription ointment.

When to call your doctor immediately

Even if it's the middle of the night, call your doctor if your baby has any of these problems:

High fever: over 100.4 degrees for infants under 3 months old, over 101.5 degrees for older babies

Trouble breathing: wheezing or gasping, bluish lips

Dehydration: can't drink or keep liquids down, hasn't urinated for 6 hours, cracked lips, sunken fontanel or eyes

Vomiting: repeated or projectile vomiting

Head injury: loses consciousness or vomits after a fall

Abdominal pain: grabs her stomach, pulls her knees to her chest and howls

Questions for your doctor

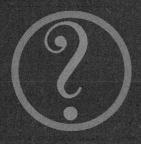

During your pregnancy, you may feel as if you see your health care provider more than your best friend. After all, you'll likely have 9 to 12 prenatal visits! Make the most of your time with your doctor by being prepared. Use these handy fill-in-the-blank sheets to track your progress, to remind yourself of important questions to ask, and to make notes of the information your doctor gives you. Don't hesitate to ask any question, no matter how small. These prenatal visits are your opportunity to learn about pregnancy, delivery, caring for a newborn, and much more.

Prenatal Visit 1

Weeks 10–12

Date _____　　Gestational Age _____　　Blood Pressure _____

Weight _____　　Heartbeat _____

If I have bleeding after today, what should I do?

_____

_____

_____

I brought in these over-the-counter products (skin care, hair care, supplements, etc.). Are they safe for me to use now that I'm pregnant?

_____

_____

What are my options for prenatal screening?

_____

_____

_____

What should I expect during the next 4 weeks?

_____

_____

_____

My uterus is "tipped." Is that a problem?

_____

_____

I have a 2-year-old at home. Is it OK to lift him up?

_____

_____

Other:

_____

_____

_____

Prenatal Visit 2

Weeks 14–16

Date _____ **Gestational Age** _____ **Blood Pressure** _____

Weight _____ **Heartbeat** _____

Should I have the multiple marker screen test?

_____
_____
_____

What will I learn from my ultrasound?

_____
_____
_____

Were my tests from my last visit OK?

_____
_____
_____

What is my blood type?

_____

What should I expect during the next 4 weeks?

_____
_____
_____
_____
_____
_____

Other:

_____
_____
_____
_____

Prenatal Visit 3

Weeks 20–22

Date _____   **Gestational Age** _____   **Blood Pressure** _____

Weight _____   **Heartbeat** _____

I have pelvic pressure. Is that normal?

_____

_____

_____

I have gained a lot of weight so far. Should I cut back on what I'm eating?

_____

_____

_____

When should I begin birthing classes?

_____

_____

_____

I had a normal ultrasound at 18–20 weeks. Will I get another one?

_____

_____

_____

Other:

_____

_____

_____

Prenatal Visit 4

Weeks 26–28

Date _____ Gestational Age _____ Blood Pressure _____

Weight _____ Heartbeat _____

Can I still travel?

_____
_____
_____

Can I continue my regular exercise routine?

_____
_____
_____

I am starting to have more heartburn. What can I do?

_____
_____
_____

Can I get a pregnancy massage?

_____
_____
_____

What should I expect during the next 4 weeks?

_____
_____
_____

Other:

_____
_____
_____

Prenatal Visit 5

Weeks 30–32

Date _____   **Gestational Age** _____   **Blood Pressure** _____

Weight _____   **Heartbeat** _____

My belly feels tight. Should I be concerned?

_____
_____
_____

If the baby seems quiet or does not move, what should I do?

_____
_____
_____

Can I take a tour of the hospital's or birth center's labor and delivery areas?

_____
_____
_____

Why are my visits more frequent in the last part of pregnancy?

_____
_____
_____

What should I expect during the next 2–3 weeks?

_____
_____
_____
_____
_____

Other:

_____
_____
_____

Prenatal Visit 6

Weeks 34–36

Date _____ **Gestational Age** _____ **Blood Pressure** _____

Weight _____ **Heartbeat** _____

Can we videotape the delivery?

_____

_____

_____

What position is the baby in?

_____

_____

_____

My mom had a cesarean delivery. Will I have one also?

_____

_____

_____

I have more swelling in my feet. Is that normal?

_____

_____

_____

Other:

_____

_____

_____

Prenatal Visit 7

Weeks 36–37

Date _____ **Gestational Age** _____ **Blood Pressure** _____

Weight _____ **Heartbeat** _____

If I do not deliver by my due date, what happens next?

_____
_____
_____

If the baby isn't moving, what should I do?

_____
_____
_____

Will I have a cervical exam? When? Why?

_____
_____
_____

Can I eat or drink when I am in labor?

_____
_____
_____

I feel fine. Can I continue to work?

_____
_____
_____

Other:

_____
_____
_____
_____
_____

Prenatal Visit 8

Weeks 37–38

Date _____ **Gestational Age** _____ **Blood Pressure** _____

Weight _____ **Heartbeat** _____

How will I know if my water broke?

_____

_____

_____

Should I call when my water breaks, even if I don't have contractions?

_____

_____

_____

How do I know if I am really in labor?

_____

_____

_____

Was my group B strep test positive or negative?

_____

_____

_____

Questions I have about labor and delivery:

_____

_____

_____

_____

Other:

_____

_____

_____

_____

_____

Prenatal Visit 9

Weeks 38–40

Date _____   **Gestational Age** _____   **Blood Pressure** _____

Weight _____   **Heartbeat** _____

What can I do to get this labor going?

_____

_____

_____

How soon after my due date can I be induced?

_____

_____

_____

Can I get an epidural when I arrive at the hospital?

_____

_____

_____

Other questions I have about labor and delivery:

_____

_____

_____

_____

Questions I have about recovery from labor and delivery:

_____

_____

_____

_____

_____

_____

_____

_____

_____

Resources

American Academy of Family Physicians
Information on mother/baby health
PO Box 11210
Shawnee Mission, KS 66207
800-274-2237
www.aafp.org

American Academy of Pediatrics
Children's health topics, clinical
resources, and research
141 Northwest Point Boulevard
Elk Grove Village, IL 60007
847-434-4000
www.aap.org

American Association of Blood Banks
Information for parents who want to
store their baby's umbilical cord blood
8101 Glenbrook Road
Bethesda, MD 20814
301-907-6977
www.aabb.org

**American College of Allergy, Asthma,
and Immunology**
Information about allergies/asthma
85 West Algonquin Road, Suite 550
Arlington Heights, IL 60005
847-427-1200
www.acaai.org

American College of Nurse-Midwives
News, information, and research on
certified nurse-midwives
8403 Colesville Road, Suite 1550
Silver Spring, MD 20910
240-485-1800
www.midwife.org

**American College of Obstetricians and
Gynecologists (ACOG)**
Information on obstetrics and gynecology issues, research, publications,
lists of providers
409 12th St., SW, PO Box 96920
Washington, DC 20090
202-638-5577
www.acog.org

American Diabetes Association
Information on gestational, juvenile,
and adult-onset diabetes
1701 North Beauregard Street
Alexandria, VA 22311
800-342-2383
www.diabetes.org

American Dietetic Association
Information on food and nutrition and
referrals to registered dietitians in
your area
120 South Riverside Plaza, Suite 2000
Chicago, IL 60606
800-877-1600
www.eatright.org

American Institute of Ultrasound in Medicine
Information about ultrasound safety, research, and guidelines for use
14750 Sweitzer Lane, Suite 100
Laurel, MD 20707
301-498-4100
www.aium.org

Doulas of North America
Information on doulas and where to find one
DONA International
PO Box 662
Jasper, IN 47547
888-788-DONA
888-788-3662
www.dona.org

Environmental Protection Agency
Information about which fish are safe to eat and other environmental/food safety issues
Fish Advisory Program
U.S. Environmental Protection Agency
Office of Science and Technology (4303T)
1200 Pennsylvania Avenue, NW
Washington, DC 20460
www.epa.gov/ost/fish

Environmental Working Group
Information on pesticides and other environmental toxins
1436 U Street, NW, Suite 100
Washington, DC 20009
202-667-6982
www.ewg.org

Genetic Alliance
Resources and information about genetic diseases and testing
4301 Connecticut Avenue, NW
Suite 404
Washington, DC 20008
202-966-5557
www.geneticalliance.org

International Childbirth Education Association and Book Center
Information on childbirth and childbirth educators
PO Box 20048
Minneapolis, MN 55420
952-854-8660
www.icea.org

March of Dimes
Information on pregnancy, genetics, birth defects, preterm birth, and related topics
1275 Mamaroneck Avenue
White Plains, NY 10605
914-428-7100
www.marchofdimes.com

Medem Online Medical Library
Physician websites and referral lists, online medical library
649 Mission Street, 2nd Floor
San Francisco, CA 94105
877-926-3336
www.medem.com

Mr. Dad
Online support for every dad, from first-time fathers to single parents
P.O. Box 16064
Oakland, CA 94610
800-647-8373
www.mrdad.com

National Highway Traffic Safety Administration

Information on child safety seats
NHTSA Headquarters
400 Seventh Street, SW
Washington, DC 20590
888-327-4236
www.nhtsa.gov

National Headache Foundation

Information about the causes and
treatment of headaches
820 N. Orleans, Suite 217
Chicago, IL 60610
888-643-5552
www.headaches.org

National Institute for Occupational Safety and Health

Workplace safety and health
information
Hubert H. Humphrey Building
200 Independence Avenue, SW
Room 715H
Washington, DC 20201
800-356-4674
www.cdc.gov/niosh

National Marrow Donor Program

Resources and information on
umbilical cord blood donation, bone
marrow diseases, transplants
3001 Broadway Street Northeast,
Suite 500
Minneapolis, MN 55413
800-627-7692
www.marrow.org

National Newborn Screening and Genetics Resource Center

Newborn screening test information
1912 W. Anderson Lane, Suite 210
Austin, TX 78757
512-454-6419
www.genes-r-us.uthscsa.edu

National Society of Genetic Counselors

Resources and information about
genetic counseling, referral lists of
counselors
233 Canterbury Drive
Wallingford, PA 19086
610-872-7608
www.nsgc.org

Special Supplemental Nutrition Program for Women, Infants, and Children (WIC)

Government agency: provides food
for low-income women and children
3101 Park Center Drive
Alexandria, VA 22302
703-305-2746
www.fns.usda.gov/wic/

State Children's Health Insurance Program (SCHIP)

Information for pregnant women
without health insurance
7500 Security Boulevard
Baltimore, MD 21244
877-267-2323
www.cms.hhs.gov/schip/

resources

U.S. Department of Labor

Information about the Family and
Medical Leave Act
Frances Perkins Building
200 Constitution Avenue, NW
Washington, DC 20210
866-487-2365
www.dol.gov/esa

U.S. Department of Labor Occupational Safety and Health Administration

Information on workplace hazards
200 Constitution Avenue, NW
Washington, DC 20210
800-321-6742
www.osha.gov

Feeding Options

African-American Breastfeeding Alliance

Resources and support for African-
American mothers who breastfeed
P.O. Box 117
Joppa, MD 21085
877-532-8535
www.aabaonline.com

International Lactation Consultant Association

Breastfeeding information, lactation
consultants, books about nursing
1500 Sunday Drive, Suite 102
Raleigh, NC 27607
919-861-5577
www.ilca.org

La Leche League

Breastfeeding information, nursing
support groups, lactation experts
1400 N. Meacham Road
Schaumburg, IL 60173
847-519-7730
www.lalecheleague.org

Medela

Breastfeeding pumps and other
nursing products
1101 Corporate Drive
McHenry, IL 60050
800-435-8316
www.medela.com

National Women's Health Information Center

Information on all women's health
topics from the U.S. Department of
Health & Human Services
8270 Willow Oaks Corporate Drive
Suite 301
Fairfax, VA 22031
800-994-9662
www.4woman.gov/breastfeeding

U.S. Food and Drug Administration Center for Food Safety and Applied Nutrition

Regulates the manufacture of infant
formula
5100 Paint Branch Parkway
HFS-555
College Park, MD 20740
888-SAFEFOOD
www.cfsan.fda.gov/~dms/inf-toc.html

Prenatal tests

During your pregnancy, your health provider may offer various routine prenatal tests to ensure that your baby is healthy and your pregnancy is progressing smoothly. Here's a guide to some of the most common prenatal tests offered in the United States.

Amniocentesis

When: Between 15 and 21 weeks

Why: To diagnose and rule out Down syndrome, Tay-Sachs disease, cystic fibrosis, sickle-cell anemia, and other genetic abnormalities. Providers generally offer this test for women over 35 (the age at which the risk of chromosomal abnormalities starts to rise), for women whose ultrasounds or blood tests indicate an increased risk for birth defects, and for women with a family history of genetic disorders.

How the test is done: Guided by an ultrasound, your practitioner will insert a thin, hollow needle into your uterus and remove a small amount of amniotic fluid. The entire procedure takes only a few minutes. Living cells from the fetus float in the amniotic fluid; these cells are grown in a laboratory for approximately 14 days, then tested for chromosomal abnormalities and markers of certain birth defects. Test results are available within 2 weeks.

Testing risks: Amniocentesis has been performed on millions of women, and in most cases it's perfectly safe. However, a small percentage of women do miscarry after the procedure; the statistics are about 1 in 200, according to the Centers for Disease Control and Prevention, although it is much less in most practices. The test is therefore performed only when you decide that the benefits definitely outweigh the risks.

Amniocentesis

When: Between 32 and 38 weeks

Why: To determine if the baby's lungs are mature. Tests on the amniotic fluid indicate whether the baby's risk of respiratory distress syndrome is less than 5 percent.

How the test is done: The procedure is the same as the amniocentesis administered at 15–21 weeks (see previous Amniocentesis entry). Chemical analysis can be completed within hours.

Testing risks: There is a small risk of bleeding, infection, onset of labor, or rupture of the membranes.

Biophysical Profile

When: Usually during the 3rd trimester

Why: To assess the overall health of a fetus. This test is usually performed when a woman is past her due date, has chronic health problems, or suffers from a pregnancy complication such as decreased amniotic fluid or placenta problems. The test might be repeated once or twice a week and it takes about 30 minutes.

How the test is done: The biophysical profile uses an ultrasound to measure fetal breathing, muscle tone, body movements, and amniotic fluid level. If your baby doesn't move within a certain amount of time, or if the ultrasound shows problems with your amniotic fluid, your health care provider might want to deliver your baby early or do other tests.

Testing risks: The test does not harm you or your baby, but approximately 20 percent of the time the test is falsely positive.

Chorionic Villus Sampling (CVS)

When: Between 10 and 12 weeks

Why: To test for Down syndrome, Tay-Sachs disease, and other genetic disorders. Your practitioner may offer this test if you're over 35, if you've had a previous child or pregnancy with a birth defect, or if your family medical history indicates that your child is at a higher-than-average risk for a genetic disorder. This test cannot be used to diagnose neural tube defects. Some women choose this test over amniocentesis, which tests for many of the same disorders, because it can be done earlier in the pregnancy.

How the test is done: Using an ultrasound as a guide, a doctor inserts a catheter (tiny tube) through the cervix or a needle through your abdomen and into the developing placenta to remove a sample of chorionic villi (small bits of tissue that attach the amniotic sac to the uterine wall). No anesthetic is required. After the sample is taken, the baby's heartbeat is checked with ultrasound. Test results are usually available within 10 days.

Testing risks: Between 1 in 200 and 1 in 100 women miscarry after CVS, according to the Centers for Disease Control and Prevention. In addition, there may be an increased risk of limb defects when CVS is done before 10 weeks. This test should be done only when you decide that the benefits clearly outweigh those risks.

Cystic Fibrosis (CF) Carrier Screening

When: Prior to pregnancy or during early pregnancy

Why: The American College of Obstetricians and Gynecologists recommends that providers make the cystic fibrosis screening test available to all couples. Cystic fibrosis is an inherited disease that affects breathing and digestion, and there is no cure; 1 in 31 Caucasian Americans carries a recessive gene for it. If you and your partner both test positive for a CF gene, your health care provider can test the baby in utero. Knowing ahead of time that your child has CF gives you a chance to learn about the disease before delivery and to find appropriate specialists to help you care for your child.

How the test is done: Blood test

Testing risks: None

Fetal Fibronectin Test

When: Between 24 and 35 weeks if you have signs of preterm labor

Why: To assess the likelihood that your contractions or cramping will progress to preterm delivery. A negative result suggests that the contractions are not changing the cervix and that delivery within the next 2 weeks is unlikely.

How the test is done: A swab obtained from vaginal discharge is tested for fibronectin, which is a substance that increases in amount as the cervix dilates.

Testing risks: None

Fetal Scalp Blood Sampling

When: During labor if electronic fetal monitoring suggests that the baby might not be tolerating labor well

Why: To assess whether the baby is getting enough oxygen during labor; if the baby is not, then the baby will be delivered.

How the test is done: The doctor will insert a thin tube through your cervix and take a few drops of blood from the baby's scalp. A laboratory analyzes the blood sample immediately for oxygen and other elements that can indicate a baby's well-being.

Testing risks: None

Genetic Carrier Testing

When: Prior to pregnancy or during early pregnancy

Why: Women may be at risk for carrying certain genetic disorders due to race and ethnicity or a family history of genetic disorders; this increases the possibility of serious illness in the baby. Examples of genetic disorders include sickle-cell anemia, thalassemias, Tay-sachs disease, fragile X (in families with a history of predominantly male mental retardation), and Canavan disease.

How the test is done: Blood test

Testing risks: None

Glucose Testing for Gestational Diabetes

When: Between 24 and 28 weeks

Why: As many as 5 percent of pregnant women are affected by gestational diabetes. In a person with gestational diabetes, the body is resistant to the effects of insulin (the hormone that converts sugar, starches, and other foods into the fuel needed for daily life). A pregnant woman with gestational diabetes may have high blood pressure, or her baby may grow large enough to require a cesarean delivery. Babies whose mothers have gestational diabetes may also be affected by breathing difficulties, low blood sugar, and jaundice during the first few days of life. If you test positive, you'll need to make diet and exercise changes; if those changes don't help enough, you may need to give yourself insulin injections or take pills to regulate your sugar.

prenatal tests

How the test is done: Your health care provider will give you a sugary liquid to drink and then take a blood sample. Determining how much sugar is in your blood will help your provider assess whether your body is breaking down sugar properly.

Testing risks: None

Group B Strep

When: Typically between 35 and 37 weeks

Why: The group B streptococcus (GBS) bacterium is relatively harmless to adults but can threaten the life of a newborn. Babies infected with GBS are at risk for pneumonia, blood infections, or meningitis. As many as 30 percent of women test positive for group B strep infections during pregnancy. If you carry GBS, your health care provider may treat you with intravenous antibiotics during labor and delivery to prevent you from transferring the infection to your new baby. If you deliver before you receive antibiotics (GBS prophylaxis) or you have a fever in labor, your newborn may have blood tests to see if he needs to be treated with antibiotics.

How the test is done: GBS may be detected with a urine culture in early pregnancy. If not, a swab from the vagina and rectum is done at 35–37 weeks.

Testing risks: None

Hematocrit/Iron Deficiency Anemia

When: Between 20 and 40 weeks

Why: Iron deficiency anemia is the most common type of anemia throughout the world. During pregnancy it can be caused by your body failing to manufacture red blood cells quickly enough to support both your muscles and your rapidly growing baby. If you test positive for iron deficiency anemia, your provider will suggest an iron supplement.

How the test is done: Blood test

Testing risks: None

HIV Test

When: Usually at the first prenatal visit

Why: To determine if a mother is infected with HIV (human immuno-deficiency virus), which could damage her immune system. The American College of Obstetricians and Gynecologists recommends that all pregnant women be tested for HIV. If an infected woman is not treated, the risk of transmitting HIV to her baby during pregnancy or delivery or postpartum is 25 percent. If HIV is diagnosed early in pregnancy, medications can be given to lower the risk of transmission to the baby to 0–2 percent.

How the test is done: Blood test

Testing risks: None

Kick Count

When: Anytime during the 3rd trimester

Why: To assess an unborn baby's health by recording his activity level. Your provider may ask you to do kick counts at home if you have a chronic health condition, are carrying multiples, or are past your due date. She may also recommend that you do a kick count if you don't feel your baby moving.

How the test is done: Your provider will ask you to lie on your side, and you'll record how long it takes for your baby to move 10 times. This test can take anywhere from a few minutes to 2 hours. A healthy baby will usually move 10 times in less than 2 hours; it may help to get your baby moving if you do the kick count immediately after eating.

Testing risks: None

Multiple Marker (Quad) Screening Test

When: Between 15 and 20 weeks

Why: To evaluate the risk for chromosomal abnormalities such as Down syndrome and neural tube defects such as spina bifida

How the test is done: A blood sample is drawn and tested in a laboratory for different biochemical markers, including alpha-fetoprotein (AFP), human chorionic gonadotropin (hCG), unconjugated estriol (uE3), and inhibin-A. Results are available within 10 days. If your test shows that your baby is at risk for a chromosomal abnormality, your provider may suggest an ultrasound and/or an amniocentesis to determine if a problem is actually present. Most women whose tests show an increased risk will have a normal baby.

Testing risks: None

Nonstress Test

When: Usually in the 3rd trimester

Why: To assess the overall health of the fetus. It is usually performed when a woman has chronic health problems, is past her due date, complains of decreased fetal movement, or has placental or amniotic fluid problems. It may be combined with a biophysical profile, and it may be done more than once a week when ongoing risk exists.

How the test is done: A small Doppler ultrasound is attached to a belt over the fetal back and measures fetal heart rate continuously for 20–30 minutes. A healthy baby will raise its heart rate with movement.

Testing risks: None

Nuchal Translucency

When: Between 11 and 14 weeks

Why: To evaluate the risk for Down syndrome

How the test is done: Your practitioner will use an ultrasound to measure the nuchal fold (a space in the tissue at the back of your baby's neck). Babies with Down syndrome tend to have a larger space than normal babies. If this test is positive, your provider may suggest an amniocentesis or CVS to determine if Down syndrome actually exists. Most often, a nuchal translucency test is combined with serum markers such as PAPP-A or free beta hCG (human chorionic gonadotropin) to improve the accuracy of the prediction of Down syndrome.

Testing risks: None

prenatal tests

PAPP-A (Pregnancy-associated plasma protein-A)

When: Between 11 and 14 weeks

Why: To detect Down syndrome

How the test is done: Blood test. It is generally combined with a nuchal translucency test and other markers to improve the accuracy of the prediction of Down syndrome.

Testing risks: None. If this test result is positive, your provider will probably recommend an amniocentesis or CVS to determine if Down syndrome really exists.

Pap Test

When: At first prenatal visit

Why: To look for abnormal cervical cells that may lead to cervical cancer

How the test is done: Cells on the surface of the cervix are removed with a special swab and evaluated in a specialized lab.

Testing risks: None. However, many pregnant women will experience spotting because the surface of the cervix is fragile.

PUBS (Percutaneous umbilical cord sampling)

When: Between 18 and 37 weeks

Why: To analyze fetal blood for disorders that can't be diagnosed through amniocentesis

How the test is done: In a procedure similar to amniocentesis, a thin needle is inserted through your abdominal wall and into the umbilical cord. A sample of the umbilical cord blood is drawn and then tested in a laboratory.

Testing risks: There is a 1 percent risk of fetal loss.

Rh Factor Screening

When: At the first prenatal visit

Why: To determine if you have a protein factor called "Rh." If you have this protein, then you are "Rh-positive"; if you do not, you are "Rh-negative." Most people are Rh-positive, but about 15 percent of Caucasian women and 7 percent of African-American women are Rh-negative. If an Rh-negative woman has an Rh-positive baby, this incompatible blood may provoke the mother's immune response and potentially harm the baby. To prevent this from happening, your provider will treat you with Rhogam (Rh-immune globulin) injections after an episode of bleeding; after a procedure such as CVS, amniocentesis, or PUBS; at 28 weeks; and immediately after childbirth.

How the test is done: Blood test

Testing risks: None

Syphilis Screen

When: At the first prenatal visit and again between weeks 28 and 32

Why: To test for syphilis bacteria. A mother who has syphilis can pass this infection on to her baby; without treatment, 40 percent of babies who are infected with syphilis while in utero die within a few days of delivery. Those who survive are at very high risk for blindness, brain damage, hearing loss, and problems with bones, skin, and teeth. If you test positive for syphilis, you will be treated with antibiotics during pregnancy, and your baby will receive antibiotic treatment shortly after birth.

How the test is done: Blood test
Testing risks: None

Tuberculosis (TB) Test

When: In the 1st or 2nd trimester
Why: To determine if a mother is infected with tuberculosis. The test is given to women who are at risk due to their country of birth, living conditions, occupation, or certain chronic illnesses. Tuberculosis can be transmitted to the fetus during pregnancy and cause neonatal death.

How the test is done: Skin test
Testing risks: The woman may have a severe skin reaction if a prior test was positive or if she had a recent TB vaccination.

Ultrasound

When: Usually between 18 and 20 weeks, but you may have earlier ultrasounds to confirm your due date, if you have any bleeding, if you have already had children with birth defects, or if another prenatal test or exam shows something abnormal.

Why: An ultrasound at 18–20 weeks will determine your baby's age, placental location, amniotic fluid level, fetal growth and heart rate, and the presence of certain birth defects.

Ultrasounds can also be used to evaluate the ovaries and cervix.

How the test is done: A technician may insert a probe into your vagina; more typically she will rub warm gel on your abdomen and then slide a transducer across your skin. (The transducer is a handheld device that looks like a microphone.) The transducer conducts sound waves that bounce off various surfaces within your body—including your baby—as vibrations. These echoes are translated into electrical signals that are then projected onto a monitor for viewing.

Testing risks: None

Urine Tests

When: At every prenatal visit
Why: To check levels of sugar and protein in your urine that could indicate health problems such as diabetes and preeclampsia

How the test is done: You will be asked to urinate into a cup at your provider's office at every visit, and a technician will test the chemical content of the urine while you're there. At the first visit, you will be asked to provide a "clean catch" urine sample after using towelettes. This sample is sent to the lab for culture to determine if any bacteria are present. Urine cultures are also done later in pregnancy if you have symptoms of infection.

Testing risks: None

Newborn tests

Newborn Screening Tests

Every U.S. state now screens newborns within the first two days of life for birth defects and chemical disorders. (Because of early-discharge policies at some hospitals, some babies have blood tests for these disorders within the first 24 hours.) Some birth defects might not be immediately visible but can cause physical problems and mental retardation unless they're diagnosed and treated early. The most common newborn screening tests offered in most states include the following:

HYPOTHYROIDISM BLOOD TEST

An underactive thyroid can retard your baby's growth and brain development. This condition affects 1 in every 3,000 babies and is the most common disorder identified by newborn screening. Hypothyroidism can be treated with oral doses of thyroid hormone.

MSUD, PKU, AND OTHER ENZYME DEFICIENCIES

Low levels of enzymes, or improperly functioning enzymes, can cause your baby to have problems regulating crucial chemical reactions in his body. If left untreated, these diseases can cause mental retardation, eye problems, or liver malfunction. Your provider will do blood tests on your baby for enzyme deficiencies such as phenylketonuria (PKU), galactosemia, and maple syrup urine disease (MSUD) within the first 48 hours after birth. If diagnosed with one of these enzyme problems, your baby can be put on a special formula to help him digest his food properly.

SICKLE-CELL ANEMIA TEST

Sickle-cell anemia affects 1 in 400 African-Americans; it is present at a lesser frequency among people of South Asian, Middle Eastern, Hispanic, and Mediterranean descent. This blood disease causes a number of health problems later in life. Young children with sickle-cell anemia are prone to certain dangerous bacterial infections, such as meningitis. Screening newborns for sickle-cell anemia offers a chance to begin antibiotic treatments early.

If you wish to do more newborn screening tests, you may have these tests conducted at a private laboratory. If so, you'll likely have to pay for them out of your own pocket. For a list of laboratories that offer advanced newborn tests, contact the National

Newborn Screening and Genetics Resource Center at 512-454-6419 or www.genes-r-us.uthscsa.edu.

Other Newborn Tests

Other tests may be ordered in the nursery by your doctor, if indicated. Unlike the newborn screening tests listed on page 426, not all of the following tests are mandated:

GLUCOSE TEST

If your baby is small or large, or if you had diabetes during your pregnancy, your doctor may test your baby's blood glucose levels. Babies with low glucose levels are typically fed immediately (breast milk or formula) or given glucose intravenously.

HEMATOCRIT (BLOOD COUNT)

If your baby is at risk for polycythemia (an abnormally high number of red blood cells) or anemia (low red blood cell count), your provider will want to measure the volume of red blood cells in your baby's blood. Blood problems of this kind in your newborn can usually be treated with a transfusion.

RH-INCOMPATIBILITY AND COOMBS' TESTS

If your blood is Rh-negative, the doctor will give your infant an Rh-incompatibility test. He may also suggest a Coombs' test to measure the presence of antibodies against your own red blood cells. Both of these blood tests look for a reaction between your newborn's blood and your own that might cause your baby to develop anemia.

BILIRUBIN SCREEN

It is becoming more common throughout pediatric practices to test for high bilirubin levels. This test may be done through blood work or by putting a special sensor on the baby's skin. It is usually done before the baby leaves the hospital after being born.

newborn tests

Labor and delivery terms

Active Labor
That time during labor when contractions are between 3 and 5 minutes apart and the cervix dilates between 4 and 8 centimeters.

Afterbirth
The membranes and placenta that are expelled after the baby is born.

Amniotic Fluid
The fluid surrounding the baby inside the amniotic sac.

Amniotic Sac
The membrane inside the uterus that surrounds the baby, the placenta, and the amniotic fluid.

Amniotomy
A common procedure that involves artificially rupturing the amniotic sac, typically because labor has stopped progressing.

Anesthesiologist
A physician whose specialty is to administer anesthesia.

Apgar Scores
Standard measurements of a baby's vital signs following birth, usually done at 1 and 5 minutes after delivery.

Back Labor
Labor pain felt in the lower back, usually because the baby is in a posterior position during labor, with the face looking up instead of down or to the side, putting greater pressure on the mother's coccyx (the triangular bone at the base of the spine).

Bilirubin
A yellow substance created by the breakdown of old red blood cells.

Bishop Score
A method of predicting the success of inducing labor by examining the cervix for dilation, effacement, position, station, and consistency.

Bloody Show
A small amount of mucus, mixed with a small amount of blood, that is expelled from the vagina immediately before or during labor.

Braxton Hicks Contractions
Irregular, usually painless (though sometimes uncomfortable) contractions occurring in the weeks before labor begins.

Breech Presentation

The baby is positioned upright in the uterus, with the buttocks or feet down toward the cervix.

Cephalopelvic Disproportion (CPD)

The baby's head is too large to pass through the mother's pelvis.

Cervix

The opening of the uterus.

Colostrum

The first fluid in the mother's breasts before her milk comes in, usually a thin yellow liquid, and most often seen near the end of pregnancy.

Contractions

A tightening of the muscles in the uterus; intervals of less than 10 minutes between contractions may signal the start of labor.

Contraction Stress Test (CST or Stress Test)

Inducing mild uterine contractions through nipple stimulation or Pitocin (an artificial oxytocin) to determine how healthy the baby is.

Crowning

The top of the baby's head appears in the vaginal opening toward the end of labor.

D&C

Surgically dilating the cervix and scraping the uterine lining to remove retained tissue.

Dilation

Opening of the cervix, typically after contractions; usually measured in centimeters. A woman's cervical opening measures 10 centimeters when it is fully dilated in preparation to deliver her baby.

Doppler

A device used to amplify the sound of a fetal heartbeat.

Doula

A woman trained to support a woman in labor and act as her advocate during the birth process.

Effacement

Thinning of the cervix and shortening of the uterus, which happens both late in pregnancy and during labor.

Engagement

The period when the baby's head descends into the mother's pelvic region; usually occurs within the last few weeks of pregnancy for first-time moms, but sometimes not until labor begins.

Epidural

An injection given in the space around the spinal cord, near the nerves in the lower back, to numb the lower body and block pain from contractions during labor.

labor and delivery terms

Episiotomy

An incision made in the perineum (the tissue between the vagina and the anus) just before birth to enlarge the vaginal opening.

External Version

Manual manipulation of a baby's position from outside the uterus, usually to turn a breech baby from a feet- or buttocks-down position to a head-down position.

Face Presentation

The baby travels facefirst through the birth canal.

False Labor

The uterus contracts without dilating the cervix.

Fetal Arrhythmia

The baby's heartbeat is irregular.

Fetal Monitor, Electronic

A device that monitors a baby's heartbeat either before or during labor. The monitor is attached to the mother's abdomen and may be used intermittently or continuously.

Fetal Scalp Electrode

A thin wire clipped to the fetus's scalp that continuously records the fetal heart rate. Used instead of an external electronic monitor.

Fontanels

Soft spots on the newborn's head where skull plates remain unfused; these allow for brain growth in the first years of life.

Forceps

An instrument that can help guide the baby through the birth canal during delivery; it looks like a giant pair of tongs and is used to grasp the head and gently guide the baby out of the vagina.

Frank Breech

A breech baby whose buttocks are closest to the cervix.

Fundus

The top part of the uterus; the height of the fundus is measured during prenatal visits as one way of monitoring fetal growth.

Hemorrhage

Excessive bleeding for any reason.

Hypnobirthing

Managing stress and pain relief during labor through hypnosis or self-hypnosis.

Incompetent Cervix

A cervix that dilates without contractions or pain, usually at less than 22 weeks' gestation.

Induction
Artificial start of labor, usually with medication, nipple stimulation, or rupture of membranes.

Intrauterine
Inside the uterus.

Intrauterine Pressure Catheter
A thin tube placed inside the uterus next to the baby's head to measure the strength of contractions.

Jaundice
A condition that makes a baby's skin and eyes appear yellow, caused by a buildup of bilirubin.

Labor
The process during which uterine contractions cause the cervix to dilate and the baby to move down and out of the birth canal.

Lamaze
A method of managing childbirth pain with breathing techniques instead of medical interventions.

Lanugo
Fine hair that covers the fetus until the final weeks of pregnancy.

Local Anesthetic
Medication that numbs a specific part of the body. Usually injected into the perineum prior to repair of an episiotomy or tear.

Lochia
Vaginal discharge of blood and the uterine lining after delivery of the placenta.

Meconium
A newborn's first bowel movement—a sticky, blackish green substance. If the bowel movement occurs in utero, the amniotic fluid is meconium-stained.

Midwife
A birth professional, usually a registered nurse with advanced training in prenatal care, labor, and delivery.

Molding
The shaping of a baby's head during the journey through the birth canal.

Mucus Plug
Thick cervical secretions that serve to protect the baby and uterus from infection; these are often released just prior to labor.

Natural Childbirth
Delivering a child with as few medications and other medical interventions as possible. Mothers instead rely on breathing techniques and other relaxation strategies to manage pain during contractions and delivery.

Obstetrician
A physician whose specialty is the care of pregnant women before, during, and immediately after childbirth.

labor and delivery terms

Occiput Anterior
Position of the baby's head in which the face is looking down.

Occiput Posterior
Also known as posterior presentation. The baby's back is aligned with the mother's back and the face is looking up.

Oligohydramnios
Insufficient amniotic fluid.

Oxytocin
A natural hormone in the body that causes muscle contractions. A synthetic version of this hormone, called Pitocin, may be administered to stimulate contractions (induce) or strengthen (augment) labor.

Perinatologist
A physician whose specialty is the care of women with high-risk pregnancies.

Perineum
The area between the anus and vagina.

Placenta
An organ that attaches to the uterine wall and grows to support and nourish the fetus.

Polyhydramnios
Increased amount of amniotic fluid.

Posterior Presentation
Also known as occiput posterior. The baby's back is aligned with the mother's back and the face is looking up.

Postmature Baby
Any baby born 2 or more weeks after the due date.

Postpartum
After childbirth.

Postpartum Blues
Mild depression in the mother after childbirth, lasting no more than 14 days.

Postpartum Depression
More severe depression or anxiety (and, rarely, psychosis) in the mother following the birth of a child or fetal loss.

Post-term Birth
Any pregnancy lasting over 42 weeks.

Premature Delivery
Delivering a baby before 37 weeks' gestation.

Premature Rupture of Membranes (PROM)
Rupture of fetal membranes at term before contractions.

Presentation
The position of the baby in utero (typically head-, feet-, or buttocks-first).

Preterm Premature Rupture of Membranes (pPROM)
Rupture of fetal membranes prior to 37 weeks' gestation.

Prolactin
One of the hormones that stimulates the breasts to produce milk.

Prolapsed Cord
A condition in which the umbilical cord emerges from the cervix before the baby.

Pudendal Block
Local anesthesia given to numb the vaginal region during labor.

Rh Factor Test
A blood test that can indicate the presence of a rhesus antibody called Rh factor.

Rh-negative
Describes the absence of the rhesus antigen on red blood cells.

Rhogam
Medication administered in an injection form during pregnancy and after childbirth to prevent an adverse reaction in the case of Rh incompatibility between mother and child.

Rupture of Membranes
Leaking of fluid from a tear in the amniotic sac, often just before or during labor. Also called "breaking of waters."

Spinal Anesthesia
Anesthesia delivered by needle to the spinal canal in order to numb the lower torso.

Station
Estimation of how low the baby's head is in the birth canal.

Stillbirth
Death of a baby before birth, but after 20 weeks' gestation.

Stripping the Membranes
Manually separating the amniotic sac from the uterine wall; this technique is sometimes used by health care providers to stimulate labor contractions.

Tachycardia
Rapid heart rate.

Term
Describes a baby who is born after at least 37 weeks of pregnancy.

Transition phase
The phase of labor when the cervix finishes dilating to a full 10 centimeters in preparation for delivery.

Vacuum Extractor
A suction device sometimes attached to a baby's head during delivery to help the baby emerge from the birth canal.

VBAC

Vaginal birth by a woman who has had a prior cesarean delivery.

Vernix Caseosa

A white, fatty substance that covers the skin of a fetus. It is sometimes still present in a newborn, especially in creases behind the knees and neck.

Index

Index

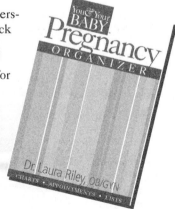